Historical Wig Styling

Historical Wig Styling: Victorian to the Present, 2nd edition, is a guide to creating beautiful, historically accurate hairstyles for theatrical productions and events.

This volume covers hairstyles from the Victorian era through the contemporary styles of today. Chapters begin with an overview of historic figures and styles that influenced the look of each period, followed by step-by-step instructions and photographs showing the finished look from every angle. The book also explores the necessary supplies and styling products needed to create the perfect coif, tips for proper wig handling, a brief history of the makeup for each historical period, and basic styling techniques useful when working with wigs or real hair. New hairstyles featured in this edition include:

– Civil War era women
– Late Victorian African-American men
– 1910s' Full width style women
– 1920s' glossy waves
– 1940s' Victory rolls
– 1950s' Poodle updos
– 1960s' flips

With over 1,000 full-color images and detailed instructions on how to create iconic hairstyles and makeup, *Historical Wig Styling: Victorian to the Present,* 2nd edition, is an excellent resource for professional costume designers and wig makers, as well as for students of Costume Design and Wig Making and Styling courses.

Allison Lowery is the Wig/Hair and Makeup Supervisor at South Coast Repertory Theatre. Previously, she was the Wig and Makeup Specialist at the University of Texas. She has created wigs and makeup for the Alabama Shakespeare Festival, the Lyric Opera of Chicago, American Players Theatre, the Utah Shakespeare Festival, and many others.

The Focal Press Costume Topics Series

Costumes are one of the most important aspects of any production. They are essential tools that create a new reality for both the actor and audience member, which is why you want them to look flawless! Luckily, we're here to help with The Focal Press Costume Topics Series; offering books that explain how to design, construct, and accessorize costumes from a variety of genres and time periods. Step-by-step projects ensure you never get lost or lose inspiration for your design. Let us lend you a hand (or a needle or a comb) with your next costume endeavor!

Draping Period Costumes: Classical Greek to Victorian
Sharon Sobel

Elizabethan Costume Design and Construction
Helen Q. Huang, Emily Home, and Kelsey Hunt

Period Reproduction Buckram Hats
The Costumer's Guide
Crystal G. Herman

Forties and Fifties Fashion for the Stage
Patterns from Vintage Clothing
Jessica Parr

Historical Wig Styling: Ancient Egypt to the 1830s
Allison Lowery

Historical Wig Styling: Victorian to the Present
Allison Lowery

For more information about this series, please visit: https://www.routledge.com/The-Focal-Press-Costume-Topics-Series/book-series/FPCTS

Historical Wig Styling

Victorian to the Present

Second Edition

Allison Lowery

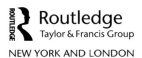

Routledge
Taylor & Francis Group

NEW YORK AND LONDON

Second edition published 2020
by Routledge
52 Vanderbilt Avenue, New York, NY 10017

and by Routledge
2 Park Square, Milton Park, Abingdon, Oxon OX14 4RN

Routledge is an imprint of the Taylor & Francis Group, an informa business

© 2020 Taylor & Francis

First edition published by Routledge 2013

Library of Congress Cataloging-in-Publication Data
Names: Lowery, Allison, author.
Title: Historical wig styling : Victorian to the present / Allison Lowery.
Description: Second edition. | New York, NY : Routledge, 2019. |
Series: The focal press costume topics series | Includes index.
Identifiers: LCCN 2019027063 (print) | LCCN 2019027064 (ebook) |
ISBN 9781138391512 (hbk) | ISBN 9781138391567 (pbk) |
ISBN 9780429422676 (ebk)
Subjects: LCSH: Wigs--Design and construction. | Hairdressing. |
Hairstyles--History. | BISAC: PERFORMING ARTS / Theater / General.
Classification: LCC TT975 .L832 2019 (print) | LCC TT975 (ebook) |
DDC 646.7/248--dc23
LC record available at https://lccn.loc.gov/2019027063
LC ebook record available at https://lccn.loc.gov/2019027064

ISBN: 978-1-138-39151-2 (hbk)
ISBN: 978-1-138-39156-7 (pbk)
ISBN: 978-0-429-42267-6 (ebk)

Typeset in Adobe Garamond
by Servis Filmsetting Ltd, Stockport, Cheshire

Printed in Canada

{ Contents }

{ *Acknowledgments* }

So many people have helped to make this book possible. Many heartfelt thanks go out to the amazing Stacey Walker, Lucia Accorsi, Lauren Ellis, Laurie Fuller, and the staff at Focal Press/Taylor & Francis; Helen Baxter, copyeditor; Kristina Tollefson, technical editor/reader of the highest quality; South Coast Repertory Theatre, especially Gillian Woodson, and Karina Moreno; Texas Performing Arts and the Texas Performing Arts Costume Shop, especially Kathy Panoff and Patricia Risser; the University of Texas Department of Theatre and Dance; Wikimedia Commons; the Bridgeman Art Library; Everything Vintage; my teachers and mentors, Martha Ruskai and Patricia Wesp; the insanely amazing Tim Babiak for the most rocking amazing photography and collaboration anyone could ask for; the models—Eric J. Black, Emma Dirks, Anna Fugate, Trevor Glenn, Leslie Hethcox, Ariel Livingston, Sabrina Lotfi, Marsherrie Madkins, Josephine McAdam, Ivy Negron, Antonia Taylor, and Linette Zare—for being incredible style chameleons; my students—Tara Cooper, Emma Dirks, Anna Fugate, Thumper Gosney, Beauty Kampf-Thibodeau, Josephine McAdam, Kara Meche, Lexi O'Reilly, Bethany Renfro, Maur Sela, Sarah Shade, Elisa Solomon, Katie Baskerville, and J. Dylan Gibson for being a constant source of inspiration; Stephanie Williams Caillabet; Darren Jinks; Rick Jarvie; Susan Branch Towne; Dennis and Jeffrey at Elsen Associates; the Friday Night Gamers—Terry, Sheena, Jeff, Sam, Charles, Brad, Chris, and Irving; the TXRD Lonestar Rollergirls; Jim's Restaurant; Mom (thank you for the never-ending love and encouragement) and Dad (how I wish you could have seen this finished); my brother Scott; fellow eccentric Dave; Barbara Klingberg and my great Uncle, the late Arthur Hall Smith, for starting me down my path in the arts; Grandma, Grandad, Patti, Mr. Oliver and Ms. Rosetta for watching over me from above, and especially to Terry, without whose love and support this book would not have been finished.

one

INTRODUCTION TO WIG STYLING TECHNIQUES

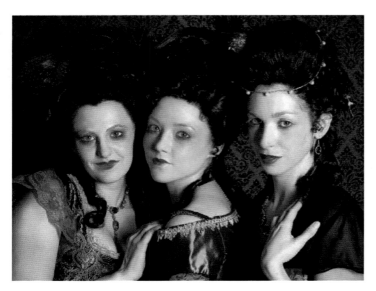

Figure 1.1 Jennifer Lynn Larsen, Josephine McAdam, and Cady Rain model a variety of elaborate wigs.

Welcome to the wonderful and sometime mysterious world of wig styling! Wigs can be a great asset to any theatrical costume or historical costume recreation. Learning the techniques of wig styling can help everyone achieve the completely authentic look they are striving for. Wigs give you the ability to create many looks that would take a long time with someone's real hair—wigs have the advantage of being able to be prepped ahead of time so that they are ready to put on at a moment's notice, which saves valuable time with your performer! This is especially helpful if you are working on a theatrical production and you only have an hour and a half to get a cast of twenty people ready in historical looks. The techniques presented in this book will help you create a wide number of different hairstyles from different eras of history. Many of these techniques can also be adapted for use on someone's real hair if a wig or hairpiece is not an option. I hope this book will be used by theatre technicians, film technicians, historical reenactors, fashion professionals, hairstylists, cosplayers, and anyone else looking to create unique and elaborate hairstyles.

Tools, Supplies, and Hair Products

There are a number of tools and products you need to assemble before you begin your journey into wig styling. For suggestions about where

to find these items, please refer to Appendix 3 in the back of the book. Here is a list of things you will need:

1. Wigs! All kinds! I most often use lace front wigs that have had their front hairline knotted by hand onto fine lace. While I prefer lace front wigs (their realistic look creates the most authentic looking hairstyles), hard front wigs (wigs that are the easiest to find commercially) can be used to great effect as well. I use equal numbers of human hair wigs and synthetic wigs. I prefer human hair wigs for men's wigs, long loose hanging wigs (human hair has weight that allows it to hang more naturally than synthetic hair), and for situations where there may only be one or two wigs in a production. Synthetic fiber holds its curl better, which makes it ideal for long running shows, outdoor theatre, or shows where there is vigorous physical activity, such as dancing or fighting. Human hair wigs are styled by a combination of wetness, heat, and styling products; synthetic wigs are set using steam.

2. A wig block (also sometimes called the head block). A wig block is a canvas head that is made for styling and making wigs. It is made of canvas and filled with sawdust so that the block is sturdy and easy to pin into. They are available in a range of head sizes. It is important to note that Styrofoam heads are not the same as wig blocks. Styrofoam heads are best used for storing a wig that has already been styled. Styrofoam shrinks (sometimes extremely) when heat is applied to it. Therefore, attempting to style a wig with heat (either with steam or by putting the head in a warm wig dryer) can cause the Styrofoam head to distort, making it very difficult to continue styling the wig. Styrofoam heads are also often smaller than a true head size, so styling on them is extra difficult.

3. A wig clamp. This is a clamp that attaches to the edge of a table so that you may work on your wig without worrying about it falling off of the table. They come in both metal and plastic—both work well.

4. Blocking tape. These are pieces of fabric or ribbon that hold the edge of a lace front wig flat while you are working. Blocking a wig is absolutely essential for wig work. It holds the wig firmly in place and evenly distributes the tension on a wig so that no one pace is in danger of pulling or even ripping. I prefer to use bias tape or twill tape. Ribbons or shoelaces will also work as blocking tape. These tapes are also sometimes used to hold a style in place as you

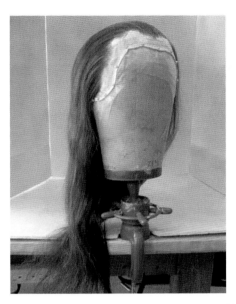

Figure 1.2　A lace front wig on a canvas wig block that is being held onto the table by a wig clamp.

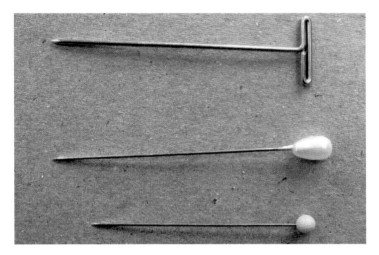

Figure 1.3　From the top: a t-pin, a corsage pin, and a quilter's pin.

work to create waves. Blocking tape can be used over and over again. Later in this chapter, you will find instructions on how to block both hard front and lace front wigs.

5. Pins. You will need two kinds of pin. Blocking pins are the pins you will use to secure the wig to the head block. I prefer to use quilter's pins with round heads, but corsage pins can also be used. These are easy to remove from the block when needed, and their round heads do not snag in the hair when you are styling the wig. You will also need t-pins. These are t-shaped pins that are used to secure rollers to the head. For both blocking pins and t-pins, the longest you can find is the most useful. Corsage pins are an excellent option as well.

6. Rollers. You will need a variety of sizes of roller. The largest size I use is 13/4 inch diameter rollers. All sizes smaller than that are the most useful. The three sizes I use most often are nickel sized (7/8 inch diameter), dime sized (5/8 inch diameter), and pencil sized (3/8 inch diameter). I use both wire rollers (sometimes called spring wire rollers) and plastic rollers. Wire rollers are easier to pin into when you are working; otherwise, I have not noticed much difference between them. Note: wire rollers usually come with

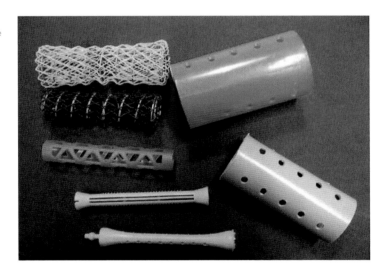

Figure 1.4　This is a good sample assortment of roller types and sizes.

a bristle brush inside of them. I always remove this little brush before using the rollers. I also like to use perm rods for tiny curls.

7. End wraps, also known as endpapers. These are used to smooth the ends of the hair so they wrap neatly around the end of the roller. Endpapers are sold by the box. One box should last you through at least fifteen hairstyles.

8. A spray bottle. You will fill the spray bottle with water so that you can wet the wig as you work. Large or small size spray bottles are fine—I prefer large so that I do not have to refill it as often. Other people are more comfortable using a smaller bottle.

9. Combs and brushes. You will also need a variety of combs and brushes to set and style the wig. I consider the following brushes essential:

   • a wide toothed comb. This is used for detangling wet wigs and for combing through hair when a brush would disturb the curl too much.

   • a rattail comb. These are used for sectioning the hair, making clean parts, and for removing all tangles from the hair.

   • a teasing/smoothing brush. This brush is absolutely essential. It is used for teasing or back combing the hair, smoothing curls around your finger, controlling flyway messy hairs, and many other things.

   • a teasing/lifting comb. This comb is not only used to tease hair, but also to lift or "pick out" a voluminous hairstyle so that it is even larger.

   • a large wire brush, often called a cushion brush. This brush is used for brushing through the entire wig once you have removed the rollers. I often use dog brushes for these. I also prefer brushes that do not have tipped bristles. I have found that the tips eventually come off and I end up wasting time picking the tips out of the wig.

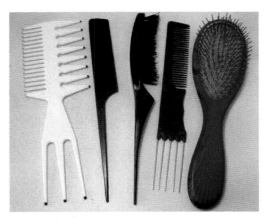

Figure 1.5   From left to right: a wide toothed comb, a rattail comb, a teasing/ smoothing brush, a teasing/lifting comb, and a large wire brush.

10. Styling clips. You will need an assortment of small, pronged curl clips (available in both single and double pronged style); long clips that are called either duckbill clips or alligator clips; and butterfly clips. The clips are used to hold sections of hair in place and for pin curl setting.

11. Hair styling pins. You will need a variety of pins once you get the point of combing out and styling your wig. Black and brown bobby pins, black and bronze hairpins, and three inch hairpins (often referred to as "wig pins") are all necessary. Silver pins can also be useful when you are working with white or gray wigs. It is a good idea to match the color of the pin to the color of the wig you are styling. When in doubt, I choose darker pins because they reflect light less.

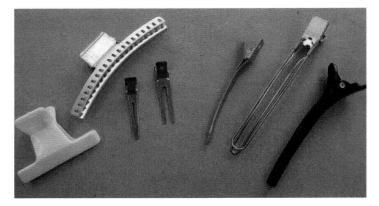

Figure 1.6   From left to right: butterfly clips, single prong curl clips, double prong curl clips, and a variety of duckbill/alligator clips.

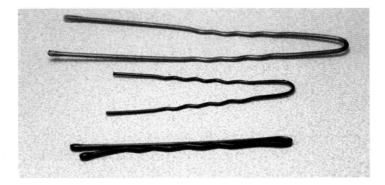

Figure 1.7   From the top: a three-inch wig pin, a hair pin, and a bobby pin.

12. A wig dryer. Once the wig has been set, it will need to be dried in a wig dryer. There are commercially available wig dryers available for purchase (Figure 1.8). You can also make your own (Figure 1.9) by putting a hair dryer in a hole cut into a large box (either cardboard or wooden—wood is preferred). An important note: if you do make your own wig dryer, you must keep an eye on it while the hair dryer is on!!! You do not want the hair dryer to overheat and start a fire. It is also important to make sure that the hair dryer is far enough away from the wig so that the heat from the dryer does not scorch or melt the hair. Angle the hair dryer so that it is not blowing directly on the wig.

13. A small hand steamer. When you are setting a synthetic wig, the curl must be set with steam. A small hand steamer makes it easy to control the direction of the steam and to ensure that every roller is attended to. There are also large commercial wig steamers available on the market, but I prefer the smaller hand steamers because they afford more control. I also like the steamers that come with a small tube to direct the steam, such as the one seen in Figure 1.10. Full size garment steamers and hat steamers also work in a pinch.

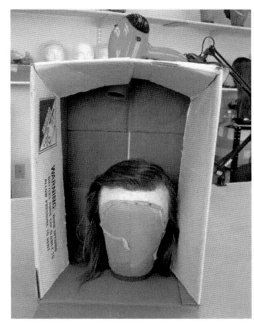

Figure 1.9 A "homemade" wig dryer, using a cardboard box and commercial hair dryer. The box flaps have been folded in so that the placement of the dryer and the placement of the head block are visible. When you are drying a wig, these flaps should be folded so that the box is closed.

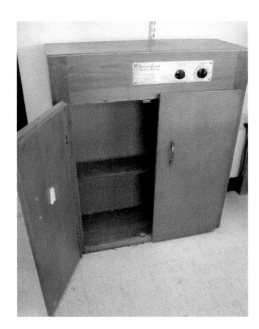

Figure 1.8 A commercial wig dryer.

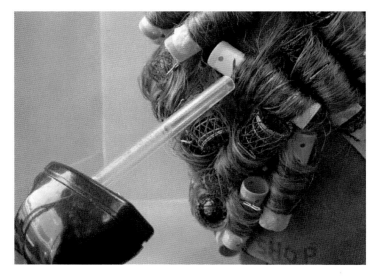

Figure 1.10 A small handheld steamer being used to steam a synthetic wig.

14. Hairnets, rubber bands/hair elastics, and rats. Hairnets in a variety of colors will enable you create long lasting, neat looking hairstyles. Rubber bands and/or hair elastics allow you to secure sections of hair and make ponytails and braids. Rats (hair pads) let you add fullness to a wig or hairstyle without having to rely on teasing. Rats can be purchased readymade, or can be created by adding loose hair inside a hairnet and rolling it up into the desired size and shape.

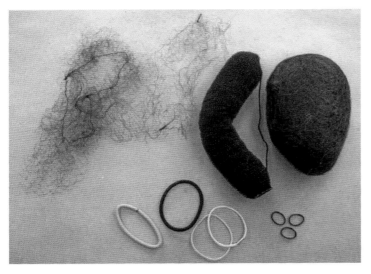

Figure 1.11   An assortment of hairnets, wig rats/pads, and hair elastics.

15. Styling products. I most often use three different kinds of hair styling product:

   • Hair spray. I prefer aerosol hairspray (as opposed to pump). Whatever brand you prefer is fine. There are sprays made specifically for wigs (particularly for synthetic wigs), but I have honestly never noticed a significant difference in the final style.

   • Setting lotion. This lotion is available at beauty supply stores and is used to hold curl and volume when it is applied to hair as it is being set. Lottabody is my preferred brand.

   • Gel. I use the cheapest readily available brand. Gel can also be used as a setting lotion in a pinch. It is also used for slicking down part of a hair style.

In general, I avoid styling products that are waxes or pomades. These tend to weigh wigs down and make them look clumpy. This can be helpful when you are creating a wig for an unsavory or dirty/greasy character, but it is more often a hindrance. Leave-in conditioners and similar products can be helpful for revitalizing a human hair wig that has become dried out over time.

16. Hair accessories. Any number of decorative combs, bows, jewelry, flowers, feathers, and other craft supplies can be used to make hair ornaments.

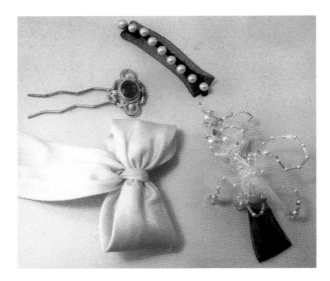

Figure 1.12   An assortment of hair accessories.

17. An apron for covering your clothes. I always wear an apron to help keep hair, water, and styling products off my clothes.

18. A selection of hairpieces. Hairpieces can be added into wigs that do not have enough hair to create a given style. A variety of colors and sizes of hairpieces is best—wiglets (small rounded hairpieces generally worn on the top of the head), switches (ponytails of hair), and falls (large hairpieces that cover ¾ of the head) are especially useful.

19. Wefting. Wefting is woven strips of hair that are used to make wigs, hairpieces, and extensions. Weft can be sewn into wigs to add length or fullness in specific areas. It is sometimes referred to as tracks or weave.

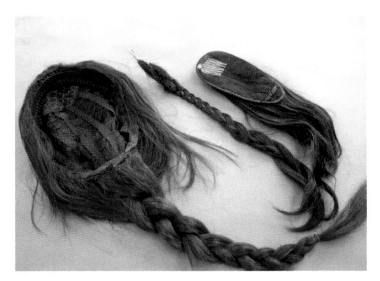

Figure 1.13 Useful hairpieces, from the left: a fall, a switch, and a wiglet.

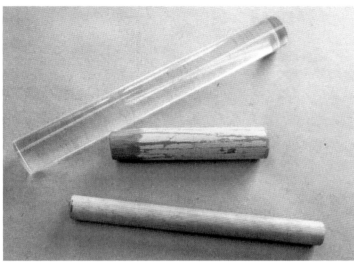

Figure 1.15 A selection of plastic and wooden dowel rods. The yellow rod is a piece of cut off broom handle—the tapered end helps it to work especially well.

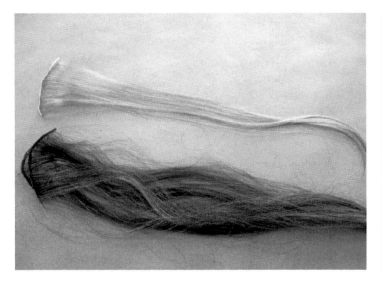

Figure 1.14 Samples of wefting.

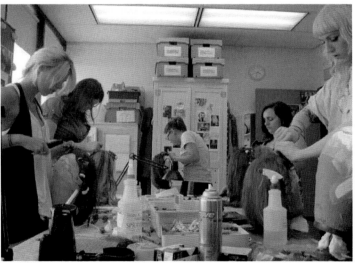

Figure 1.16 University of Texas students Emma Dirks, Bethany Renfro, Lexi O'Reilly, Sarah Thornell, and Lola Hylton at work in the wig room.

20. A selection of wooden or plastic dowel rods, in similar diameter to the rollers you assembled. Dowel rods can be used for pin curl setting, or for helping to shape finished ringlets and curls.

21. A space to work in. Ideally, this space will be well ventilated, well lit, and have a good sized table for your supplies. You can organize your supplies however best suits you. Some people like shelves, some like cabinets, some like rolling carts.

Handling Wigs

Once you have assembled all your supplies and done your research so that you know all about the style you want to create, you will be ready to begin styling. But where do you start? First, you must learn some basic things about handling wigs.

Human Hair vs Synthetic Hair

The two main materials that the wigs you will be using are made of are human hair and synthetic hair. (Yak wigs are also sometimes used; follow the same rules for handling them as you would for human hair.)

Human hair wigs are made of the hair from, yes, humans. Human hair wigs are set by getting them very wet and then drying them with heat. Hot tools, such as curling irons, flat irons, and crimping irons may be used on human hair wigs. Human hair wigs move more like a real head of hair. Their sheen is more like that of a real head of hair. They are, however, susceptible to bad hair days, sweat, and humidity just like a real person's hair. Human hair wigs are good choices for short men's wigs, long women's wigs that need to look very natural, and wigs that need to last in your stock for a long time. Human hair wigs are also a good choice if you are in a situation where only one or two people in a production need wigs and everyone else is using their own hair. In that instance, you want the wigs to be a close to a real head of hair as possible so that they blend with the other looks.

Synthetic wigs are made of plastic hair that is extruded through a machine. Because of this, synthetic hair can be made in any number of lengths and colors. *Synthetic wigs must always be styled with steam!* This includes any kind of curling, waving, or straightening. *No hot tools must ever touch synthetic wigs!* Flat irons, curling irons, and other hot tools will cause the plastic hair of the wig to melt, which will make it useless. Once the hair has been fried, there is nothing you can do to bring it back. All you can do is cut the fried hair out of the wig and replace it with new hair. There are new types of synthetic hair being developed that can withstand styling with hot tools, but unless the wig explicitly says that it can be styled with heat, you should assume that you cannot do this. Also, pay strict attention to the stated temperature listed on a "heat resistant" synthetic that it can tolerate. Better safe than sorry! Synthetic wigs are a good choice for when you need unusual colors or excessive length. They are also good for a hairstyle that needs to last—this makes them an excellent choice for vigorous musicals or outdoor theatre. Synthetic wigs hold their style very well. They are also significantly cheaper than human hair wigs.

Hard Front Wigs vs Lace Front Wigs

Both synthetic and human hair wigs will come with one of two kinds of front: a hard front or a lace front. A hard front wig is the most common front for the wig to have. This wig has a bound off fabric edge that finishes off the entire front part of the wig. This often looks artificial and hard, which is why is called a hard front. If you are using a hard front wig, you will need to do some tricks to soften the hairstyle around the face so that it looks more natural on the performer. Lace front wigs are wigs that have had the hard front of the wig cut off. The front edge of the wig then has a piece of an almost invisible fine lace, known as wig lace, sewn to the front of the wig. Individual hairs are then knotted into this wig lace with a hook, creating the illusion of hair that is growing directly out of the wearer's skin. These wigs look much more realistic. They are also more delicate and must be handled carefully—you should never hold a lace front wig by the lace! A lace front wig can also be a wig that has been made completely from scratch, with all the hair in the wig being knotted into the lace. These wigs are very lightweight and very natural looking; they are also the most delicate of all kinds of wigs.

Blocking the Wig

Blocking a wig is the act of securing a wig to a wig block with pins before you begin the styling process. Both hard front and lace front wigs must be blocked before you begin working on them. You should never work on a wig that is not properly secured to a wig block—this will cause the wig to slip around on the block or to get stretched out of place—possibly even torn.

To block a hard front wig:

1. Place the wig block on a wig clamp that is secured to the table.
2. Place the wig on the block. Be sure it is in the proper place on the head—not too far forward or too far back. Check to make sure the side tabs are even.

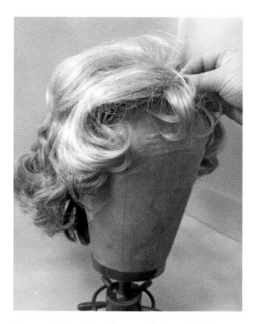 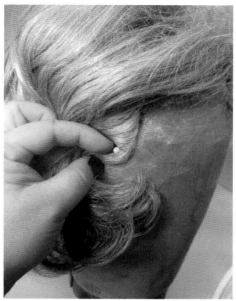 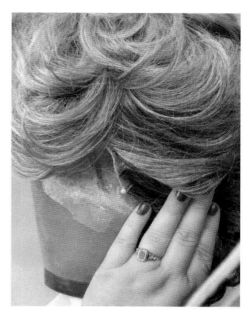

Figures 1.17, 1.18, and 1.19   Blocking a hard front wig: place a pin at the center front hairline (left); at each ear tab (center); and at either side of the nape of the neck (right).

3. Place a blocking pin at the center front edge, at each ear tab, and at either side of the nape of the neck. All these pins should be about an 1/8 of an inch from the front of the wig. It is also helpful to place the pins in at a slight angle so that they are less likely to slip out of the wig while you are working.

To block a lace front wig:

1. Place the wig block on a wig clamp that is secured to a table.

2. Place the wig on the block, again making sure it is in the right place. Check to make sure that the sides of the hairline are even.

3. Place a blocking pin at either side of the head above each ear, and at either side of the nape of the neck.

4. Use a piece of blocking tape to smooth and hold the lace front in place. The tape should be placed just above the edge of the wig lace. Begin at the center front of the wig and place a blocking pin in the blocking tape. Continue pinning along the hairline, placing a blocking pin every inch or so. Be sure to pin around the hair at the sideburns as well.

5. Secure any loose blocking tape you may have out of the way. This will keep it from getting caught by combs or brushes while you are working.

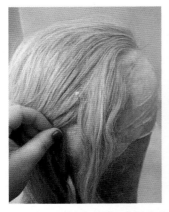
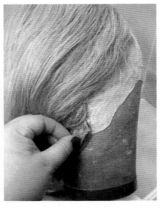
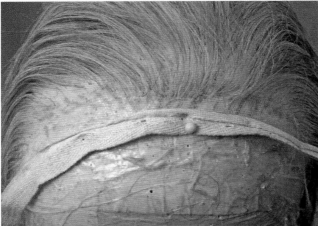
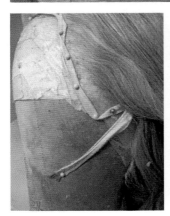
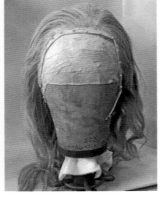

Figures 1.20 to 1.24 Blocking a lace front wig. Notice the placement of the blocking pins. Also notice how the tape is secured around the sideburn area.

Basic Styling Techniques

Hairstyles are made up of four elements: straight hair, wavy hair, curly hair, and braids/coils/buns. There are a number of ways these different textures can be achieved.

Straight Hair

A human hair wig can be thoroughly wet, combed through, and dried to become straight (unless you are working with naturally curly or permed hair). Human hair can also be ironed with a flat iron. To do this, section the hair on the wig into five sections. Begin at the nape of the neck, and run the flat iron through the hair from root to tip. Move from the nape of the neck gradually up to the front hairline of the wig. Work in small sections to get the hair thoroughly straight.

A synthetic wig that is not already straight is straightened by steam. Again, section the wig hair into five sections (the hair should be damp for this). Begin at the nape of the neck. Use a rattail comb to pull a small section of hair taut. Direct the nozzle of the steamer towards the section of hair at the roots. You should be able to see the hair shaft straighten itself out under the steam. Pull the comb through the hair, moving the steamer along with it until you reach the ends of the hair. Repeat this for every section of the hair, working your way up the wig from the nape of the neck to the front of the hairline. Once the wig is straight, place it in a wig dryer to dry, or allow it to air dry on a shelf.

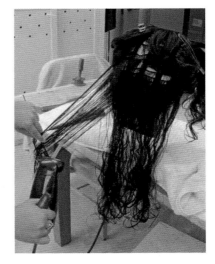

Figure 1.25 Thumper Gosney demonstrates how to properly steam a synthetic wig.

Wavy Hair

Wavy hair is hair that ripples in an "S" shape. There are three main methods to achieve wavy hair: water waving (also known as finger waving); pin curling, and roller setting. The kind of waves and how much volume you wish for the end result to have will determine which method of waving you choose. Here, all three methods of waving will be demonstrated on one wig.

Water Waving

Water waving, or finger waving, creates a wave that is extremely flat to the head. When combed out, these waves will be larger and softer than those created by the other waving methods.

To create water waves:

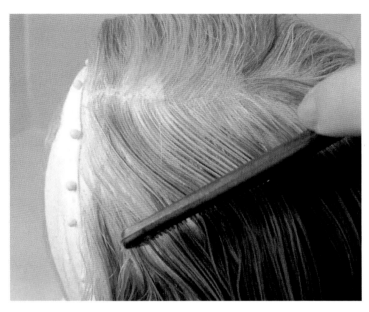

Figure 1.27 Step 2. Place the part in the wig wherever you wish for it to be. Comb the hair by the part in one direction (either towards or away from the hairline).

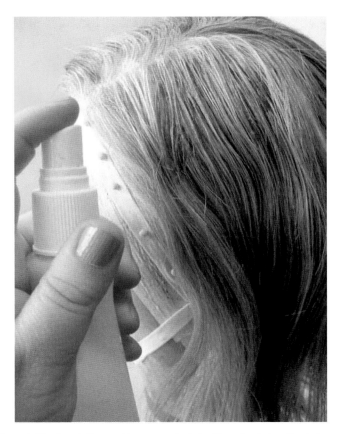

Figure 1.26 Step 1. Thoroughly saturate the hair with setting lotion. Comb the setting lotion through the hair to make sure it gets all the way to the ends.

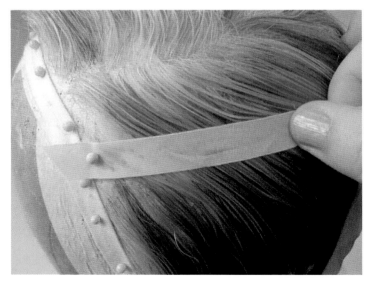

Figure 1.28 Step 3. Once you have the hair combed in the direction you want, secure it by pinning a long piece of blocking tape down the center of the wave. The blocking tape will hold the waves in place as you work.

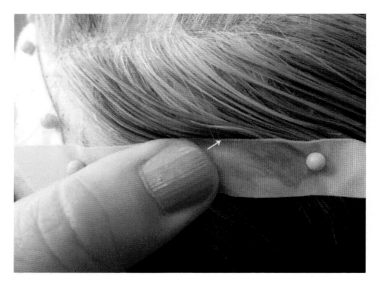

Figure 1.29   Step 4. To create a more defined ridge in the wave, push up with the ribbon before you pin it down.

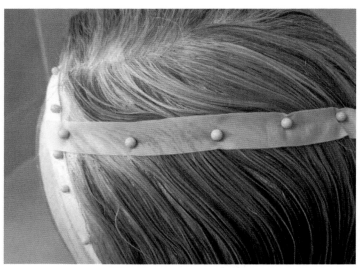

Figure 1.30   Step 5. The first half of the wave is pinned in place. Pin the ribbon all along the wave.

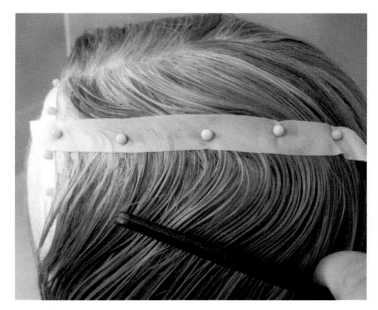

Figure 1.31   Step 6. Next, comb the length of the hair in the opposite direction from the direction you started with.

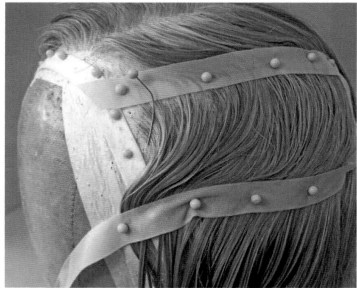

Figure 1.32   Step 7. Use the blocking tape to secure the center of this part of the wave. The first "S" of the wave has been formed.

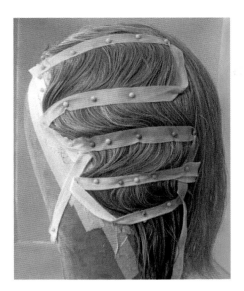

Figure 1.33 Step 8. Continue working your way down the head, alternating directions. You may need to continue to rewet the hair as you working—it is important that the hair be thoroughly saturated as you are shaping the waves. You can do waves that go all the way around the head, or you can wave a small section of the hair—it all depends on the style you want!

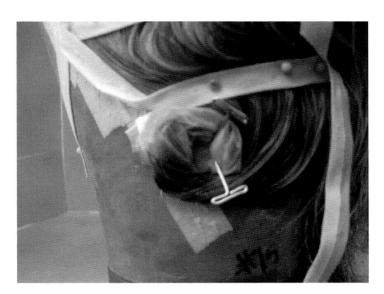

Figure 1.34 Step 9. For a nice finish at the bottom of a water wave, I will often arrange the hair into a pin curl.

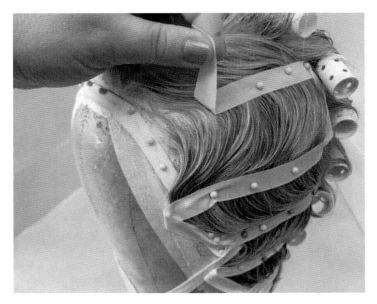

Figure 1.35 Step 10. Dry the wig in the wig dryer for at least 75 minutes. When you are ready to comb out the wig, begin by removing the tape. You should start removing the tape at the top of the wig, not the bottom.

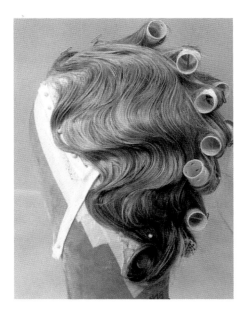

Figure 1.36 Step 11. For a slicker, more shellacked look, you can leave the wig as it is, without combing through the hair.

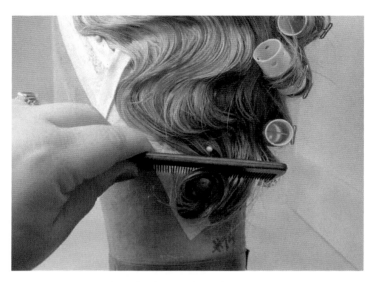

Figure 1.37 Step 12. If you decide to comb out the waves, begin at the bottom ends of the hair and work your way up.

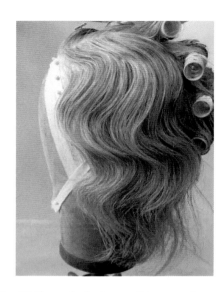

Figure 1.38 Step 13. The combed out wave will be very soft.

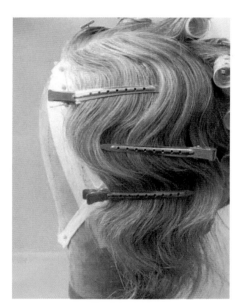

Figure 1.39 Step 14. Use duckbill clips to add more definition to the waves, if desired.

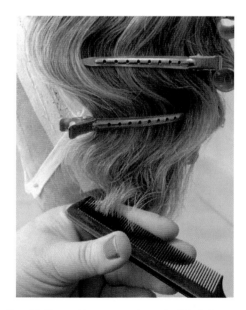

Figure 1.40 Step 15. If you wish to neaten the ends of the hair, use a rattail to comb to smooth the ends around your finger.

Once you have completed arranging the waves, mist the wig with hairspray and let it sit overnight. Remove the duckbill clips and the wig should be ready to be worn.

Pin Curling

Pin curling is the traditional method of hair setting that was so popular in the 1930s, 40s, and 50s.

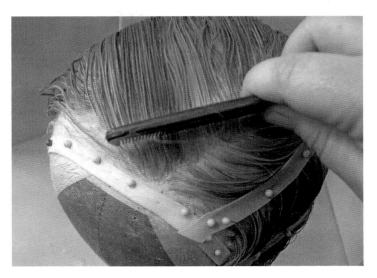

Figure 1.41   Step 1. Again, begin by saturating the hair with setting lotion and combing all the hair in one direction, starting at the part.

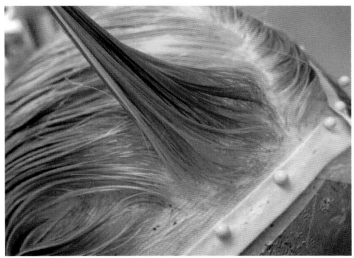

Figure 1.42   Step 2. Use your rattail comb to separate a square section of hair, about one inch by once inch.

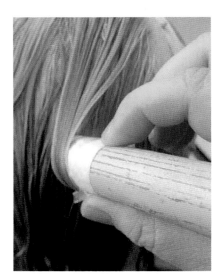

Figure 1.43   Step 3. Use a dowel rod or other kind of stick to shape your curl and keep it perfectly round. Place an endpaper over the ends of the hair, and begin rolling the hair at the tip.

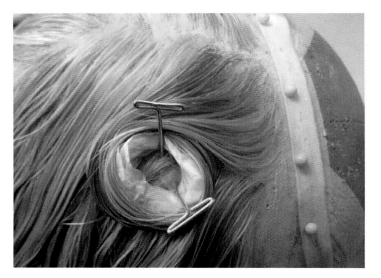

Figure 1.44   Step 4. Once you have wound the hair all the way up to the roots, slide the stick out and secure the curl with pins or clips. (I prefer pins because they do not leave as much of a crimp in the hair.)

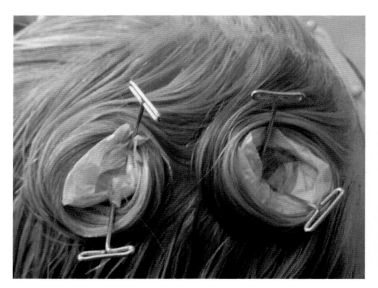

Figure 1.45 Step 5. To achieve a perfect wave, the next curls in the row (working down the head from the crown) should go in the same direction. Both of these curls have been wound counterclockwise.

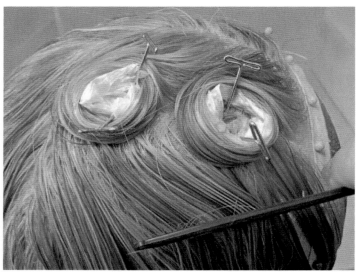

Figure 1.46 Step 6. When you are ready to do the next row, comb all the hair in the opposite direction from the first row. (In this example, the first row had the hair combed away from the face, so the second row will be combed towards the face.)

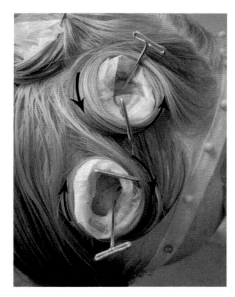

Figure 1.47 Step 7. The next row of pin curls should be wound in the opposite direction as the row above. In this case, the first row was curled counterclockwise, so the second row is wound clockwise. The arrows indicate the direction.

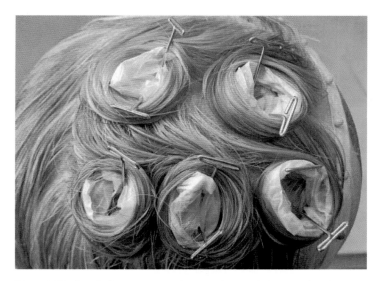

Figure 1.48 Step 8. Continue setting the second row with the pin curls going clockwise. Again, you may need to rewet the hair as you are working.

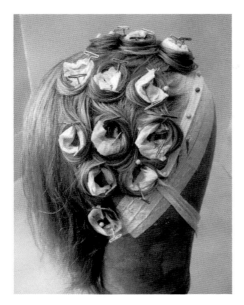

Figure 1.49 Step 9. As you work your way down the head, the curl direction will continue to alternate between counterclockwise and clockwise. When you are done setting the wig, dry it in the wig dryer for at least 75 minutes.

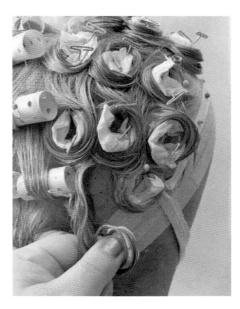

Figure 1.50 Step 10. To comb out the pin curl set, begin by removing the pin curls from the bottom up.

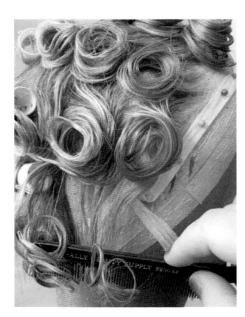

Figure 1.51 Step 11. Use a rattail comb to comb through all the curls.

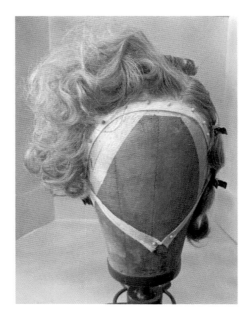

Figure 1.52 Step 12. Notice how much more voluminous the pin curl set is compared to the water wave set.

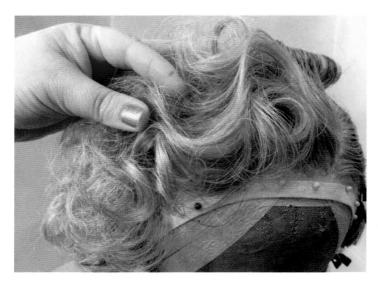

Figure 1.53   Step 13. Begin pinching the waves with your fingers and pushing the hair around until the waves start to fall into place.

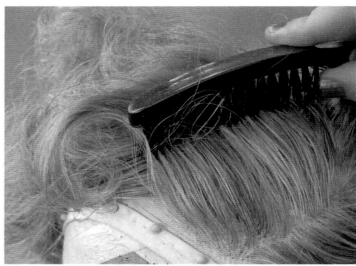

Figure 1.54   Step 14. Use a smoothing brush to flatten down the hair and push the waves into place.

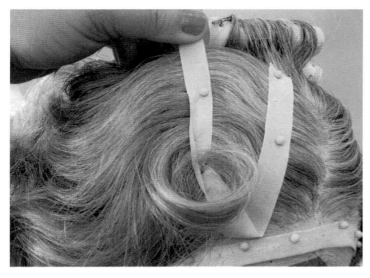

Figure 1.55   Step 15. Pin bias tape in the center of the curve of each section of the wave to set it in place.

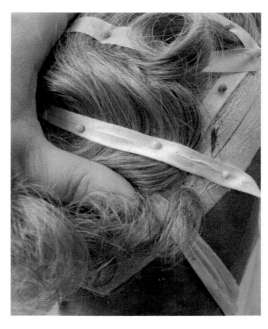

Figure 1.56   Step 16. Use the bias tape and your fingers to push up on the wave to make the ridges more defined.

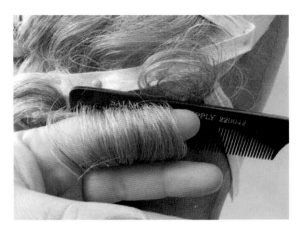

Figure 1.57 Step 17. When you reach the ends of the hair, use the rattail comb or the smoothing brush to smooth the curls around your fingers. This will create a clean, neat curl.

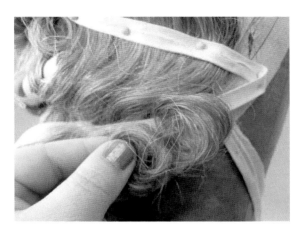

Figure 1.58 Step 18. Slide the finished curl off of your finger and arrange it in an attractive way.

Just like with the water wave set, when you are finished arranging the curls you should mist the wig with hairspray and let it sit overnight. Remove the bias tape when you are ready for the wig to be worn

Roller Setting

Using rollers to set the hair is the most effective way to get a round neat curl. If you push the curl flat, it becomes a wave.

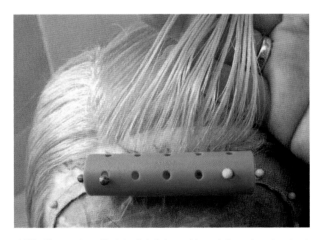

Figure 1.59 The section of hair is slightly less wide and deep than the plastic roller.

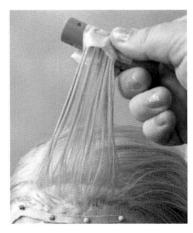

Figure 1.60 The section of hair should be held taut.

A few notes about roller setting:

1. The section of hair that you are going to set on the roller should never be wider or deeper than the roller itself.

2. When you are rolling a section of hair, be sure to maintain tension on the hair in order to get a nice smooth set. Letting the hair go slack while the wig is being set will result in a messy wig.

3. A roller can be set on base (Figure 1.61), forward of base (Figure 1.62), or off base with drag (Figure 1.63). Under most circumstances, you will want to set with the roller on base. For a pompadour effect that adds lots of volume, you will set the roller forward of base. For a flatter look that sits closer to the head, you may need to set the wig off base with drag.

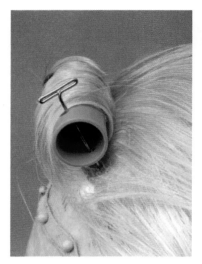 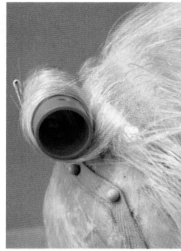 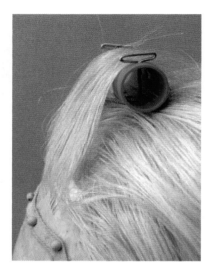

Figures 1.61, 1.62, and 1.63   A roller set on base (Figure 1.61); forward of base (Figure 1.62); and off base with drag (Figure 1.63)

4. Use a t-pin to secure each roller in place. Turn the t-pin so that it is parallel to the hair in the roller. This will help you avoid snagging hair in the t-pin.

5. Using an endpaper will give your curls much less frizzy ends. To use an endpaper, slip it behind the section of hair (Figure 1.64) fold each side of the endpaper over towards the center (Figure 1.65), spritz the endpaper with water, and slide it down until the ends of the hair are encased (Figure 1.66).

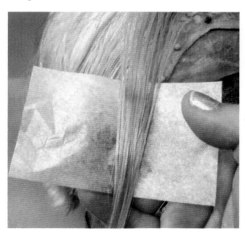 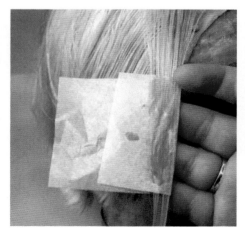 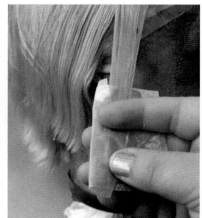

Figures 1.64, 1.65, and 1.66

Roller Setting for Waves

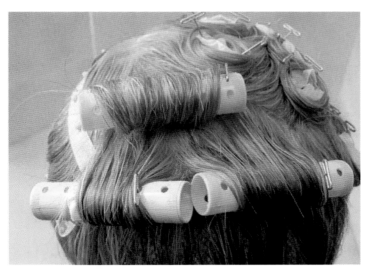

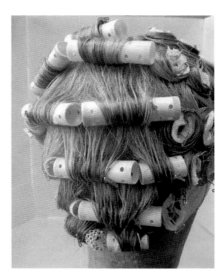

Figure 1.67   Step 1. Begin setting the rollers at the part of the wig. These rollers are be set off base with a small amount of drag. As you work your way down, make sure that the roller in one row sits over where two rows come together in the next row down. This is called a brick set, because the rollers are offset like bricks in a wall.

Figure 1.68   Step 2. Set the wig from top to bottom.

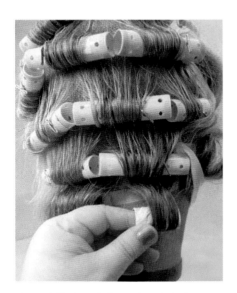

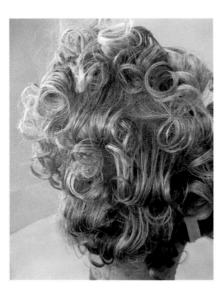

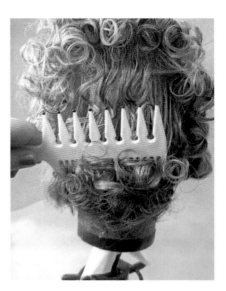

Figure 1.69   Step 3. Steam the wig if it is synthetic hair and put it in the wig dryer for at least 75 minutes. When you are ready to comb out the set, begin removing the rollers from the bottom.

Figure 1.70   Step 4. After you have removed all the rollers, you will see gaps in the hair. These are called roller breaks.

Figure 1.71   Step 5. Use a wide toothed comb to gently pick through all the curls. This will help get rid of the roller breaks.

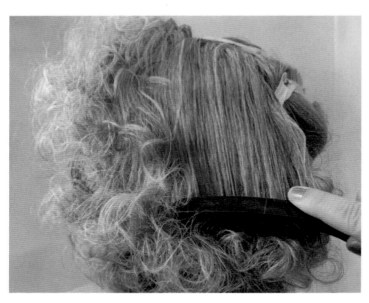

Figure 1.72   Step 6. Run a smoothing brush through the curls to begin shaping the hair into waves.

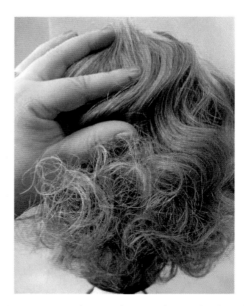

Figure 1.73   Step 7. Use your fingers to begin pinching and pushing the waves into shape.

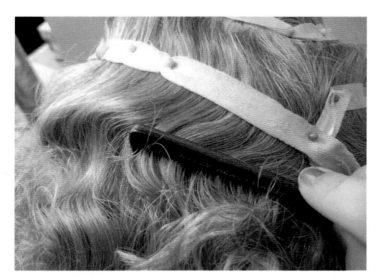

Figure 1.74   Step 8. Use a rattail comb to push the waves in place. Secure them with bias tape.

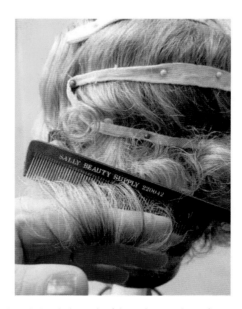

Figure 1.75   Step 9. Comb the ends of the curls around your fingers to make them smooth and neat.

When you are done, mist the wig with hairspray and let it sit overnight. Remove the bias tape when you are ready for the wig to be worn.

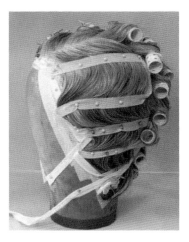 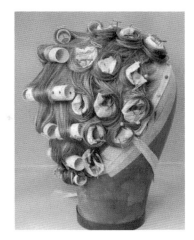 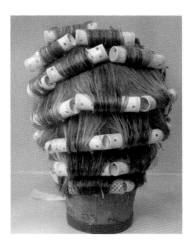

Figure 1.76, 1.77, and 1.78 One wig, set three ways: a water wave set (Figure 1.76); a pin curl set (Figure 1.77); and a roller set (Figure 1.78).

Curly Hair

Just as there are different sizes and shapes of waved hair, there are also different kinds of curly hair. I will now discuss a variety of methods for creating curly hair.

Roller Setting

Hair can be made curly by setting it on rollers, using the same technique as described above in the wavy hair section. The comb out is different, however. Instead of pressing the hair flat into waves, you want to work with the hair in a looser way.

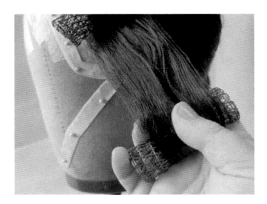

Figure 1.79 Step 1. Unroll the rollers straight out horizontally.

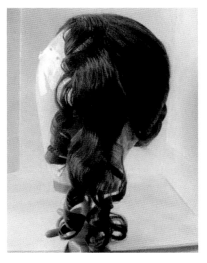

Figure 1.80 Step 2. If you do not brush the curls out, they will be loose and somewhat clumped together.

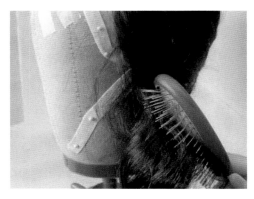

Figure 1.81 Step 3. Use a large wooden brush to smooth out the curls and get rid of the clumps.

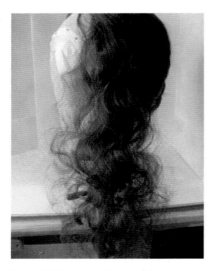

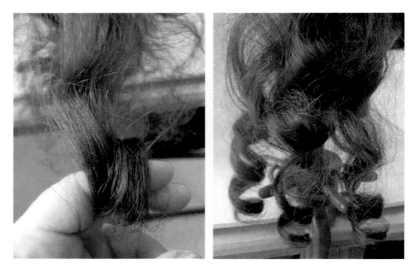

Figure 1.82   Step 4. After brushing, the curls become loose and soft.

Figure 1.83 and 1.84   Step 5. If you want more defined curls, you can brush the ends around your fingers.

Sausage Curls/Ringlets

Sausage curls, or ringlets, are those curls that form a smooth tube or column of hair. Ideally, there are no gaps in the column of hair. This is a rigid kind of curl that was especially popular in hairstyles in parts of the 19th century.

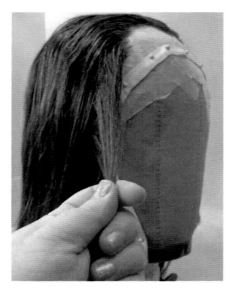

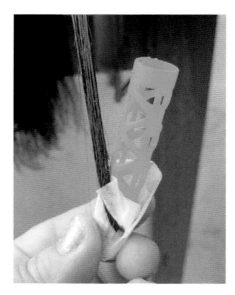

Figure 1.85   Step 1. Separate out a small vertical section of hair and thoroughly wet it.

Figure 1.86   Step 2. Begin rolling the hair around the bottom of the roller.

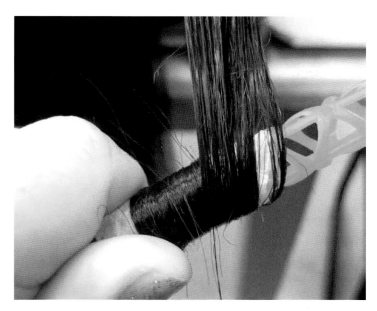

Figure 1.87   Step 3. As you wind the hair around the roller, make sure you overlap some of the hair every time the hair goes around the roller.

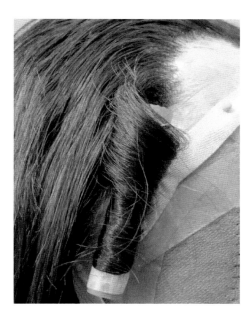

Figure 1.88   Step 4. Pin the roller vertically. Once you have set all your curls, steam the hair if it is synthetic and dry it in the wig dryer for at least 75 minutes.

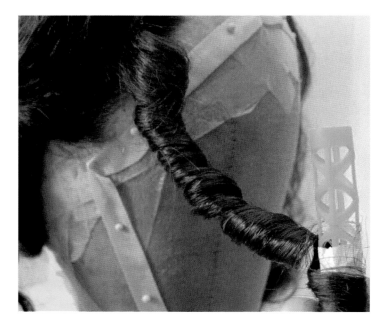

Figure 1.89   Step 5. After the hair is dry, unwind it from the roller.

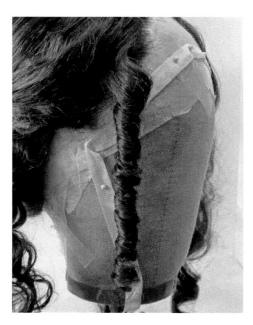

Figure 1.90   Step 6. You will have a column of hair at this point, but it usually not as neat and tidy as it could be.

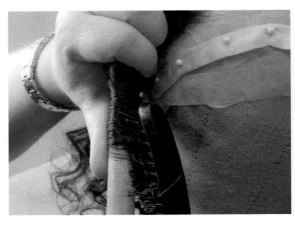 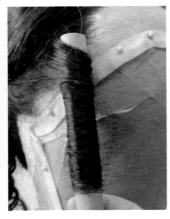

Figures 1.91 and 1.92   Step 7. Use an appropriate size of dowel rod and shape the curl by brushing it around the rod.

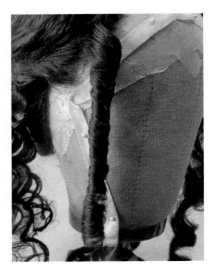

Figure 1.93   Step 8. Gently slide the dowel rod out of the bottom of the ringlet. You will be left with a smoother, neater sausage curl.

Spiral Curls

Spiral curls are more of a combination of a wave and a curl. This is a very natural looking curl that is useful for styling many historical looks.

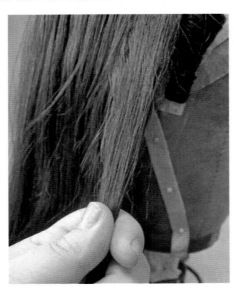 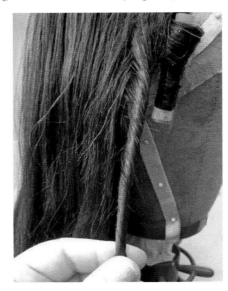

Figure 1.94   Step 1. Again, separate out a vertical section of hair. This section of hair should be of fairly substantial thickness. The size of the section will depend a little on how dense the hair is in your wig, but a section that is at least one inch wide by two inches high is a good starting point. If you make this curl with a section of hair that is too thin, you will end up with a lot of tangled frizz.

Figure 1.95   Step 2. Twist the hair in the direction you want the roller to face. Twist the section of hair tightly, but not so tightly that the hair begins to twist back up on itself.

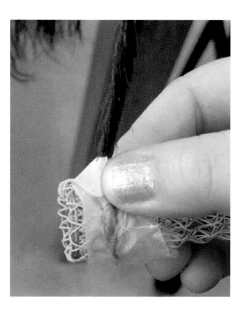

Figure 1.96   Step 3. Begin rolling the twisted section onto the roller at the bottom.

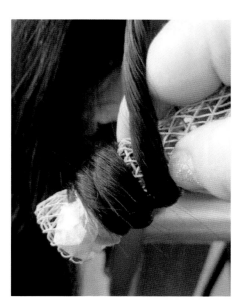

Figure 1.97   Step 4. As you wind the hair up on the roller, the twisted coils should stack up on top of each other.

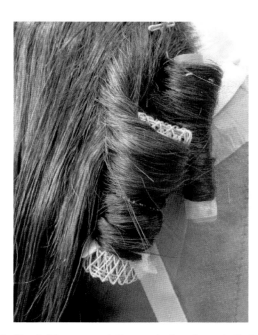

Figure 1.98   Step 5. When you reach the top, pin the roller vertically. Steam the hair if necessary and dry it in the wig dryer for 75 minutes.

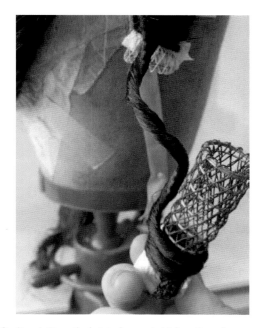

Figure 1.99   Step 6. Once the hair is dry, unwind it from the roller.

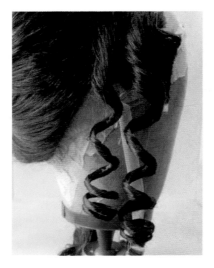

Figure 1.100   Step 7. Notice the snaky look of the hair as it comes off of the roller.

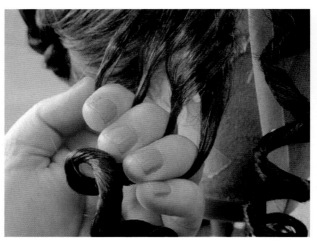

Figure 1.101   Step 8. Use your fingers to comb through each section of hair. Each time you comb through the hair, the curls will get softer and less defined. You can also use a wide toothed comb to comb through the curl.

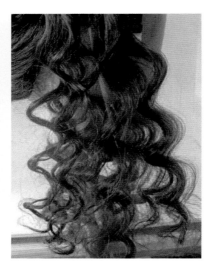

Figure 1.102   Step 9. The finished curl will be very soft and natural looking.

Curl Clusters

Sometimes, you will discover that you need a cluster of curls in a hairstyle.

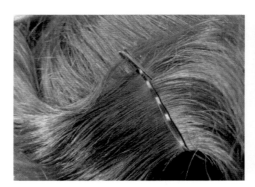

Figure 1.103   Step 1. Firmly secure the base of the section where you want it by interlocking two bobby pins. This done by crossing two bobby pins in an "X" shape. Also make sure that you pin into the base of the wig and not just into the hair itself for a really firm hold.

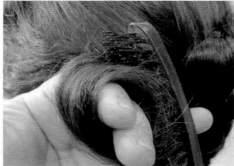

Figure 1.104   Step 2. Brush the hair around your finger with a smoothing brush.

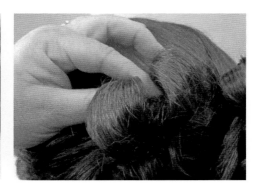

Figure 1.105   Step 3. Loosely bring the bottom of the curl up towards the base and drape it until it looks pretty.

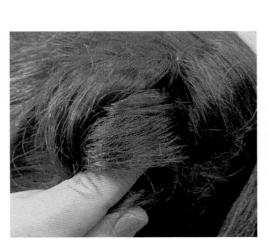
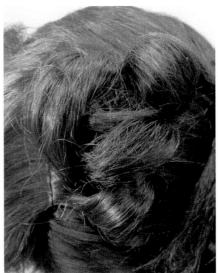

Figures 1.106 and 1.107   Step 4. Secure the arrangement with a couple of bobby pins.

Being able to hide your bobby pins as you work is an important skill. When you are pinning a curl, always place your pins on the inside of a curl (Figure 1.108). When you are pinning a twisted section of hair, insert the pin on the outside of the twist with the bobby pin pointing up (Figure 1.109). Twist the bobby pin up and around into the twist, locking the pin in the inside of the twist (Figure 1.110). Hiding your pins is important whether you are using bobby pins, hair pins, or wig pins. It is also important to not try to pin too much hair at once. If your pin wants to slide back out of a section of hair, it probably means that you are attempting to put too much hair in your pin.

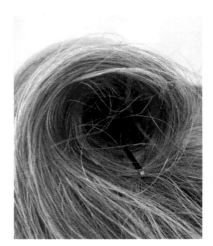
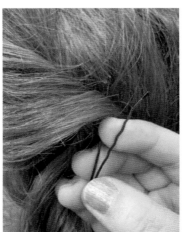
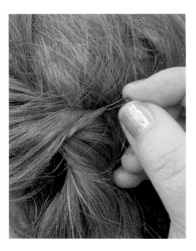

Figures 1.108, 1.109, and 1.110   From the left: Figure 1.108 Hiding a bobby pin inside a curl. Figure 1.109 Hiding your bobby pin inside a twist. Figure 1.110 Hiding your bobby pin inside a twist.

Braided Hair

Another commonly used style element is the braid. Braids are a simple, quick way to create a period look.

Traditional Three Strand Braid

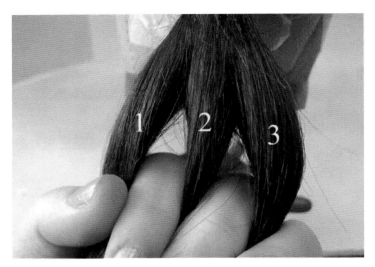

Figure 1.111   Step 1. Separate the section of hair into three strands.

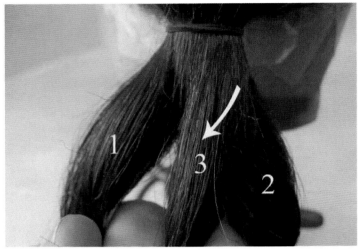

Figure 1.112   Step 2. Cross one of the outside sections over the middle section so that it becomes the new middle section.

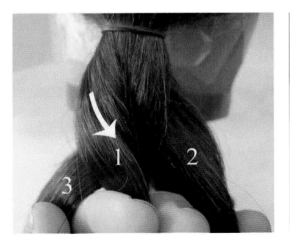

Figure 1.113   Step 3. Cross the other outside section over into the middle.

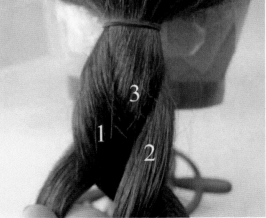
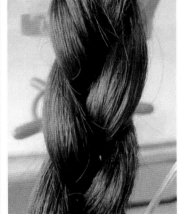

Figures 1.114 and 1.115   Step 4. Repeat this process until you reach the ends of the hair. Secure the end of the braid with a rubber band or elastic that matches the hair color.

French Braid/Reverse French Braid

A French braid is a braid where not all the hair is braided at once, and pieces of hair are added into the three sections as you make the braid. This results in a braid that sits very flat to the head and does not create a lot of bulk.

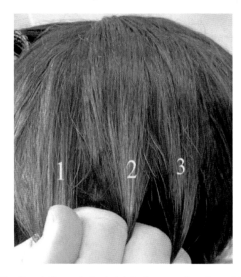

Figure 1.116   Step 1. Separate the hair into three small sections at the top of where you want the braid to begin. The size of the sections will be determined by how intricate you wish for the braid to look.

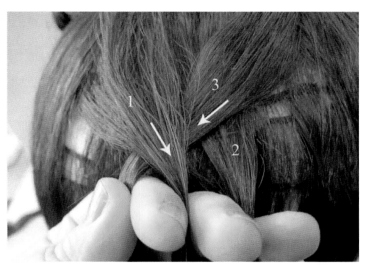

Figure 1.117   Step 2. Braid the hair the same way you did for the traditional braid, crossing the outside sections over to the middle section.

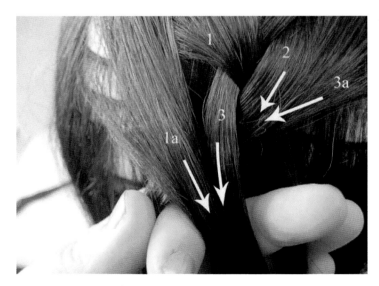

Figure 1.118   Step 3. After making the initial pass through the original hair sections, begin adding more hair to the braid by picking up small sections of hair to add in as you work.

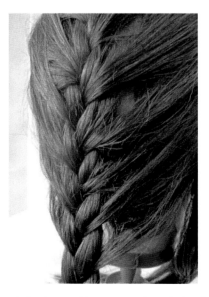

Figure 1.119   Step 4. Continue working your way down the braid, adding sections as you go. The finished braid will sit neatly against the head.

In a reverse French braid (sometimes called a *Dutch braid*), instead of crossing the section over to the center, you will instead cross them underneath to the center. This will cause the finished braid to look like it is sitting on top of the hair, but still allows the braid to sit very close to the head.

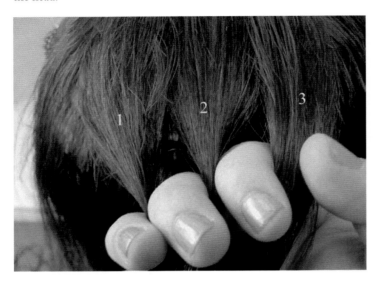

Figure 1.120   Step 1. Again, begin by dividing the hair into three sections.

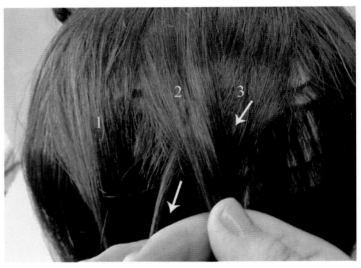

Figure 1.121   Step 2. Cross the outside section under the middle section to begin the braid.

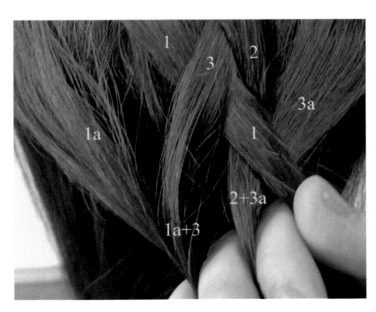

Figure 1.122   Step 3. After you make the initial pass through the first three sections of hair, begin picking up small sections of hair to add into the braid.

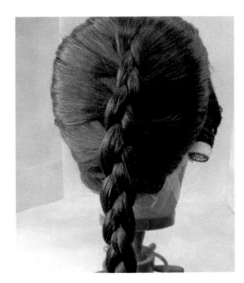

Figure 1.123   Step 4. Continue adding sections of hair to the braid until you run out of hair, continuing to cross the sections underneath as you work. Secure the end of the braid with an elastic. The finished braid will look as though it is sitting on top of the hair.

Rope Braids

A rope braid is a two-strand braid where the sections are twisted together. It is an especially nice braid to use in period hairstyles.

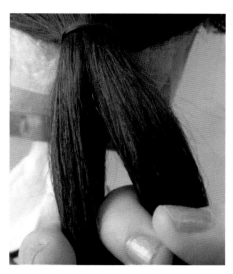

Figure 1.124   Step 1. Separate the hair into two sections. You can either begin with the hair in a ponytail, or with two loose sections of hair.

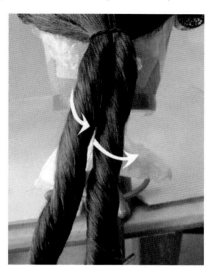

Figure 1.125   Step 2. Twist each section of hair in the same direction. For example, if you twist one section to the right, you must also twist the second section to the right. Do not twist the sections so tightly that they begin to twist back up on themselves.

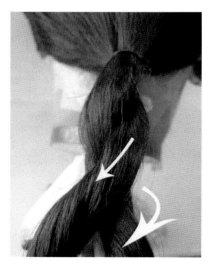

Figure 1.126   Step 3. Twist the coiled sections of hair together in the opposite direction from the one you did the initial twisting in. For example, if you twisted each section to the right in step 2, you would then twist the two sections together to the left. Secure the end of the braid with an elastic.

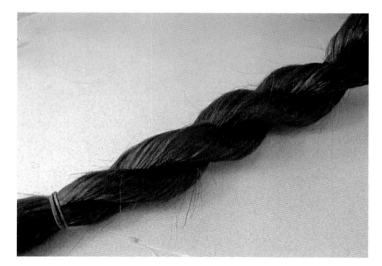

Figure 1.127   Step 4. The finished rope braid.

Fishtail/Herringbone Braids
The fishtail (or herringbone) braid is another braid that begins with two sections of hair. It is another nice braid to use in period hairstyling.

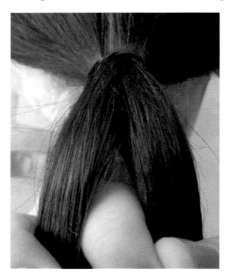

Figure 1.128 Step 1. Divide the hair into two sections. Again, you either start with the hair already in a ponytail, or with two sections of loose hair.

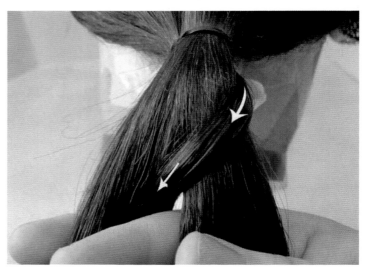

Figure 1.129 Step 2. Take a small section of hair from the outside of one section, and cross it over to the inside of the opposite section. The smaller the section of hair you cross over, the more intricate the finished braid will look.

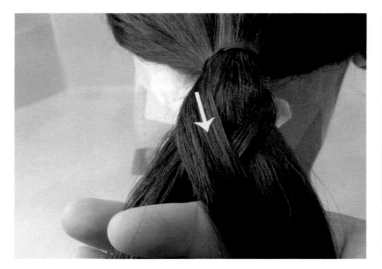

Figure 1.130 Step 3. Take a section from the outside of the opposite section of hair and cross it over to the inside of the first section. Continue working from side to side until you reach the bottom of the braid. Secure the bottom of the braid with an elastic.

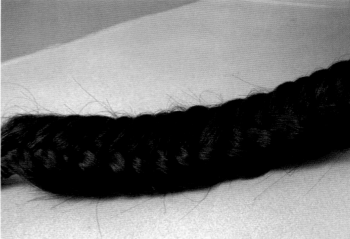

Figure 1.131 Step 4. The finished fishtail/herringbone braid.

Basic French Twist

One other styling skill that is very useful to know how to do is the basic French twist. Many of the styles in this book incorporate a French twist as a part of the finished style. A French twist is an elegant way to get all the hair up to the crown of the head.

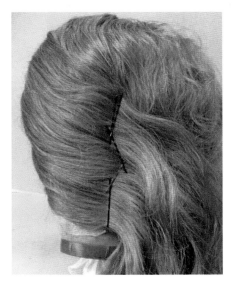

Figure 1.132   Step 1. Sweep all the hair in the back of the wig off to one side. Secure the hair with a row of interlocking bobby pins going up the center of the head.

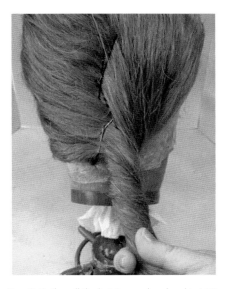

Figure 1.133   Step 2. Gather all the hair in your hand and twist it.

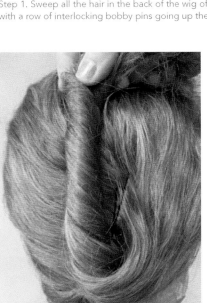

Figure 1.134   Step 3. Pull the twisted hair up alongside the row of bobby pins.

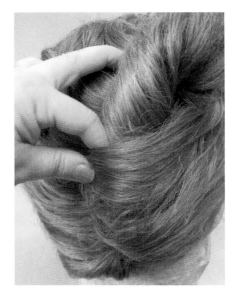

Figure 1.135   Step 4. Pull the twisted base of the ponytail up over the ponytail.

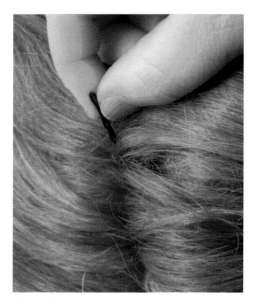

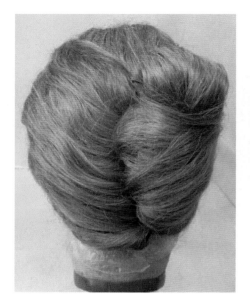

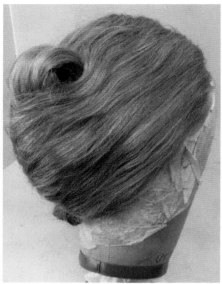

Figure 1.136   Step 5. Secure the roll by tucking and pinning bobby pins all along the roll.

Figures 1.137 and 1.138   Step 6. What you do with the loose ends of the hair will depend on what they style you are creating needs to look like. Here, I simply rolled the ends under to form a curl that completes the French twist.

Using Your Own Hair

All the styles in this book could be done on a real person's hair if their hair was the appropriate length. Obviously, you cannot pin rollers directly into a living person's head, but you can recreate the setting pattern with plastic rollers that are allowed to dry overnight or under a bonnet hair dryer (like you might see at a hair salon),with hot rollers, or with a curling iron. Pin curls (secured with clips or hairpins) and braids can also be done on real hair. One thing to keep in mind when approaching styling real hair is that you will need the same supplies to be readily available to you as you would for styling wigs. If the set illustrated is done with twenty rollers, trying to achieve it with six hot rollers of the wrong size is not realistic. Also keep in mind that many historical hairstyles were either wigs or they incorporated hairpieces. You may also need to use added hairpieces to achieve the look you are going for. These hairpieces would need to be styled in advance of styling the person's hair, using the techniques outlined in this chapter (waving, curling, or braiding.)

Breaking Down/Putting Together a Hairstyle

Once you have mastered all the basic styling techniques, you must then figure out how to put them all together to make a hairstyle. Following the steps for each period in this book will give you a good starting point, but you are going to want to do variations on each period in order to ensure that you do not create a production full of clones.

The best way to approach putting together a hairstyle is to break the hairstyle down into five sections: the front, the left side, the right side, the crown, and the nape. If you examine what each section of hair needs to look like, it becomes much easier to form a plan of attack for the hairstyle. For example, let's look at this detail of a hairstyle from Sandro Botticelli's painting *Primavera* (Figure 1.139). By breaking this style down into sections (Figure 1.140), you can begin to plan how you might style a wig in this hairstyle.

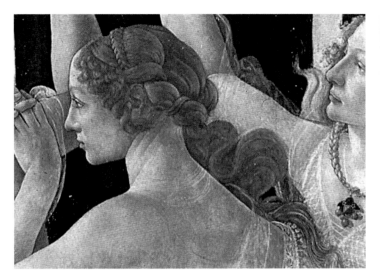

Figure 1.139 Sandro Botticelli's painting *Primavera*.

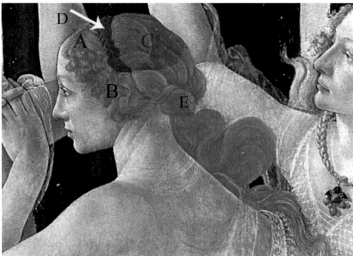

Figure 1.140 The Botticelli hairstyle broken down in sections.

The top/front of the hairstyle (A) is very flat with a center part. The side sections (B) have a tighter, wavier curl. This look could be achieved by setting this section of the hair on dime sized rollers set in spiral curls. Setting these curls with drag at the roots would help keep section A flat and without much volume. The crown of the wig (C) is also flat, with the ends of the hair going into large, soft curls. There is also a small braid (D) over the crown of the head. At the nape of the neck (E), the large soft curls continue from the crown of the head. These large soft curls in sections C and E could be achieved by setting the hair on quarter sized rollers, set off base with drag. In Figure 1.141, a recreation of this hairstyle styled and modeled by Josephine McAdam, she has added an additional small switch of hair in order to create the braid circling the crown of the head.

Always refer back to your period research and ask yourself "Is this section of the hair curly?"; "Are there ringlets hanging down in the back?"; "Should the bun be at the crown of the head or at the nape?" Other similar questions will help you figure out the hairstyle.

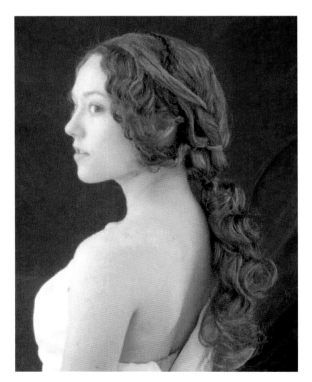

Figure 1.141 Student Josephine McAdam models her version of Botticelli's hairstyle.

Hairstyling Tips

Some other tips for putting together a successful hairstyle:

1. Do not try to make your hairstyle too perfect. Wigs look better when they have a slightly more natural look. Humans aren't perfect, and their hair is rarely perfect either. This is not an excuse to style the hair sloppily. Rather, think about putting the style together in a realistic way—real people have hairs that are a bit out of place or not perfectly curled.

2. Have a small bit of the hair break the hairline of the wig somewhere. We rarely see every bit of someone's hairline. Adding little wisps and tendrils helps to both disguise the fact that the hair is a wig and to make the style look more natural.

3. Hairnets are your friend! Use hairnets to secure sections of a hairstyle in place. This will make the section hold better, look neater, and cut down on wig maintenance.

4. The wig will look more natural if it reveals the shape of the skull somewhere. It does not need to be a large section of hair that is plastered down to the head. Rather, even the smallest section of the style that is close to the head will make the wig look more realistic. There are exceptions to this rule—1960s' hairstyles, for examples, do not generally hug the head anywhere (maybe this is why 60s' hair often looks so … *wiggy*!).

5. Consider the weight and balance of the wig as you style. A wig that is extremely top heavy or back heavy will be uncomfortable for the performer who has to wear it. Also consider whether the wig will need to be worn with a hat or headpiece. Try the hat or headpiece on the wig as you are styling it in order to be sure everything works together.

6. The audience does not wish to see all the effort that went into styling your wig. Do not overwork the wig so much that it looks like a product encrusted, tortured wig held together with 100 carefully placed bobby pins. A proper set and careful hiding of pins will go a long way towards making the hairstyle look graceful.

7. Consider the character. The hair on a character's head says a lot about who they are. It reveals things like social status, environment, and personality. As a wig designer, you can help the actor develop their character by making appropriate hair choices.

Is the character a buttoned up librarian whose hair has not moved in twenty years? Is she a social climber whose hair is ridiculously overdone? Is he a Restoration era fop who slavishly follows every trend of the day? Make good choices so that the audience knows exactly who the character is.

8. Period is in the silhouette; character is in the details. The overall shape of the hairstyle will let the audience know what period in which the play or film is taking place. The details within that hairstyle determine the character. This includes not only the details of the style itself, but also the details of the hair decorations.

Wig Sizes and Fitting

In a perfect world, all wigs would be custom made for the person who will be wearing them. Of course, we do not live in a perfect world. Fortunately, there are many great options available for purchase and use as they are. But which wig to order?

Many available wigs come labeled with a general cap size. While every brand is slightly different, here is a general guide to wig cap sizes that are based on the horizontal circumference of the head (the widest part of the head, usually just above the ears, measured parallel to the floor):

Child—19/20 inches

Petite—21 inches

Petite/Average—22 inches

Average—22 inches

Average/Large—22 ½ inches

Large—23 inches

There are other measurements that are also very useful to know if you are working with wigs. A comprehensive chart of these measurements and their locations has been included in Figure 1.142. Once taken, you can then transfer these measurements to a wig block, constantly checking your accuracy as you go.

Another way to make sure of a good fit is to take a head tracing of the person who will be wearing the wig. A head tracing is done by covering the hair with a wig cap, then covering the head with clear plastic wrap (Figure 1.143). Clear tape is then used to cover the plastic

HAIR & MAKEUP INFORMATION

DATE _____ PRODUCTION _____

CHARACTER _____ PERFORMER _____

Makeup Experience: None   Basic   Intermediate   Professional
Have you ever worn a wig? Yes   No   Lace Front?   Yes   No
Any Allergies to makeup & /or spirit gum?   Yes   No
If yes, Please list _____
Do you sweat a lot on stage? Yes   No
Do you wear contacts or glasses?   Yes   No

HEAD MEASUREMENTS

A. _____ CIRCUMFERENCE OF HEAD

B. _____ NAPE TO FRONT

C. _____ EAR TO EAR

D. _____ TEMPLE TO TEMPLE (BACK)

E. _____ SIDEBURN TO SIDEBURN (OVER CROWN)

F. _____ SIDEBURN TO SIDEBURN (OVER TOP)

G. _____ ACROSS NAPE

H. _____ WIDTH OF SIDEBURN

I. _____ EAR TO EAR (AROUND BACK)

J. _____ TEMPLE TO TEMPLE (FRONT)

K. _____ BRIDGE OF NOSE TO HAIRLINE

L. _____ BRIDGE OF NOSE TO RECEDING POINT

M. _____ EAR TO NAPE

N. _____ TEMPLE TO SIDEBURN

O. _____ BACK OF EAR TO BACK OF EAR

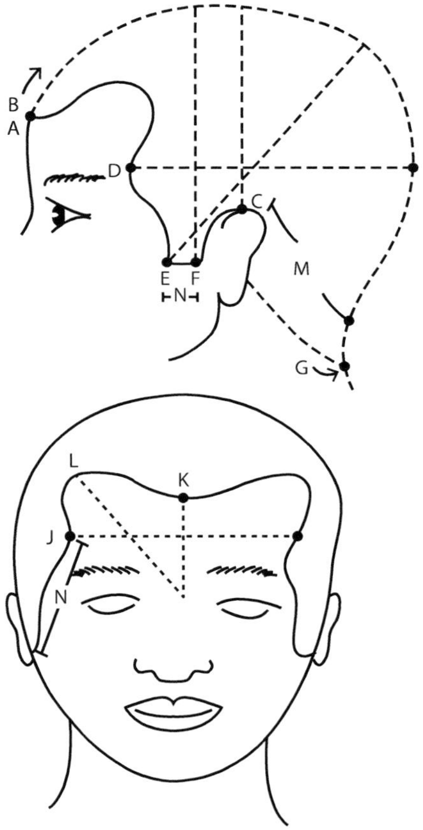

Natural Hair Color _____
Naturally Straight / Curly / Wavy / Permed
Length of hair _____

Figure 1.142 Wig measurement chart.

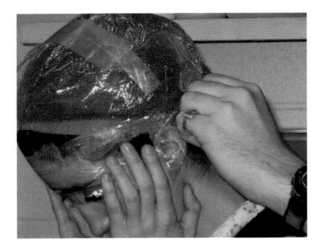

Figure 1.143   Cover the subject's hair and wig cap with plastic wrap.

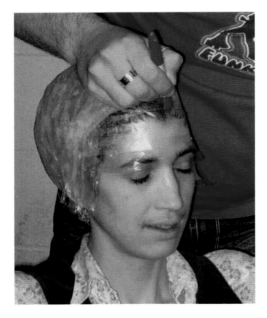

Figure 1.144   Once you have covered the head with clear tape, trace the exact hairline with a permanent marker.

wrap. This holds the plastic wrap in the exact shape of the head. You can then trace the exact hairline of the person with a permanent marker (Figure 1.144). Once you are done, you can then transfer the plastic tracing to a canvas block.

Once you put the plastic tracing on the block, you may find that you need to pad out the head so it is the exact shape of the wearer's head. To do this, choose a block where the plastic sits snugly at the hairline all the way around the head. Secure the hairline with tape (Figure 1.145). Once the tracing is secure, cut small slits in the wig and stuff the empty areas (Figure 1.146). You can use tissue, newspaper, paper towels, or cotton batting as a stuffing material. Once the empty area is full, retape

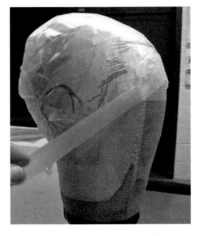

Figure 1.145   Secure the edge of the plastic tracing all the way around the head with clear tape.

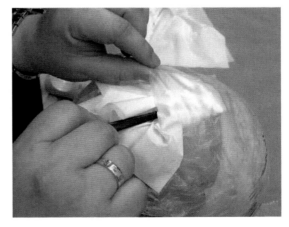

Figure 1.146   Cut small slits in the plastic tracing wherever there is empty space inside. Stuff with your chosen stuffing material, and then tape it back closed once the plastic is full.

the slit closed. But be careful not to overstuff the tracing—you don't want to distort the head shape.

Having an exact copy of the head that will be wearing the wig is useful even if you do not have the time or the ability to custom make a wig. The tracing can guide you when you are styling the wig. For example, you can strategically place sections of hair or curls to conceal small areas where the person's hair might show under the wig.

Working With Less Than Ideal Wigs

Sometimes a wig simply does not fit or cannot do the style you want it to do. Don't despair! There are still a few tricks you can try to make a less than ideal wig work.

Often, the bottom edge of a wig is unfinished, with exposed elastic or ribbon along the nape edge. While this is fine for a style where the hair hangs down, it is very problematic if you want to create an updo. If this is the case, first remove a couple of pieces of the weft (most wigs have way too much hair in them anyway, so a couple of tracks will not be missed). To do this, turn the wig inside out and use a pair of small sharp scissors to carefully snip the stitches holding the weft in

place (Figure 1.147). Select rows that are not holding important pieces of the wig's structure together. Once you have snipped the stitches, turn the wig back right side out and remove the loose weft by pulling it gently out of the wig.

Once you have removed the weft, turn the wig inside out and pin it to the canvas block, making sure to stretch the elastic behind the ears (if you don't stretch it, the wig will become too small). Pin the pieces of weft around the bottom of the wig, going from the back of one ear, down and around the nape, to the back of the other ear (Figure 1.148). Use a curved needle to stitch the weft in place. Once you have finished, turn the wig back right side out. The hair you added underneath will now cover the nape edge of the wig when you pull it up to make an updo.

Sometimes, even the largest wig will not be large enough for the person who needs to wear it. One solution to this problem is to buy two of the same wig and piece them together. Two good places to add to the wig are the center front (Figure 1.149) and the center back nape area (Figure 1.150).

To add to the center front, cut off the front section of one wig and stitch it to the front of the second wig. This will add length from front to back, which is where the wig is often too small. You may also need to cut a slit in the center of the second wig so

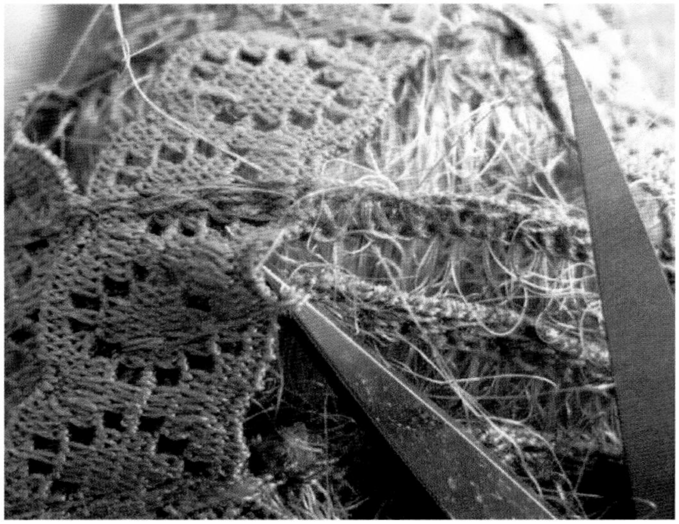

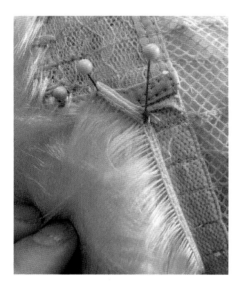

Figure 1.147   Carefully snip the stitches holding the weft in place on the inside cap of the wig.

Figure 1.148   Pin the weft on the inside nape edge of the wig and stitch it in place.

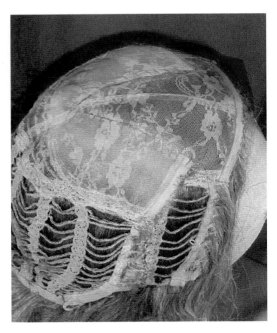

Figure 1.149 The blue highlighted area shows where the piece of the first wig should be added to the second wig at the center front.

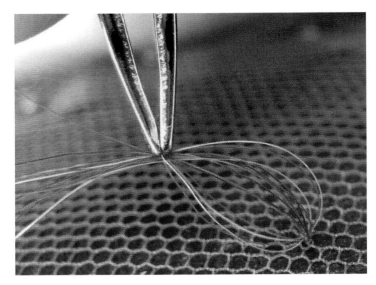

Figure 1.151 Use slant-tipped tweezers to pluck/untie knots from a too densely knotted piece.

that it opens up wider. This is helpful if the wig is too short across the top.

To add to the nape section of the wig, simply cut the nape section off of the first wig and add it to the nape of the second wig. This will create more length from front to back, and is a little bit simpler of an alteration to perform.

Even a commercially made lace front will often require a little bit of adjusting. These wigs are usually sold with a very generic, artificial looking hairline. Going into the wig with a pair of slant tipped tweezers and plucking out some of the knots will create a much more believable hairline. Pay attention to where the subject's hairline sweeps forward and dips back; let that guide you to which knots to pluck out. This can also be done on commercially made facial hairpieces. These are made with very dense hair; thinning out some of the knots can create a more natural appearance for the facial hairpiece. In either case, make sure to firmly secure the wig or facial hair to the canvas block before beginning to pluck it.

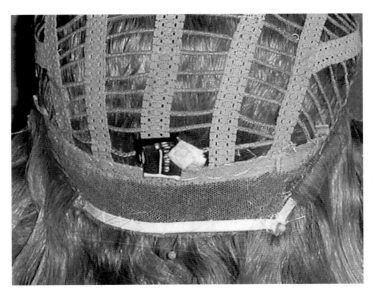

Figure 1.150 The orange highlighted area shows where the nape section cut off the first wig is to be added to the second wig.

Wig Washing and Care

Taking care of your wigs when you are finished with a particular hairstyle will insure that your wig stock has a long and happy life. Too many places simply toss their used wigs, full of styling products and pins, into a box until the next time they are needed. Doing this allows sweat, moisture, and product to sit in the wig, breaking it down, until the next time it needs to be styled. Taking the time to care for your wigs can make all the difference in the world for the next time.

Wigs should be washed after they have been used. Some wig professionals like to use shampoos and conditioners specifically designed for wigs; others (including myself) often wash wigs with baby shampoo and condition with a good moisturizing conditioner. Sometimes, you may also need to remove product buildup from a wig. This can be done by using a clarifying shampoo, or, in more extreme cases, baking soda. (To do this, make a paste by adding a little water to the baking soda in the palm of your hand. Gently rub the paste into the section of hair you are trying to remove the buildup from. The baking soda will act as an abrasive to remove the hairspray. Once the buildup is removed, take the time to rinse the wig thoroughly until all the baking soda is gone.)

Wigs can be washed either on the wig block or off the wig block in a sink or plastic tub. Before washing, remove all decorations, hairnets, hair pins, rubber bands, and elastics from the wig. Brush the wig thoroughly until all the tangles have been removed.

Washing the Wig off the Wig Block

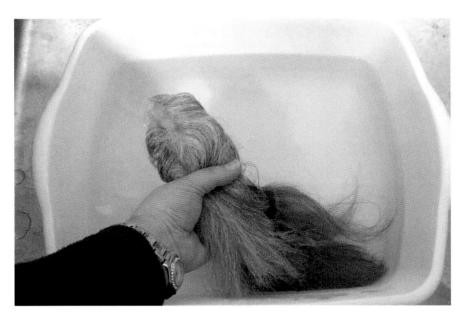

Figure 1.152 Step 1. Wet the wig by dipping it into a sink or tub, using a smooth sideways motion. Do not ever hold the wig by the front lace—wet lace can easily be damaged or stretched out of shape. Also, do not soak the wig in the tub or swish it around—this can lead to tangling.

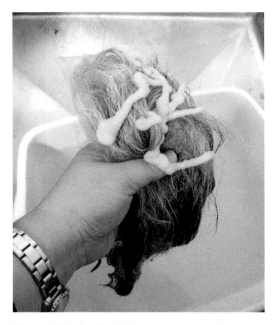

Figure 1.153 Step 2. Add the shampoo or conditioner to the top of the wig. Add a little water. Work the product into the wig using smooth downward strokes. Do not tousle the wig hair.

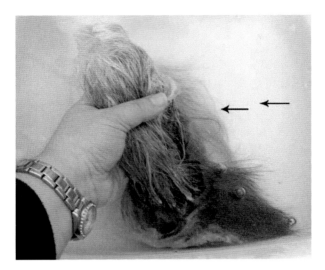

Figure 1.154   Step 3. Rinse the product out of the hair by dipping it through the tub, again using a sideways dipping motion. You may need to replace the water in the tub after you have rinsed a few times in order to get all the cleanser out of the hair. You can also rinse the wig using a hose attachment for your faucet, making sure to support the wig from the inside as you do so.

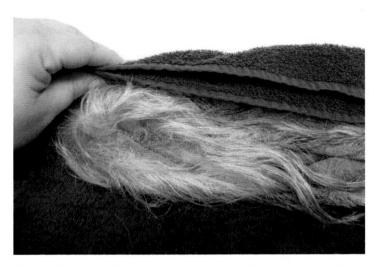

Figure 1.155   Step 4. Once you have shampooed, conditioned, and thoroughly rinsed the wig, lay it out on a clean dry towel. Roll the wig up in the towel.

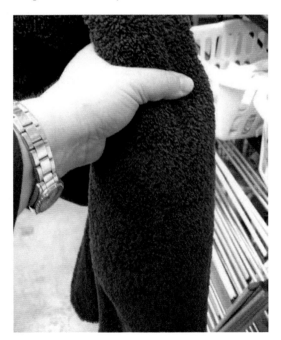

Figure 1.156   Step 5. Gently squeeze the excess water out of the wig into the towel using a downward motion with your hands.

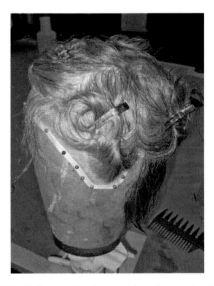

Figure 1.157   Step 6. Remove the damp wig from the towel and block it back on a canvas wig block. Spray the wig with detangling spray if needed. Divide the hair into sections and use a wide toothed comb to begin detangling the wig at the nape, working your way up to the top and hairline. Once the wig is detangled (take your time!) either put it in the wig dryer to dry or let it air dry. If the wig is synthetic, steam it straight before letting it dry. This will give you a nice straight wig ready for styling the next time you need to use it.

Washing the Wig on the Wig Block

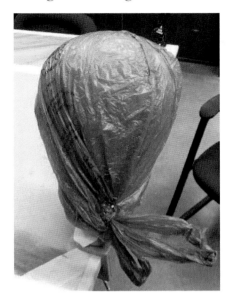

Figure 1.158   Step 1. Cover the wig with either plastic wrap or a plastic bag. Block the wig on top of the plastic.

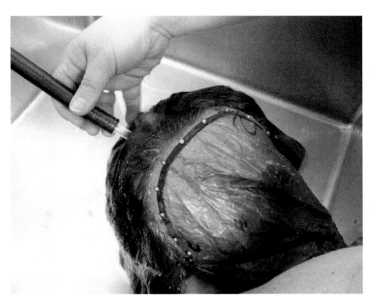

Figure 1.159   Step 2. Use a hose attachment for your sink to wet the wig thoroughly with lukewarm water.

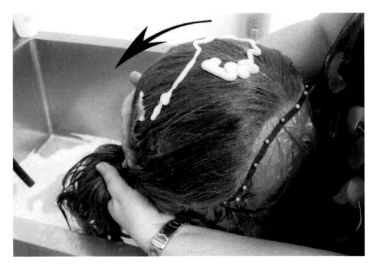

Figure 1.160   Step 3. Place a small amount of your shampoo or conditioner on top of your wig and use a smooth downward motion to work it through the hair. Rinse the hair using the hose, taking care not to tousle the wig.

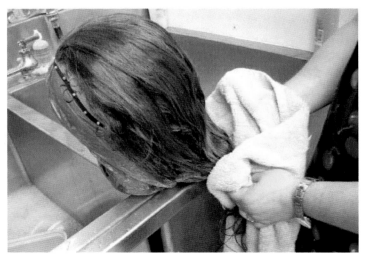

Figure 1.161   Step 4. Once the wig is washed, conditioned, and rinsed, use a clean dry towel to blot excess water out of the wig. Section the wig and detangle it with a wide toothed comb, beginning from the bottom of the wig.

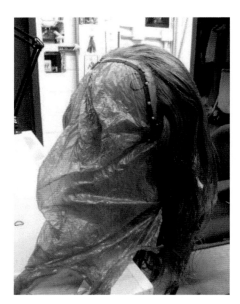

Figure 1.162 Step 5. Steam the damp wig straight if it is a synthetic wig. Put the wig in the wig dryer to dry. If you are using a plastic bag to cover the block, untie the bottom so that air can get in to dry the canvas block.

Storing Your Wigs

It is very helpful to have some sort of system for storing your wig stock. This will make sure that you can find any wig you are looking for and also keep the wig in the best possible condition. I prefer to store my wig in individual plastic storage bags. I braid all wigs that are long enough to keep them from tangling. These bags can be stored in bins, boxes, or drawers. It is also helpful to keep an inventory of your wigs so that you always know what you have.

Tips for Using This Book

In each chapter, I have discussed basic looks for each period, including period research. For each major period in fashion history, I have taken you through the steps to create at least one hairstyle representative of that period. Sometimes the style will be a direct copy of particular reference picture; other styles will be styles that I have created by combining several references in order to show you specific techniques. I will note which reference I am working from when applicable. As you become more comfortable with wig styling, you will begin to be able

to create different hairstyles based on the basic techniques that were discussed. I have listed in each chapter ideas about variations on these styles. I have also included in the beginning of each chapter a list of artists, designers, and style icons/important people to help start you on your research into each period.

In the styling examples, I use rollers that are the same size in diameter, but different colors. Different colors do not have any significance in the styling—they just happen to be the colors of the rollers I have. I also do not make any distinction between spring wire rollers or plastic rollers—I use them interchangeably. I will note the size of roller you need to use in order to make the instructions more clear.

For almost every wig style I style, I set a small tendril of hair on a pencil sized (or smaller) roller in front of the ear (Figure 1.163). I also often (especially when styling an updo) set short tendrils or curls around the nape of the wig, starting back behind the ears (Figure 1.164). These small wispy curls help both hard front wigs and lace front wigs look more realistic by camouflaging the edge of the wig.

For most of the styling examples, I use lace front wigs because they are the ideal choice. If you do not have lace front wigs, you can still create most of the styles in this book. You can adapt wigs in many

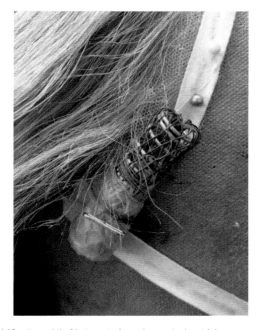

Figure 1.163 A tendril of hair set in front the ear in the sideburn area of the wig.

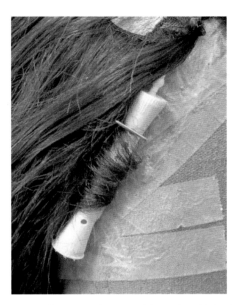

Figure 1.164   Tendrils of hair set at the nape of the neck and behind the ears help conceal the back edge of the wig.

ways—you can add wefting to them to add volume or length, you can incorporate hairpieces in order to add to the style of your wig. If you are using a hard front wig, you may need to take extra steps in order to conceal the front edge of the wig. For example, you may need to set additional small tendrils of hair going forward onto the forehead. Other styles have the hair coming onto the face in such a way that the hairline would be covered already. Still other styles are from historical periods where wigs would have been worn, so the wig looking like a wig instead of like natural hair is not an issue. Look carefully at the wigs you have available to you and the style you are trying to create in order to make good choices about what wig will work best for your project.

Practice all the wig techniques, do a lot of historical period research, and think about your characters. You are now ready to begin creating period hairstyles. The following chapters will guide you through the basics of styling in periods throughout history.

Good luck making many fantastic creations!

two

EARLY VICTORIAN ERA

(1835–1860)

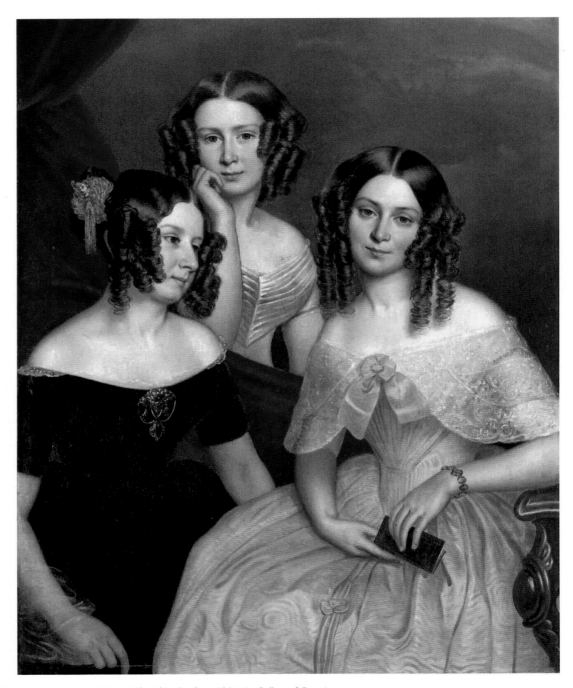

Figure 2.1   *The Three Robinson Sisters*, George Theodore Berthon, 1846, Art Gallery of Ontario.

Important Events

1837	Queen Victoria takes the throne of England
1837	Samuel Morse develops the telegraph
1839	Louis Daguerre and J.N. Nièpce coinvent Daguerreotype photography
1845	Elias Howe invents the sewing machine
1845	Irish famine begins
1848	The pre-Raphaelite Brotherhood is founded
1849	The American Gold Rush
1851	The Great Exhibition/the first World's Fair is held
1854–1856	The Crimean War

Important Artists/Designers

William Blake, Dominique Ingres, John Everett Millais, Joseph Karl Stieler, Franz Xaver Winterhalter

Important People/Style Icons

Prince Albert and Queen Victoria, Charles Dickens, Empress Eugenie, Franz Joseph I, Jenny Lind, Victoire de Nemours

Early Victorian Women

Following the excess and height of 1830s' hairstyles, Victorian hairstyles became more subdued. Queen Victoria took the throne and her more conservative sensibilities set the tone for the fashions in her era. *Godey's Ladies Book* (1830–1878), a periodical that featured pictures of fashions and hairstyles, was also exerting great influence over popular fashion. The high buns of the 1830s moved down to the back of the head just below the crown. The hair remained parted in the center, with a second hair parting often going from ear to ear over the top of the head, separating the front of the hairstyle from the back.

The area of hair around a lady's ears was a particular focal point in this era. The ears might be entirely covered with long ringlets, as in Figures 2.2 and 2.4. These ringlets might consist of looser curls, or they might be defined columns of hair known as sausage curls. The hair might also be braided or coiled and looped around the ears, as in Figure 2.3.

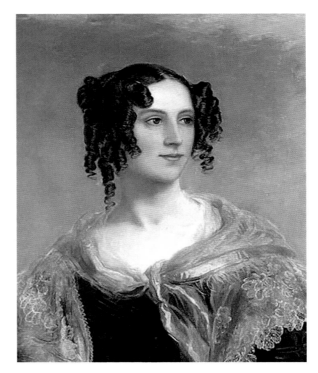

Figure 2.2 Detail from *Portrait of a Lady, Thought to be Clementine Metternich*, a follower of Franz Xaver Winterhalter.

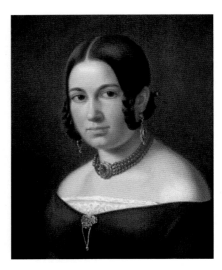

Figure 2.3 *Portrait of Christine Dieckhoff*, Georg Wittemann, 1846. Notice how this lady's braids loop around her ears.

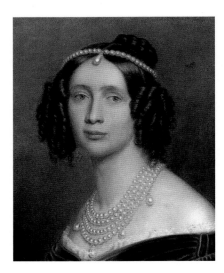

Figure 2.4 *Maria Anna of Bavaria, Queen of Saxony*, Joseph Karl Stieler, circa 1842.

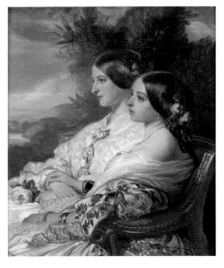

Figure 2.5 *Queen Victoria and Her Cousin, the Duchess of Nemours*, Franz Xaver Winterhaler, 1852, Royal Collection of the United Kingdom.

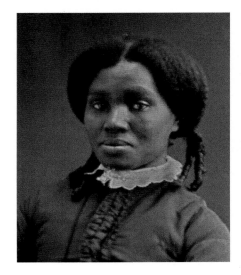

Figure 2.6 Daguerrotype of an unidentified African-American woman, circa 1850, George Eastman House Collection.

More simple styles can also be found later in this period, with hair simply being smoothed down from a center part, and then smoothed back to cover the ears. Figures 2.5 and 2.6 show examples of this style. Sometimes the hair was puffed out over the ears to add volume to the sides of the hair. This helped visually balance the head with the large hoopskirts women were beginning to wear at this time.

It was also very important at this time for a woman's hair to look shiny and healthy. Figures 2.1 and 2.5 are good examples of shining hair. Pomades and oils were used to heighten this effect.

Early Victorian Men

Men's hair in the Victorian era was becoming longer on top, so that it could be formed into romantic windswept curls and waves. These hairstyles often had a deep side part. The top of these hairstyles was often quite flat to the head, then increasing in fullness over the ears (Figure 2.7).

Men's facial hair was still enjoying great popularity at this time. All sorts of styles were fashionable, including sculptured full sideburns, neat mustaches, and long square goatees (see Figures 2.6 and 2.7). Men's hair was also expected to be shiny at this time.

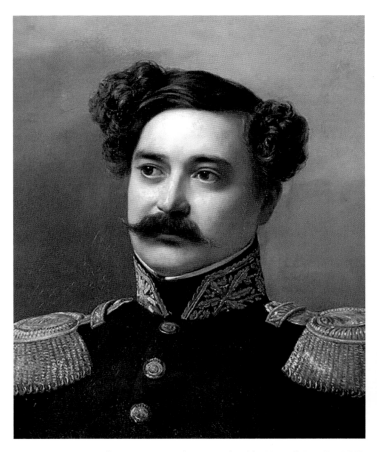

Figure 2.7 *Portrait of Simon Anton Freiherr von Tubeuf*, by Heinrich Brandes, 1840. This gentleman's hair has been arranged in elaborate curls over his ears.

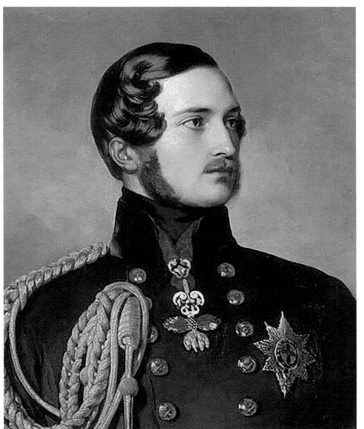

Figure 2.8 Detail from *Prince Albert of Saxe-Coburg and Gotha, Wearing the Golden Fleece*, by Franz Xaver Winterhalter, 1842, Royal Collection of the United Kingdom. This portrait shows off a longer men's hairstyle with a deep side part in the hair, a mustache, and dramatic sideburns.

Victorian Woman's Styling— Step by Step

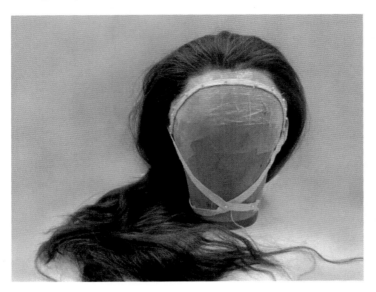

Figure 2.9 Step 1. Begin with a wig that is long (16 inches long at the nape of the neck) and mostly all one length. There could be some shorter layers (10 inches long) around the face. Here, I used a lace front synthetic.

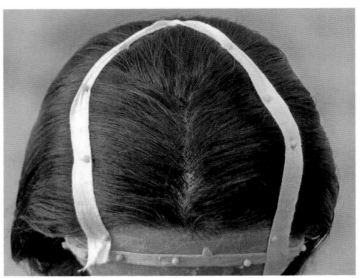

Figure 2.10 Step 2. Part the hair in the center with a rattail comb. Next, pin blocking tape around the top of the head a few inches away from the part. This will help keep the hair in the front section of the wig flat and smooth.

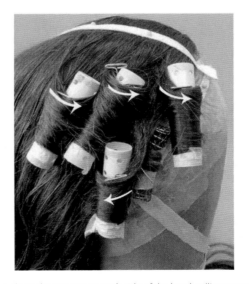

Figure 2.11 Step 3. Set three sausage curls on the top row on each side of the head, rolling towards the face. For the second, lower row, set one sausage curl rolling away from the face. Use dime sized rollers for all these curls. Also set a small tendril rolling towards the face.

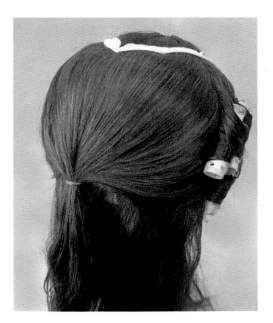

Figure 2.12   Step 4. Pull most of the rest of the hair in the wig into a ponytail at the back of the head. Leave a section of hair hanging loose at the nape of the neck.

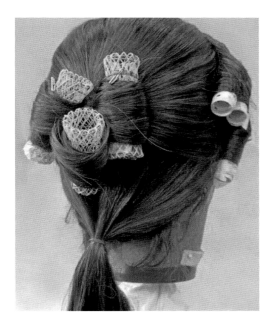

Figure 2.13   Step 5. Set the hair in the ponytail on three nickel sized rollers.

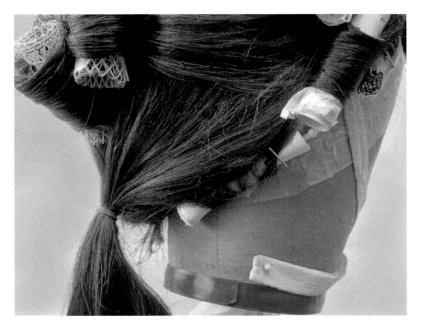

Figure 2.14   Step 6. Pull the hair at the nape of the neck into a second, lower ponytail. You will then roll the hair in the low ponytail onto four nickel sized rollers.

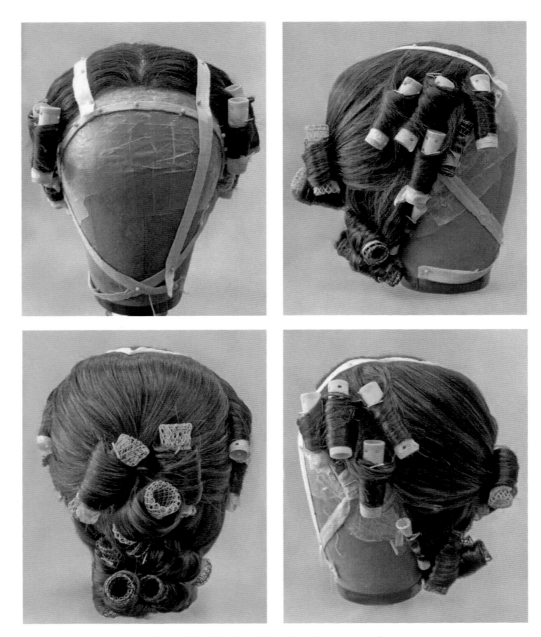

Figures 2.15–2.18   The finished Victorian woman's style set.

Once you have finished setting the wig, steam each roller thoroughly if the wig is made of synthetic hair. If the wig is human hair, soak each roller with water sprayed from a spray bottle. After steaming or wetting, place the wig in a wig dryer for 75 minutes.

To style:

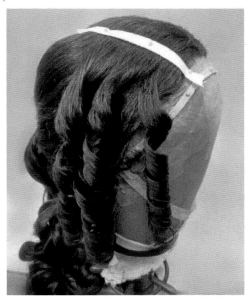

Figure 2.19   Step 7. Remove all the rollers in the wig, beginning at the nape of the neck. Take extra care when you unwind the ringlets at the sides of the face.

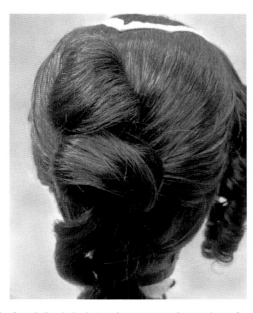

Figure 2.20   Step 8. Brush the hair in the top ponytail around your fingers to form four looped curls. Pin two of these curls in place with bobby pins.

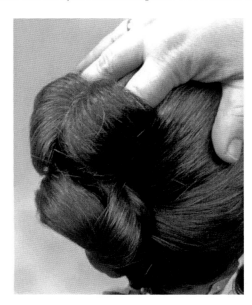

Figure 2.21   Step 9. Bring the second two curls up and on top of the first two curls you pinned in place. Use your fingers to arrange the curls in a pretty way and pin them in place.

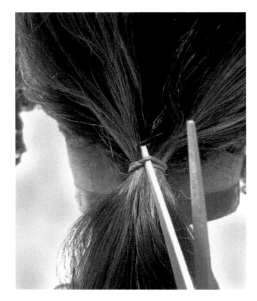

Figure 2.22   Step 10. Snip through the rubber band holding the lower ponytail. This will allow you to get rid of the rubber band without tangling the hair.

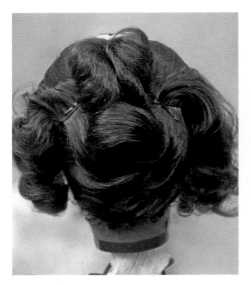

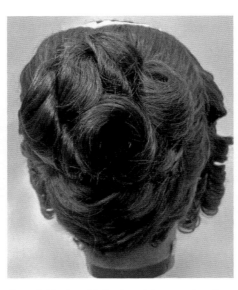

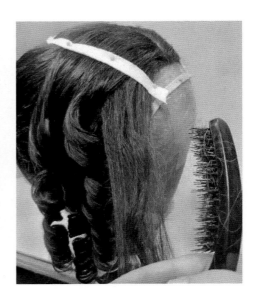

Figure 2.23 Step 11. Divide the hair at the nape of the neck in half. Drape each half section up the back of the head, and pin it on the side of the bun. (The lower left section should be pulled up and pinned on the right side of the bun, and the lower right section should be pulled up and pinned to the left side of the bun.)

Figure 2.24 Step 12. Brush each loose section of hair around your finger to form another curl. Pin these curls in place and incorporate them into the bun. You can cover the bun with a hairnet to make it even more secure and neat.

Figure 2.25 Step 13. Move to the ringlets in the front of the hairstyle. Brush through each ringlet section with a teasing/smoothing brush.

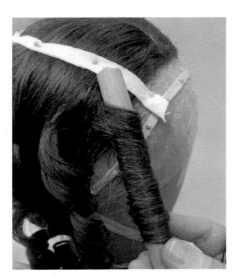

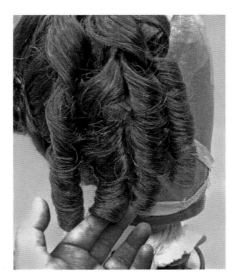

Figure 2.26 Step 14. Brush each sausage curl around a dowel rod, then slide the dowel rod out of the curl. Misting the hair with hairspray before you brush it around the dowel rod will help the ringlet stay in place even better. Be sure not to put so much hairspray on the section that it sticks to the dowel rod.

Figure 2.27 Step 15. If the bottom of the ringlet begins to separate, use your finger to push the bottom bit of hair up inside the rest of the ringlet.

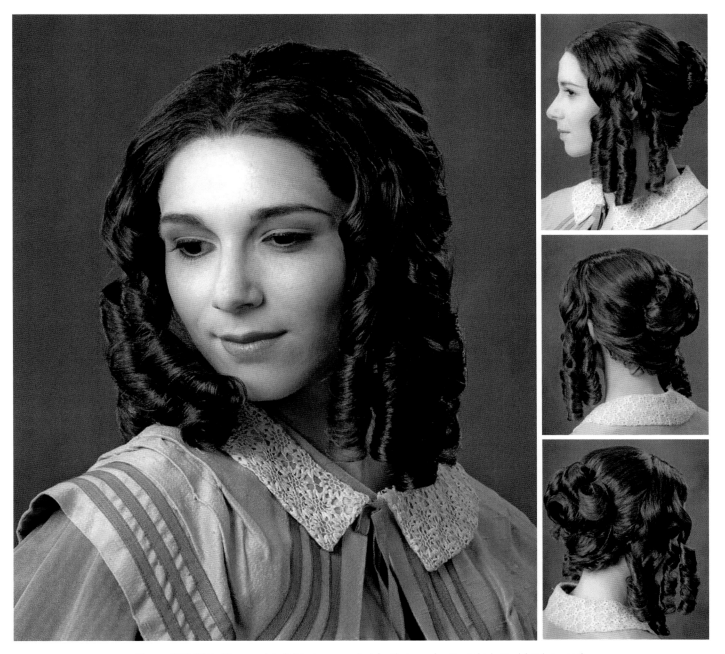

Figures 2.28–2.31 The completed Victorian woman's style. Photography: Tim Babiak. Model: Sabrina Lotfi.

Victorian Woman's Fuller Styling— Step by Step

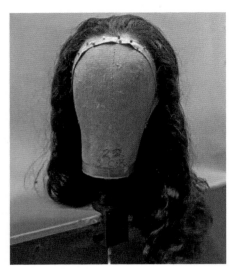

Figure 2.32 Step 1. I used Figure 2.6 as a reference for this style. Therefore, I decided to use a long human hair wig that has been permed to have a natural curly texture.

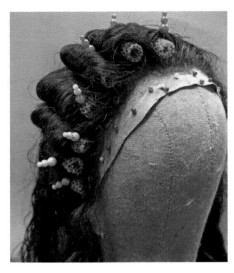

Figure 2.33 Step 2. Make a center part in the wig and use pencil sized rollers to roll straight down the side front section.

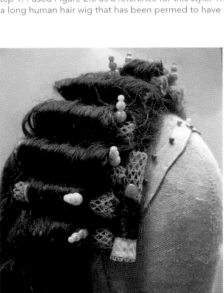

Figure 2.34 Step 3. Set another pencil size roller rolling towards the face to make a small sausage curl.

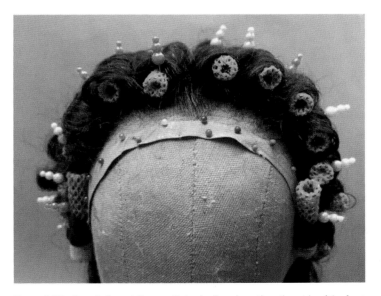

Figure 2.35 Step 4. Repeat the pencil sized rollers down the other side of the front section.

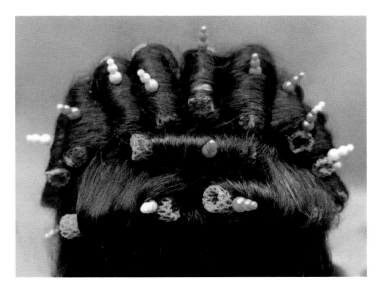

Figure 2.36 Step 5. Beginning right behind the center part, set several pencil sized rollers going straight back.

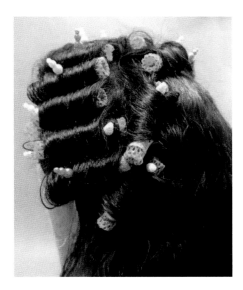

Figure 2.37 Step 6. Set several more rollers angling back from the front section towards the center back of the head.

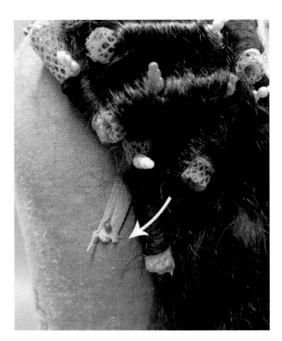

Figure 2.38 Step 7. Add a second small sausage curl rolling towards the face behind each ear.

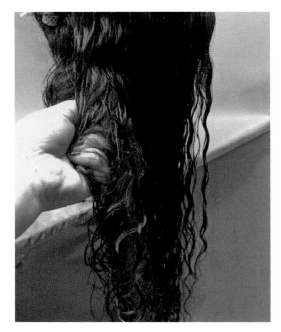

Figure 2.39 Step 8. For the remainder of the wig, we are going to take advantage of the texture the wig has. Thoroughly wet the wig and comb through it with a wide toothed comb. Scrunch handfuls of the hair to accentuate the texture.

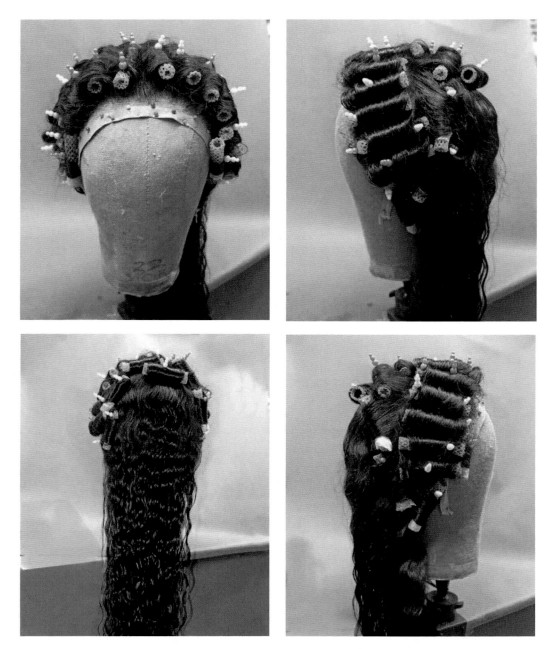

Figures 2.40–2.43   The finished Victorian woman's fuller style set.

Once you have finished setting the wig, steam each roller thoroughly if the wig is made of synthetic hair. If the wig is human hair, soak each roller with water sprayed from a spray bottle. After steaming or wetting, place the wig in a wig dryer for 75 minutes.

To style:

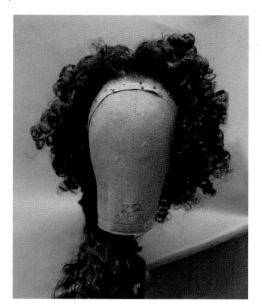

Figure 2.44   Step 9. Remove all the rollers in the wig. Take extra care when you unwind the ringlets at the sides of the face.

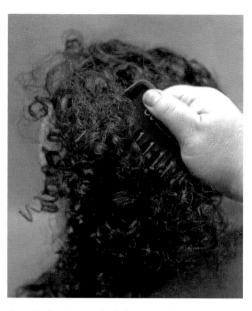

Figure 2.45   Step 10. Comb through all the hair with a wide toothed comb.

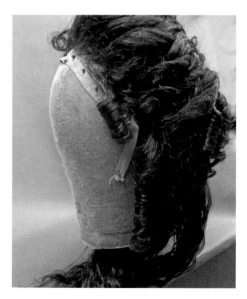

Figure 2.46   Step 11. Take care to move aside the two sausage curls around each ear. These will be smoothed later in the process.

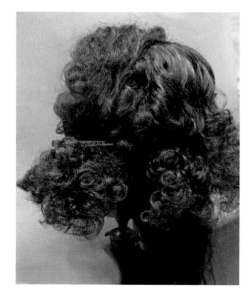

Figure 2.47   Step 12. Separate out the side front sections and pin them out of the way with duckbill clips.

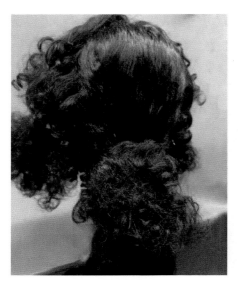

Figure 2.48 Step 13. Add the hair from the center section that was in rollers to the large section of textured hair and pull all this hair into a low ponytail.

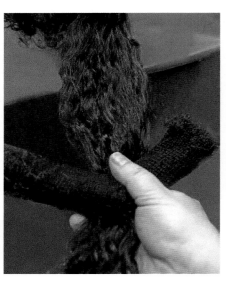

Figure 2.49 Step 14. Take a long cylindrical hair pad and roll the hair in the ponytail around it up towards the nape of the neck.

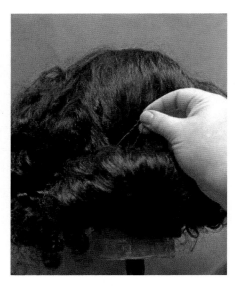

Figure 2.50 Step 15. Use large hairpins to secure the roll in the center.

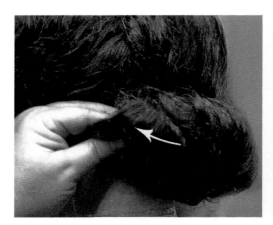

Figure 2.51 Step 16. Pull the hair in the roll around to each side in order to cover the ends of the hair pad. Pin in place.

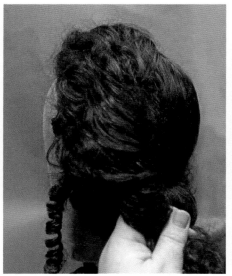

Figure 2.52 Step 17. Gather each side section into your hand and twist it twice. Push the twist towards the ear and slightly upwards in order to create maximum volume over the ears. Pin each side in place.

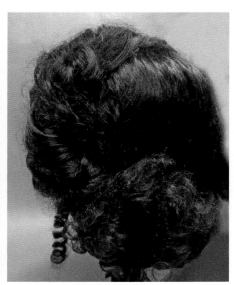

Figure 2.53 Step 18. Gently smooth out the ends of each side section with a wide toothed comb.

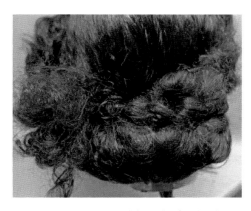

Figure 2.54 Step 19. Braid the ends of each side section and cross them over the top of the rolled bun.

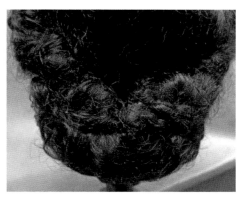

Figure 2.55 Step 20. Make sure to tuck in the ends of each braid and pin so that no bits of hair are sticking out.

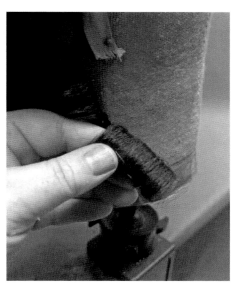

Figure 2.56 Step 21. Brush the small sausage curls around your finger in order to smooth them.

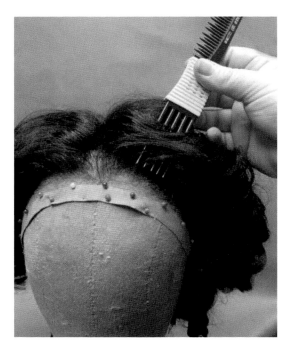

Figure 2.57 Step 22. Use a lifting comb/pick to lift the side sections for maximum volume.

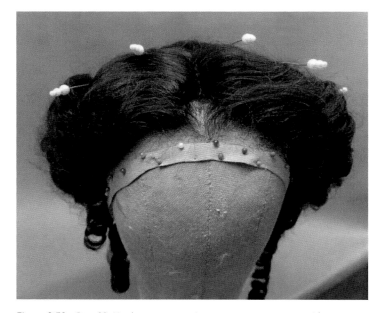

Figure 2.58 Step 23. Use large corsage pins to urge any waves you wish to accentuate in place. Mist with hairspray and allow to sit for several hours.

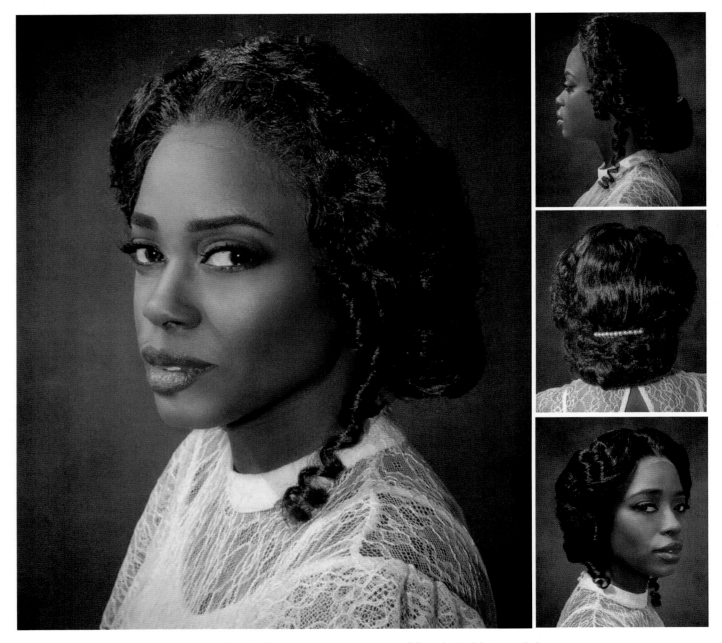

Figures 2.59–2.62   The completed Victorian woman's fuller style. Model: Antonia Taylor.

Variations

To create variety in your Victorian/Romantic women's hairstyles, follow the examples in Figure 2.63. Some of the hairstyles in the painting have ringlets around the face, some have the hair smoothed back over the ears. Some of the styles have buns only in the back, while some of the styles have a few ringlets hanging down. Some of the hairstyles are decorated with ribbons, some with flowers. You can experiment with head coverings such a small lacy caps or knitted snoods (Figure 2.64). You can also dress the hair in loops or braids around the ears as in Figure 2.3.

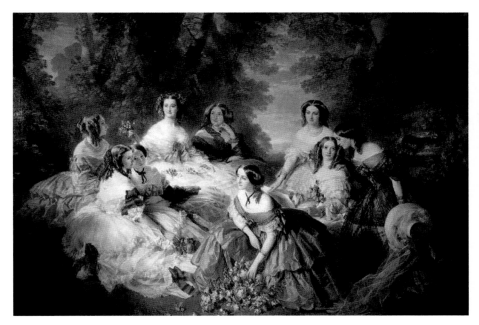

Figure 2.63 *Eugenie, Empress of the French, and Her Ladies,* by Franz Xaver Winterhalter, 1855, Musée National de Palais de Compiegne.

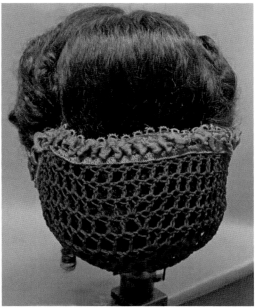

Figure 2.64 The Victorian woman's wider style wig has been dressed with a snood over the low chignon at the nape.

Victorian Makeup

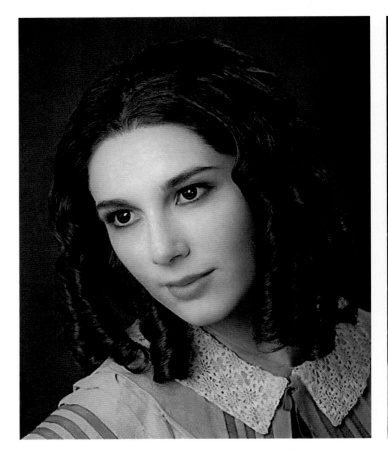

Figure 2.65   A typical Victorian beauty look. Model: Sabrina Lotfi.

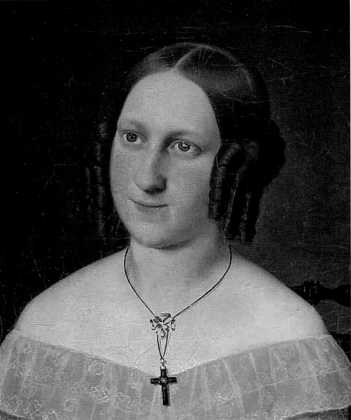

Figure 2.66   Portrait of a young woman wearing a blue dress and lace gloves, Andreas Hunaeus, 1841. This woman is an example of the ideal "English rose" with rosy cheeks and minimal makeup.

Queen Victoria believed that painted faces were "vulgar," so Victorian era women had to be very discreet in their use of cosmetics. Many women hid their cosmetics in portable toilet chests, many of which had secret compartments. The Victorian woman might use "Crème Celeste" to achieve perfectly pale skin. Eyebrows would be neatly plucked. Eyelashes were accented with castor oil or beeswax, with a little soot rubbed in to darken them. Beet juice or carmine dye might be rubbed into the cheeks for color. Lip salves might have a hint of color mixed in to color the lips. Large liquid eyes were esteemed, and were often achieved by adding drops of belladonna to dilate the pupils. The look would be finished off with a dusting of rice powder or powder of crushed pearls.

Victorian Man's Styling— Step by Step

This hairstyle is based on a combination of the styles seen in Figures 2.7 and 2.8.

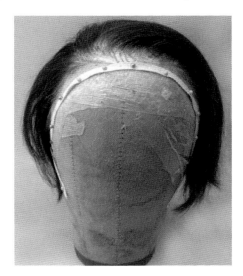

Figure 2.67 Step 1. Begin with a short wig that has longer hair (at least five inches long) on top and shorter hair in the back and nape areas. A fully ventilated, human hair lace wig is best for this kind of hairstyle. I used a fully ventilated lace front wig made of human hair.

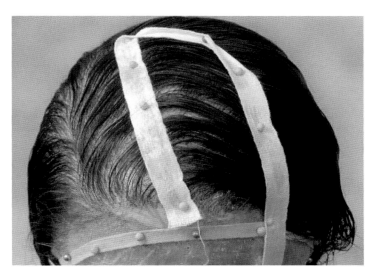

Figure 2.68 Step 2. Make a deep side part in the wig with a comb. Saturate the top section of the wig with setting lotion. Form a flat wave on the top of the wig by combing the hair away from the face and pinning the center of the wave with a piece of blocking tape. Next, comb the hair towards the face to form the second half of the wave, and pin it in place with the blocking tape.

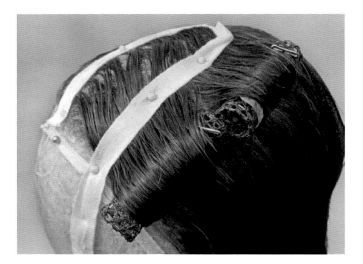

Figure 2.69 Step 3. Use dime sized rollers to set curls at the end of the waved section of hair.

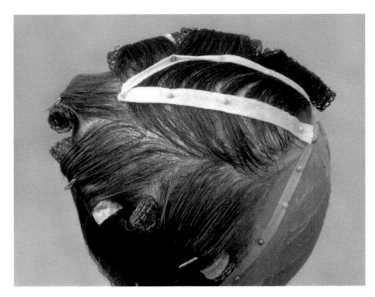

Figure 2.70   Step 4. Continue working your way around the head with dime sized rollers.

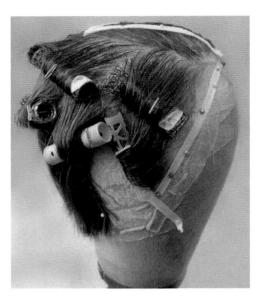

Figure 2.71   Step 5. Drop down to the next row of rollers. Set the first roller (pencil sized) going away from the face in the temple/sideburn area. The rest of the row should be rolled towards the ears on dime sized rollers.

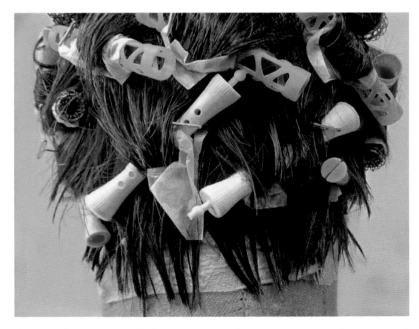

Figure 2.72   Step 6. Continue setting the wig on decreasing sizes of rollers, ending on small perm rods. Also alternate the rows in diagonal directions. Do not worry if some of the hair is too short to fit around a roller. We will curl this hair by hand later.

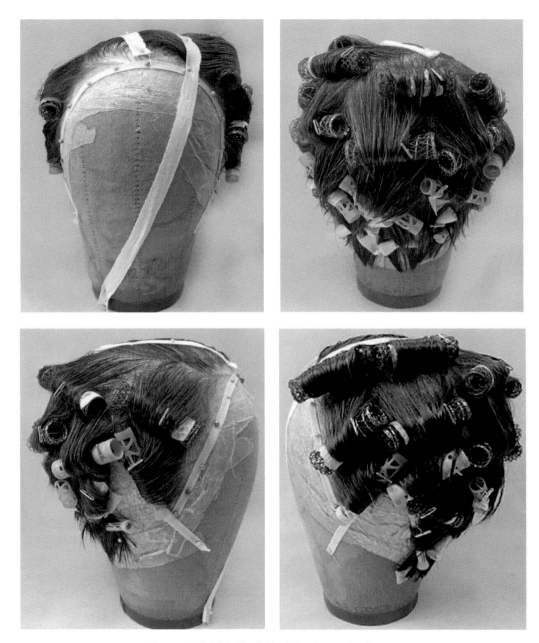

Figures 2.73–2.76 The finished Victorian man's style set.

Once you have finished setting the wig, steam each roller thoroughly if the wig is made of synthetic hair. If the wig is human hair, soak each roller with water sprayed from a spray bottle. After steaming or wetting, place the wig in a wig dryer for 75 minutes.

To style:

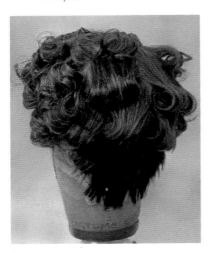

Figure 2.77 Step 7. Remove all the rollers from the wig, beginning at the nape of the neck.

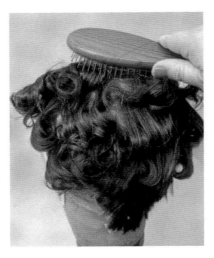

Figure 2.78 Step 8. Use a large brush to thoroughly brush through all the hair in the wig.

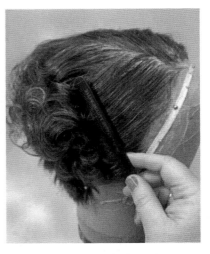

Figure 2.79 Step 9. Go back into the wig with a rattail comb. Use the comb to smooth out the waves and curls in the hairstyle and to push them into place.

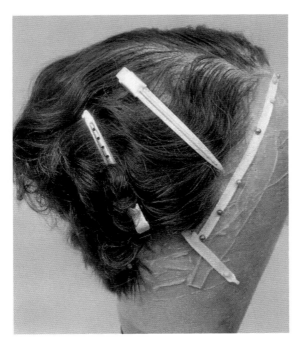

Figure 2.80 Step 10. Use duckbill clips to hold the waves in place. Mist this section with hairspray.

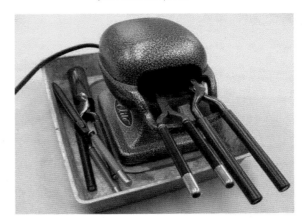

Figure 2.81 Step 11. Plug in a Marcel oven and allow it to heat up. A Marcel oven is a small oven into which you place metal curling irons. This heats them to very high temperatures. Marcel irons come in very small sizes that make them ideal for styling short lengths of hair. Once it becomes warm, place a couple of small Marcel irons inside. Once the irons are hot, test them on a scrap piece of human hair in order to ensure that they will not scorch the hair. **Always test a Marcel iron's heat before using it on a wig!!!!** Marcel irons should never be used on a synthetic hair wig—they will scorch the hair beyond repair. If you are using a synthetic wig or do not have access to a Marcel oven, style the short hairs by rolling them on a bobby pin if the hair is long enough. If the hair is not long enough, comb the short hairs in the direction you wish for them to go, spray them with hairspray, and allow them to set overnight.

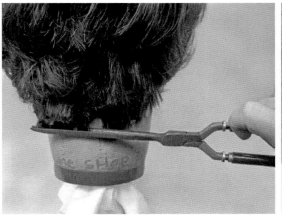
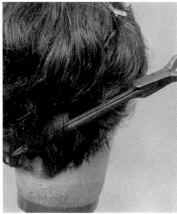

Figures 2.82 and 2.83   Step 12. Use the Marcel irons to curl any bits of hair that have not already been curled.

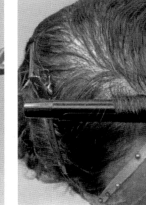

Figure 2.84   Step 13. Use a regular electric curling iron to curl small sections of hair at the front of the wig. Letting a small section of the hair fall in front of the hairline will help the wig look much more natural.

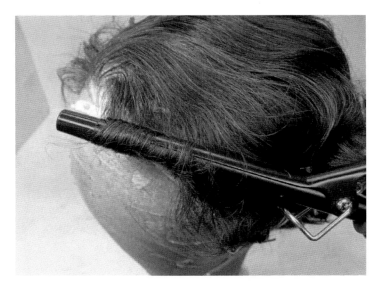

Figure 2.85   Step 14. Use the curling iron on the longer side of the part to curl the hair up and away from the face.

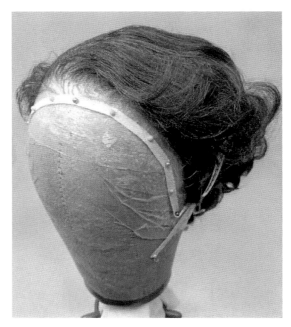

Figure 2.86   Step 15. Brush through the hair that you have just curled so that it forms a sweeping flip up. You can add facial hair to your performer—here, I added a pair of mutton chops to complete the final look.

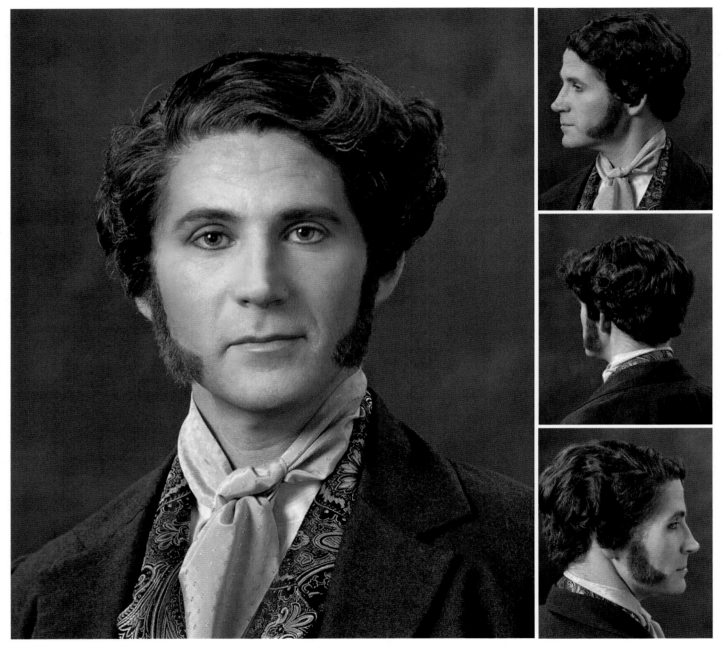

Figures 2.87–2.90   The completed Victorian man's style. Photography: Tim Babiak. Model: Leslie Hethcox.

Variations

Experiment with different lengths of hair to create men's looks for this period. The hair might be longer and smoother, or shorter and curlier. Change up the facial hair looks to really play up the differences in this period—make good use of various sizes of sideburns, mustaches, and goatees.

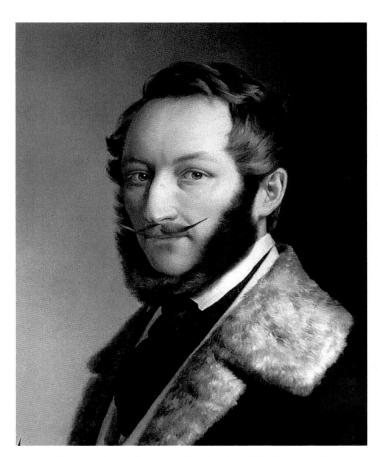

Figure 2.91 Detail from *Self-portrait*, Miklos Barabas, 1841, Hungarian National Gallery. The artist is seen wearing shorter hair, but also unusual and dramatic facial hair.

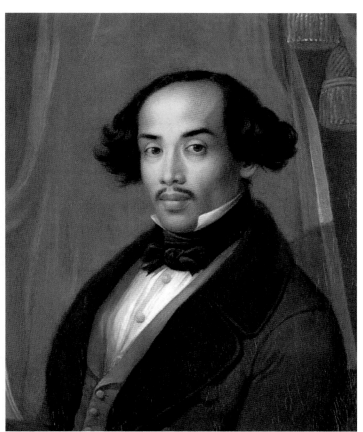

Figure 2.92 Detail from *Portrait of Raden Saleh, Painter*, attributed to either Raden Saleh or Friederich Carl Albert Schreuel, circa 1840, Rijksmuseum, Amsterdam. This artist wears a hairstyle that is very flat on top, wider at the sides around the ears, and a simple mustache.

three

MID-/LATE VICTORIAN

(1860–1885)

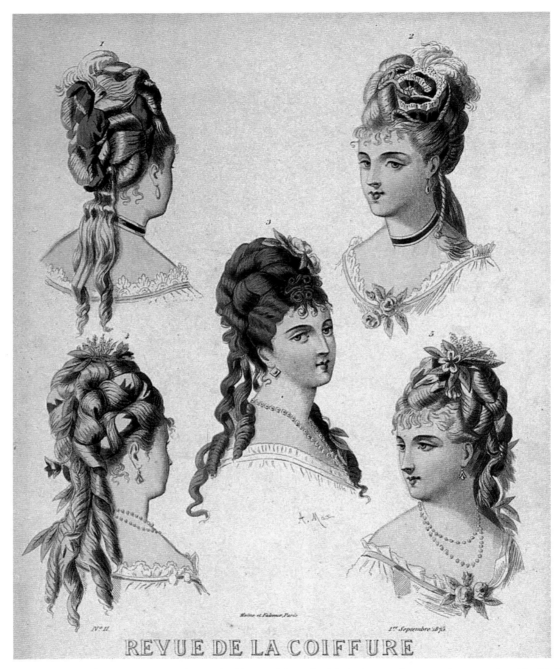

Figure 3.1   The heads and shoulders of five women with their hair combed back and dressed with high chignons, flowers, and scarves, colored line block, 1875, Wellcome Images Collection.

Important Artists/Designers

Edward Burne-Jones, Honoré Daumier, Edgar Degas, Edouard Manet, Claude Monet, Camille Pissarro, Pierre Auguste Renoir, Dante Gabriel Rossetti, Charles Frederick Worth

Important People/Style Icons

Empress Elisabeth of Austria, Jesse James, Lillie Langtry, Franz Liszt, Queen Victoria

Mid-/Late Victorian Women

Women's hair in the Civil War/late Victorian era shifted in shape. The width and fullness around the face moved up to a higher position on the head. The ears were also being exposed again for the first time in decades.

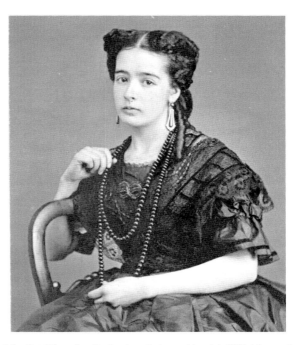

Figure 3.2　Detail from Sra. De Sancha, photographic print, 1870, Library of Congress. Notice how the fullness in this hairstyle is nearly at the top of the head and that the ears are exposed.

At the nape of the neck, the hair was still often pulled into a heavy roll or chignon. The crown of the head was usually left smooth. The roll of hair on the nape was sometimes contained by a snood (a decorative hair net).

The clean, rounded shapes of the hairstyles complemented the full hoopskirts of the dresses from that era. Later in this era, the fullness in the skirts shifted to the back of the dresses as the bustle became a popular fashion. Just as the fashion became more streamlined on the sides, so did the hairstyles. The hair became very tight on the sides and the fullness moved up to the top of the head (Figure 3.4). In many ways, the silhouette of the time period made women resemble horses.

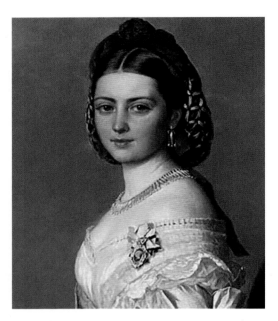

Figures 3.3 Detail from *Victoria, Princess Royal, Crown Princess of Prussia (Vicky)*, Albert Grafle, 1863, Royal Collection of the United Kingdom. Victoria wears a decorative snood in this painting.

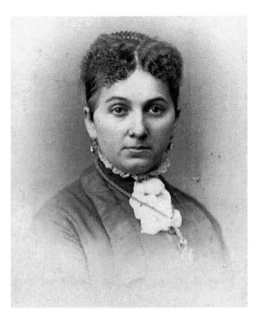

Figure 3.5 Nellie M. Jones Myers, photograph taken at the Cornell Photography Studio in Waterville NY, circa 1870s. Notice the slightly frizzed, waved texture present in the front of the hair in this typical daytime hairstyle.

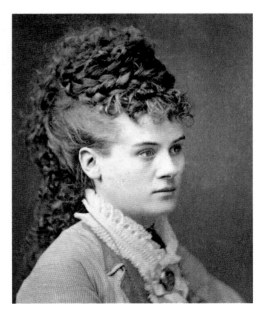

Figure 3.4 Mimmi Malmqvist, actor in William Abjornsson's theatre company, 1877, Swedish Performing Arts Agency.

The bustles gave the illusion of a second set of legs, and the shape of the hair was very like that of a horse's mane.

For daytime, the hair was sleek on the sides with a simple high bun. In 1872, French hairdresser Marcel Grateau pioneered a technique of using hot tongs to semi-permanently wave hair. Soon, people all over Europe were seeking to have their hair styled in this fashion. The deep waves created by this technique were incorporated into hairstyles of this time in a variety of ways. The heat from this type of styling was hard on the hair, however. Looking at photographs of women from this time often reveals hair that has taken on a frizzed, fried texture (Figure 3.5).

For evening affairs, the hair was dressed very high on the top of the head with long ringlets hanging down the back. The hairstyles would be elaborately decorated with ribbons and flowers, such as those shown in Figure 3.1 at the beginning of the chapter and in Figure 3.6. Large braids, barrel rolls, and coils were often wrapped around the top and crown of the head. Several different things could be happening at the center front of the hairstyle. They could be simply cut into a short fringe, such as in the figure on the bottom right of Figure 3.1. The style could have a small, tightly marcel waved section at the center front,

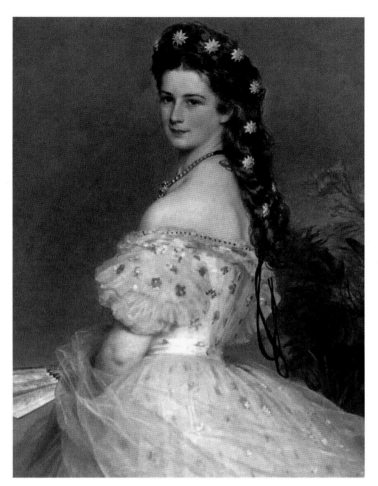

Figure 3.6 Detail from *Empress Elisabeth of Austria in Courtly Gala Dress with Diamond Stars*, Franz Xaver Winterhalter, 1865.

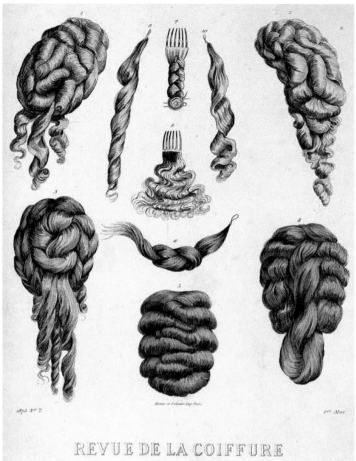

Figure 3.7 Ten illustrations of different types of wig and hairpiece from a French magazine, May 1875.

such as on the Figure 3.5. A third option was for the hair to be arranged in a clump of small tight curls at the center front, such as in Figure 3.4.

These elaborate styles showed off the mid/late Victorian fascination with women's hair. Empress Elisabeth of Austria (Figure 3.6) was so renowned for her luxurious long hair that many portraits were painted of her with her hair worn down and featured. Because these styles were so elaborate, they often required a greater amount of hair than most people can grow. The use of artificial hairpieces became very common and necessary to achieve this fashion. Large tortoiseshell combs were also very popular during this time period.

Mid-/Late Victorian Men

Men's hairstyles at this time are slightly shorter than those found in the previous decades. They still often had a deep side part, sometimes with an asymmetrical pouf on top.

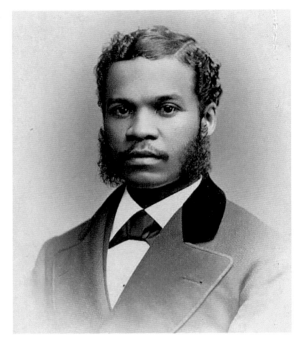

Figure 3.8   Photographic print of an unidentified African-American man, Broadbent and Phillips, 1206 Chestnut Street, Philadelphia, 1870. This gentleman wears a typical deep side part in his hair and elaborate side whiskers.

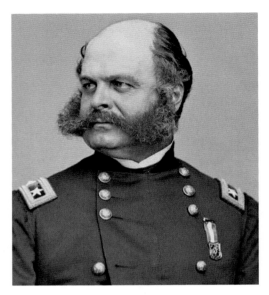

Figure 3.9   Portrait of Maj. Gen. Ambrose E. Burnside, officer of the Federal Army, by Matthew Brady, negative, glass, wet collodion, between 1860 and 1865. Restored by Michel Vuijlsteke.

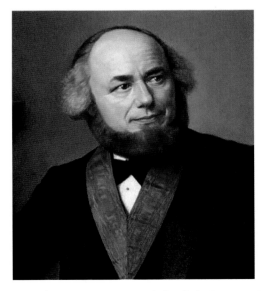

Figure 3.10   Detail from *Wichard Lange*, Friedrich Wilhelm Graupenstein, 1873, Hamburg Museum.

This era continued the heyday of extravagance in men's facial hair. In the 1860s, American general Ambrose Burnside wore a distinctive fashion of facial hair. His look consisted of full side whiskers that were connected by a mustache. These side whiskers are now often referred to as "sideburns" in reference to his name.

Almost any variation on facial hair can be found in this period if one looks hard enough. Figure 3.10 shows a beard that exists under the chin only. The man in Figure 3.8 has bristly side whiskers and a mustache, but no chin hair.

Whatever the late Victorian era man's facial hair choice might be, it was shown off to advantage by the high collars and elaborate neckwear of the period.

Mid-/Late Victorian Woman's Styling— Step by Step

This wig was inspired by the style in Figure 3.6, with the small, tightly waved bangs seen on a couple of the styles in Figure 3.1.

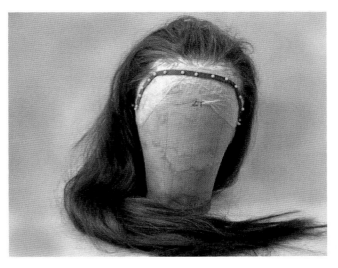

Figure 3.11 Step 1. Begin with a wig that is long (at least 16 inches at the nape of the neck) with a generous amount of hair. A wig with bangs also works well for this style. The wig in this picture is synthetic hair with a lace front.

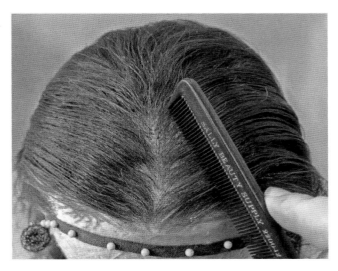

Figure 3.12 Step 2. Make a clean center part in the front section of the hair.

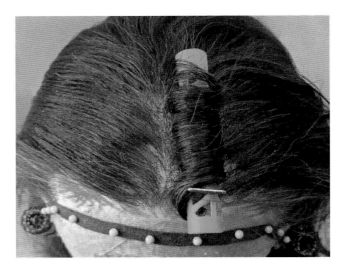

Figure 3.13 Step 3. Set the front section on base on small, pencil sized rollers, rolling away from the center part.

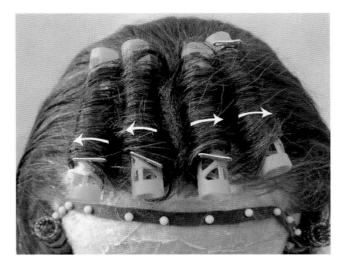

Figure 3.14 Step 4. Set two rollers on either side of the center part.

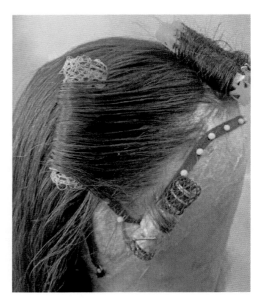

Figure 3.15   Step 5. Set the sides of the wig on quarter sized rollers, rolling back away from the face. Notice how the wig has been set with a lot of drag—the straight hair at the root of this curl will keep the sides of the hairstyle from becoming too voluminous.

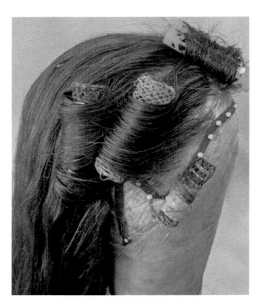

Figure 3.16   Step 6. Set a second quarter sized roller behind the first roller on each side.

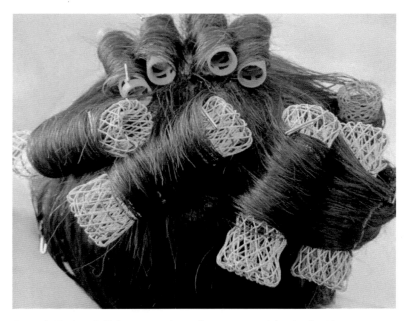

Figure 3.17   Step 7. Shift your attention to the crown area of the wig. Set this area on quarter sized rollers in a diagonal row with a little bit of drag at the roots.

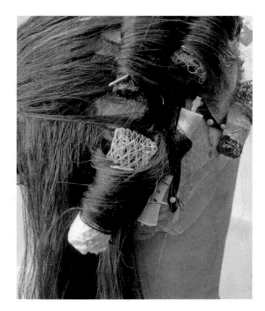

Figure 3.18   Step 8. Drop down behind the ear and set another quarter sized roller rolling away from the nape of the neck. A small tendril of hair has also been set on a perm rod.

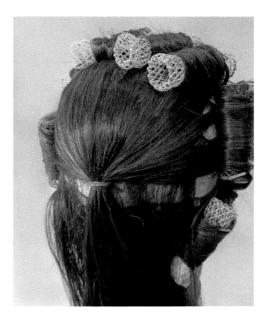

Figure 3.19   Step 9. Pull a section of the hair from the crown and back of the head into a ponytail.

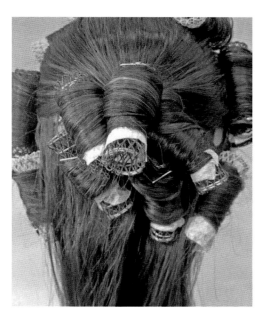

Figure 3.20   Step 10. Set the hair in the ponytail on quarter sized rollers.

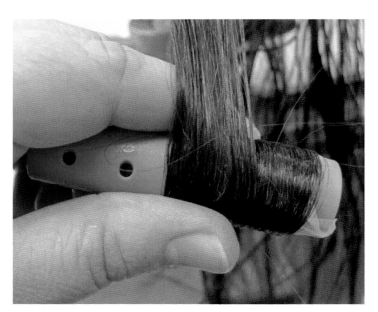

Figure 3.21   Step 11. The remaining hair at the back of the wig should be set in sausage curls on dime sized rollers. As you roll the ringlets, make sure the hair in each turn of the roller overlaps some of the hair from the previous turn.

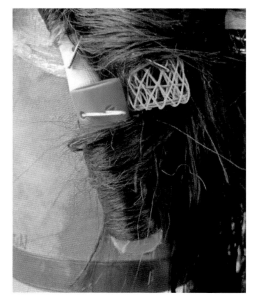

Figure 3.22   Step 12. Once you finish rolling the sausage curl, turn the roller vertical and pin it in place.

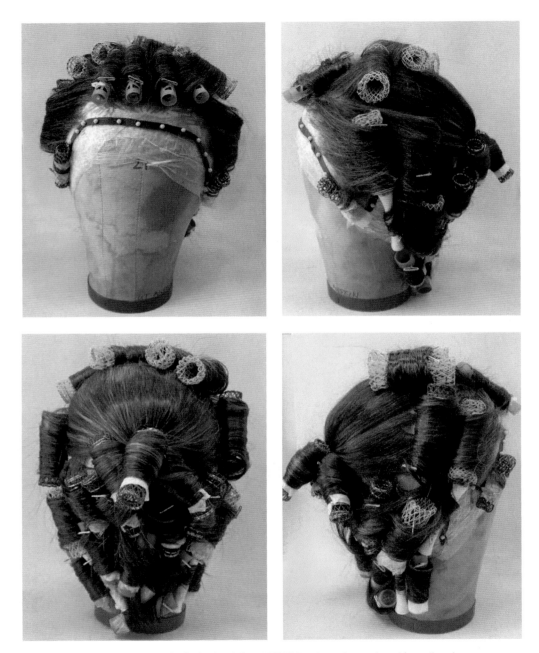

Figures 3.23–3.26   The finished mid-/late (1870's) Victorian style set, viewed from all angles.

Once you have finished setting the wig, steam it if it is synthetic. If it is human hair, spray the hair through with water. Put the wig in the wig dryer after you have finished steaming and/or spraying, and dry it for 75 minutes.

To style:

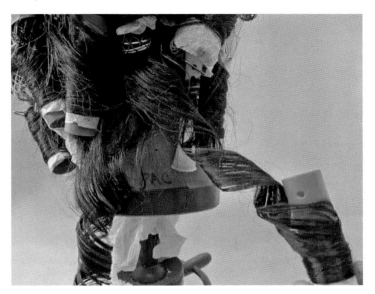

Figure 3.27   Step 13. To style, remove all of the rollers, beginning at the nape of the wig. Carefully unwind the sausage curls.

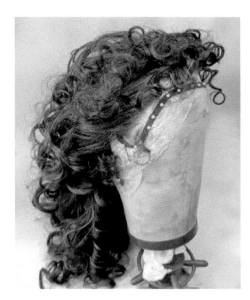

Figure 3.28   Step 14. The wig, with all the rollers removed.

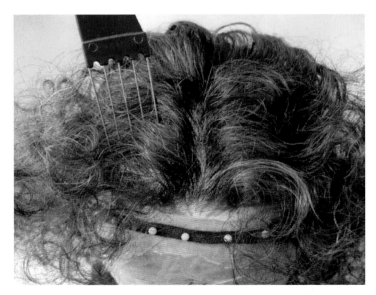

Figure 3.29   Step 15. Use a wire teasing comb to pick through and fluff the hair at the center front section of the wig. This will break up the curls and help to hide any roller breaks you may have.

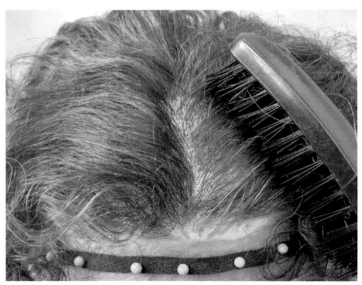

Figure 3.30   Step 16. Next, brush through and smooth this section of hair with a teasing/smoothing brush.

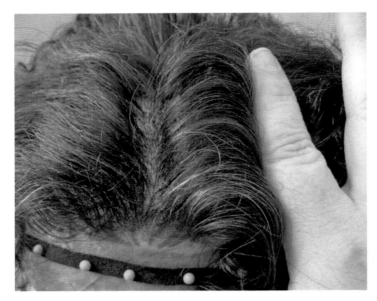

Figure 3.31   Step 17. Push the small waves in this section into shape with your fingers.

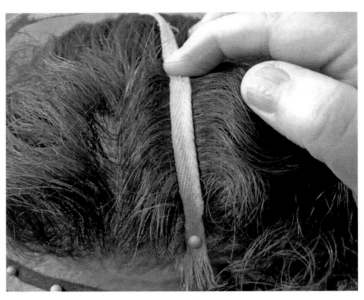

Figure 3.32   Step 18. Pin blocking tape in place to help you hold and shape these waves.

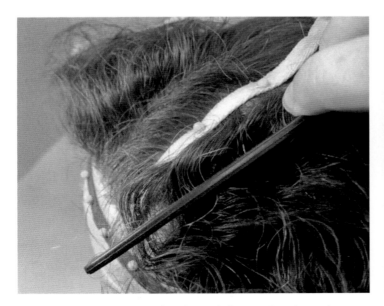

Figure 3.33   Step 19. Use a rattail comb to push the waves into place and to create ridges between each crest of the wave.

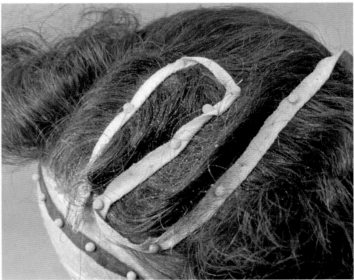

Figure 3.34   Step 20. The full wave, pinned in place and sprayed with hairspray.

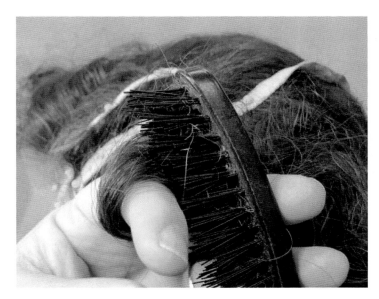

Figure 3.35 Step 21. Shape the ends of the hair from the section by brushing them into small curls around your finger.

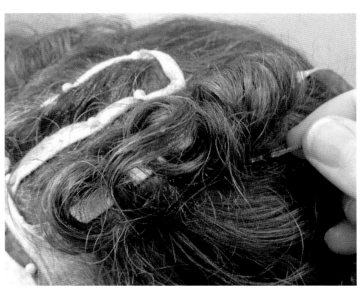

Figure 3.36 Step 22. Arrange the small curls in place and secure with a bobby pin.

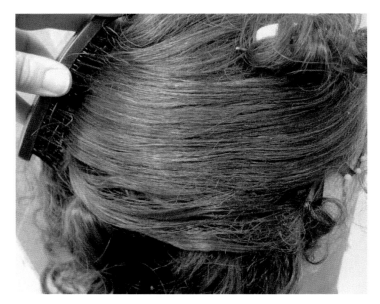

Figure 3.37 Step 23. Move down to the side sections of the wig. Brush through these sections with your teasing/smoothing brush.

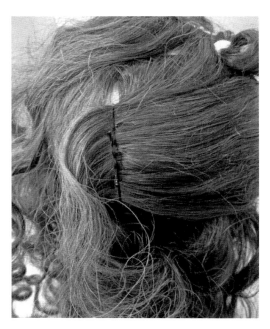

Figure 3.38 Step 24. Secure the side sections near the base of the ponytail with crossed bobby pins.

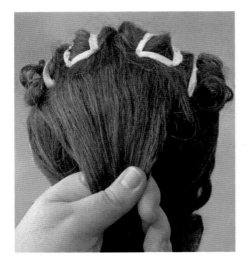

Figure 3.39   Step 25. Move to the crown of the head. Brush through this entire section of hair with your teasing/smoothing brush and gather all the hair into your hand.

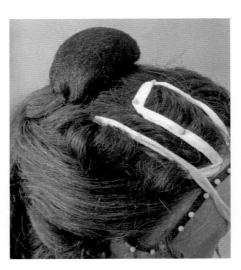

Figure 3.40   Step 26. Pin a small hair rat at the middle on the crown of the head. Secure the rat with bobby pins.

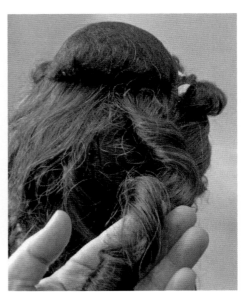

Figure 3.41   Step 27. Form some of the hair underneath the rat into a large ringlet.

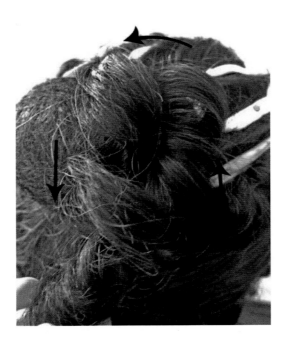

Figure 3.42   Step 28. Drape the hair in the ringlet up alongside the hair rat. Fold it in half and pin the ringlet in the center. Pin the other half of the ringlet back down in the direction you started from.

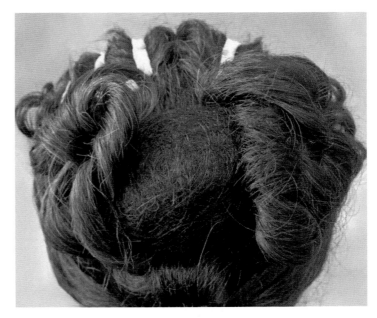

Figure 3.43   Step 29. Ringlets pinned on both sides of the hair rat.

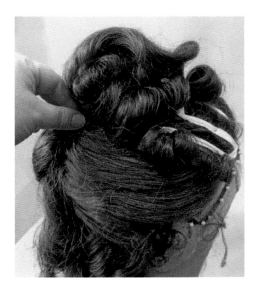

Figure 3.44 Step 30. Take a small section of hair from the ponytail in the back of the wig, form it into a ringlet, and use it to cover the rest of the small rat.

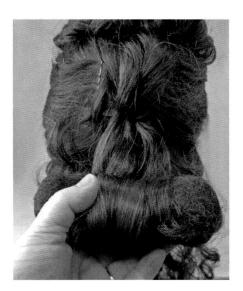

Figure 3.45 Step 31. Brush through the rest of the hair in the ponytail, and roll it up in a second rat or hair pad.

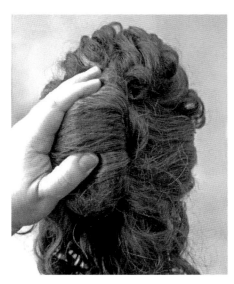

Figure 3.46 Step 32. Turn the hair rat that has been rolled with hair sideways and pin it so that it sits vertically along the back of the head.

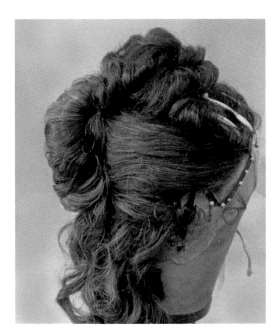

Figure 3.47 Step 33. The roll, pinned in place with large wig pins. The hair has been adjusted so that the entire rat is covered.

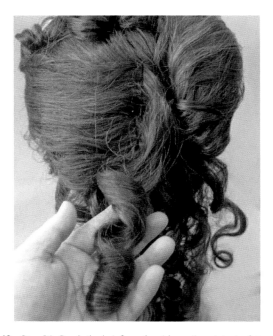

Figure 3.48 Step 34. Comb the hair from the side sections into ringlets.

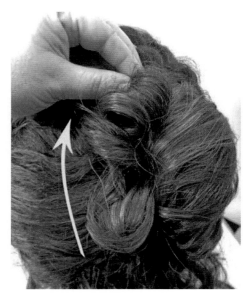

Figure 3.49   Step 35. Pin these ringlets on either side of the roll.

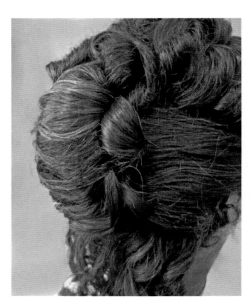

Figure 3.50   Step 36. Finished view of the ringlets pinned in place.

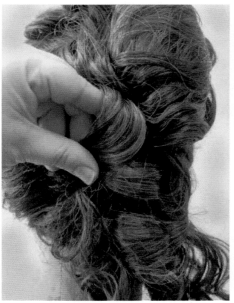

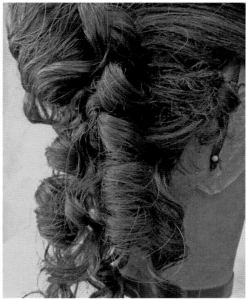

Figure 3.51 and 3.52   Step 37. Continue shaping the hair in the back into ringlets and arranging them in a pretty way.

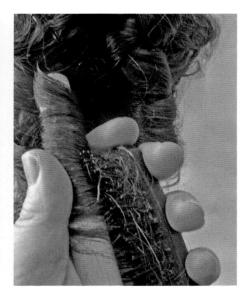

Figure 3.53   Step 38. To form the long sausage curls hanging down in the back, use a dowel rod to brush the curls around. Once you remove the rod, you will have a nice smooth curl.

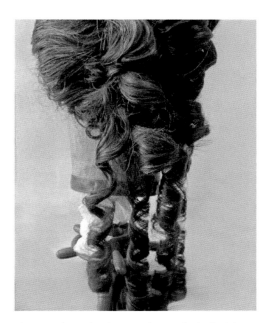

Figure 3.54 Step 39. The ringlets hanging down in the back of the wig, once they have been smoothed and formed into shape.

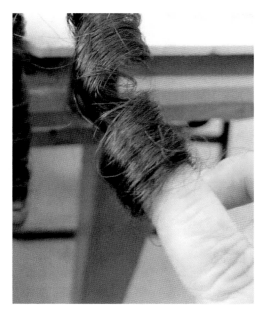

Figure 3.55 Step 40. If the ends of your ringlets stick out irregularly, shove the end of the ringlet up into itself with your finger.

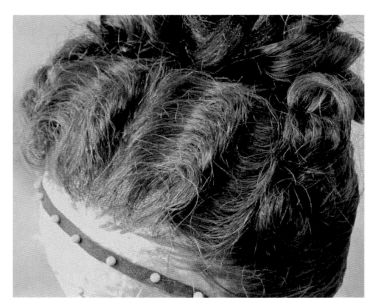

Figure 3.56 Step 41. When you are ready for the wig to be worn, remove the blocking tape that was holding the waves in place in the front of the wig.

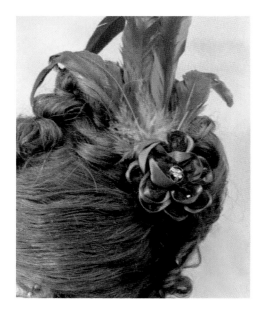

Figure 3.57 Step 42. Add some decorative accents to complete the period look of this wig.

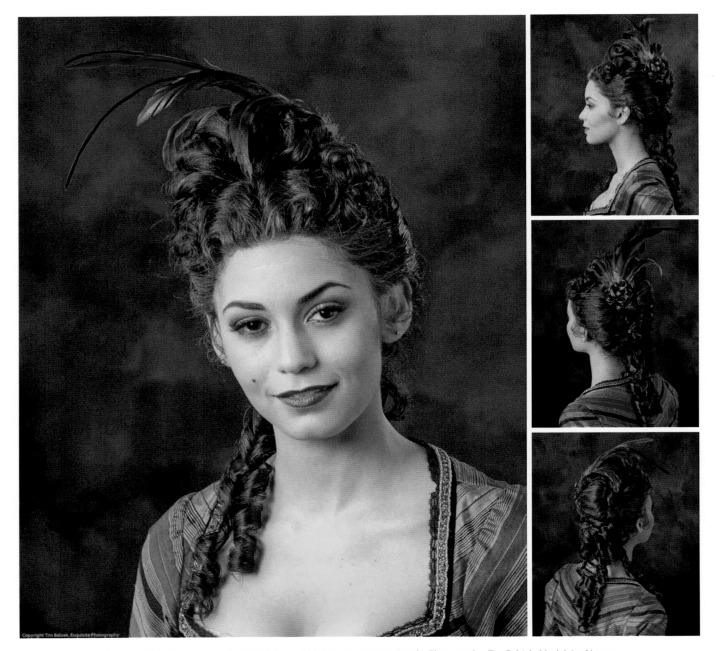

Figures 3.58–3.61   The completed mid-/late (1870's) Victorian woman's style. Photography: Tim Babiak. Model: Ivy Negron.

Variations

For styles from the early part of this era, you could do any number of variations of a wig with a center part and waves or rolls smoothed back above the ears. In the back, these wigs could be ringlets, rolls, or loose curls caught up in a snood.

In the later part of this era, there are many possibilities for variety just in the decoration alone. Experiment with ribbons, flowers, combs, birds, and jewels to create many different looks. You can also use variety in the center front of the wig. You can do either small sculpted finger waves (such as in the demonstrated style) or you can do a cluster of tight frizzled curls, such as in Figure 3.62.

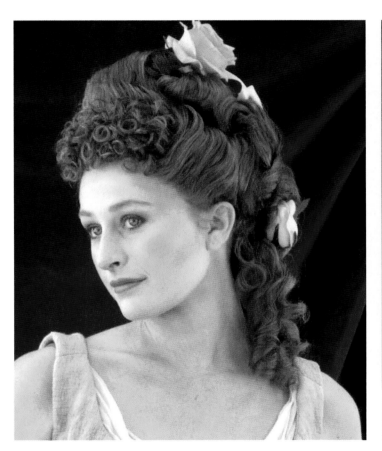
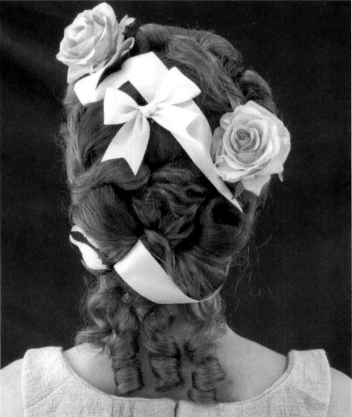

Figures 3.62 and 3.63   A late Victorian wig styled by Thumper Gosney. Notice the section of small tight curls in the center front of the wig. Model: Juliet Robb.

Mid-/Late Victorian Makeup

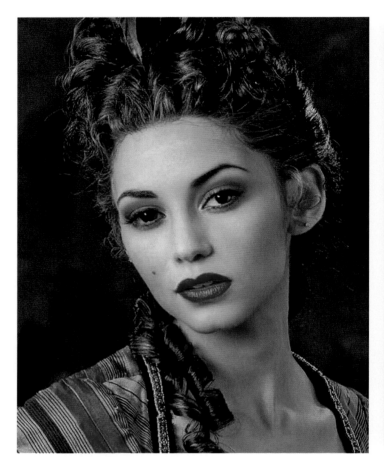

Figure 3.64 A typical "professional beauty" look of the late Victorian era. Model: Ivy Negron.

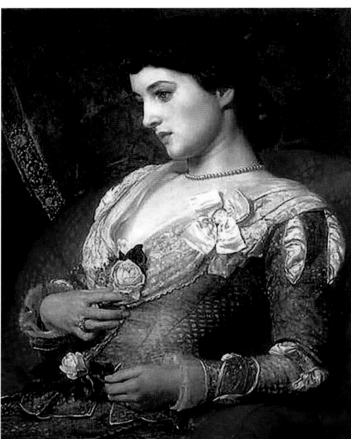

Figure 3.65 *Portrait of Lillie Langtry*, Edward John Poynter, 1877.

Mid-/late Victorian culture gave rise to the phenomenon known as "professional beauties." Pictures of society beauties were exhibited in store windows, creating one of the first celebrity cultures. Lillie Langtry (Figure 3.89) was a particularly noted professional beauty. Use of cosmetics became more open. Zinc oxide replaced lead in face powder, ending many years of toxic lead use. Powders with blue or lavender tints were available to help women look unearthly pale even in the golden glow of candles and lamps. Women were also tracing their veins with blue pencils. Rouge and lip color became more popular, as did a darkly accented eye.

Mid-/Late Victorian African-American Man's Styling— Step by Step

This wig was inspired by the style in Figure 3.8.

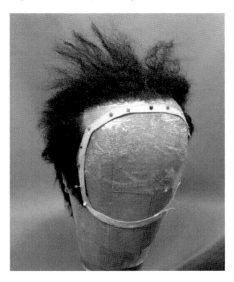

Figure 3.66 Step 1. For this style, I began with a wig that was made with tightly textured hair. This wig is fully hand tied, with tighter hair being knotted into the front.

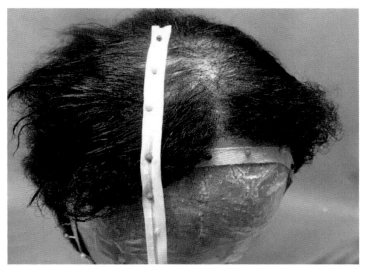

Figure 3.67 Step 2. Make an off-center part in the wig. Saturate the top of the wig with setting lotion. Comb the hair forwards towards the face. Use a blocking tape to hold the wave in place.

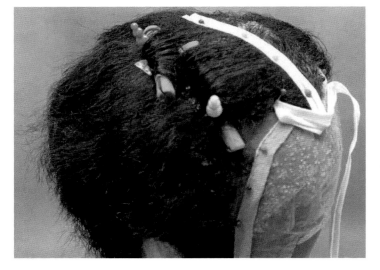

Figure 3.68 Step 3. Comb that section of hair back away from the face, sculpting the wave. Use small perm rods to set the ends of the hair.

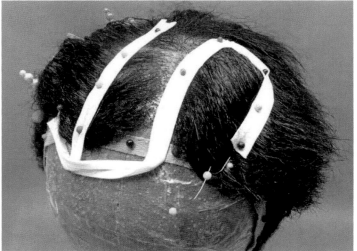

Figure 3.69 Step 4. Make a second wave on the opposite side of the part, again saturating the hair with setting lotion.

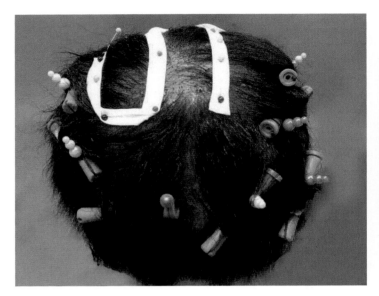

Figure 3.70 Step 5. Use small perm rods to set diagonal rows around the crown of the wig.

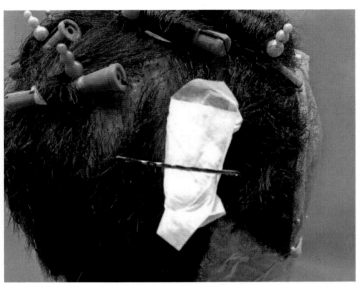

Figure 3.71 Step 6. When the sections of hair become too short to wrap around a perm rod, I move to using bobby pins as though they were a very small roller. Use an end paper on the section off. Slide the open bobby pin over the end paper, and then roll it under just as you would a roller or perm rod.

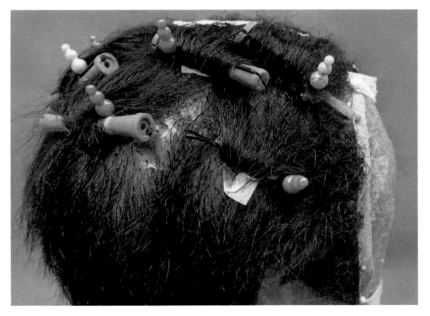

Figure 3.72 Step 7. Pin the bobby pinned section in place. Continue to use bobby pins in diagonal rows down the back of the wig.

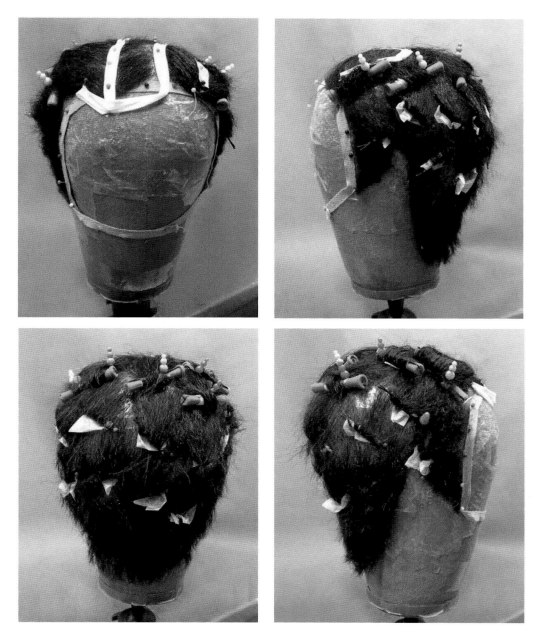

Figures 3.73–3.76 The finished late Victorian African-American man's style set, viewed from all angles.

Once you have finished setting the wig, steam it if it is synthetic. If it is human hair, spray the hair through with water. Put the wig in the wig dryer after you have finished steaming and/or spraying, and dry it for 75 minutes.

To style:

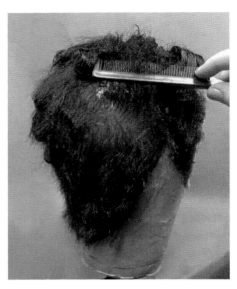

Figure 3.77   Step 8. Remove all perm rods and bobby pins from the wig. Leave the blocking tape in place in the front. Comb through the wig, breaking up all of the curls. I find it helpful to comb both up and down the wig.

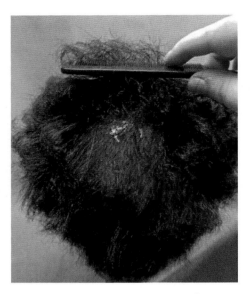

Figure 3.78   Step 9. Lightly tease small sections of hair to get rid of any roller breaks.

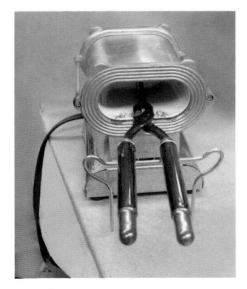

Figure 3.79   Step 10. Use a Marcel oven and small iron to curl the sections of hair that were too small to roll. Place the iron in the oven and allow it to get hot. *NB:* Marcel ovens are not recommended for use on synthetic hair.

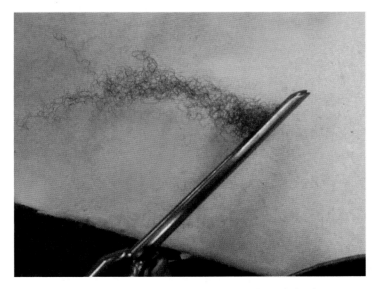

Figure 3.80   Step 11. Always test the iron on some loose hair (ideally, the same hair the wig is made of) before touching the iron to the wig. If the test sample burns, allow the iron to cool before using it. Keep testing it until it is a safe temperature.

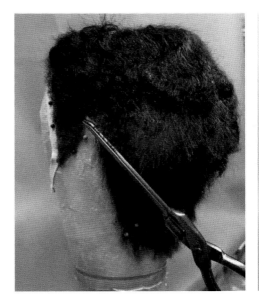

Figure 3.81 Step 12. Curl tiny sections of hair with the iron. Work in multiple directions so that you do not create lines in the hairstyle.

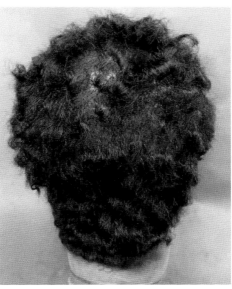

Figure 3.82 Step 13. Make sure to curl the entire back and top of the wig. You can even work into the sections of hair that were rolled if they are too straight at the roots.

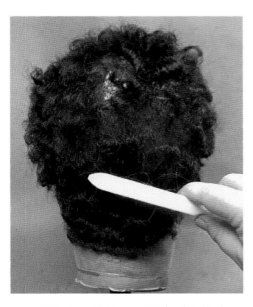

Figure 3.83 Step 14. Use a teasing brush to brush through the back and top of the wig. Again, brush both up and down to integrate the sections of hair.

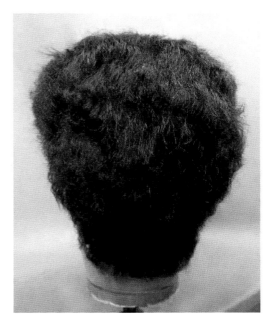

Figure 3.84 Step 15. To finish, use the brush to smooth the back of the wig.

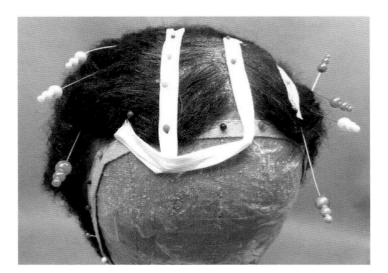

Figure 3.85 Step 16. Use large corsage pins to shape the waves around the face. Mist with hairspray. Leave the pins and blocking tape in place until it is time for the wig to be worn.

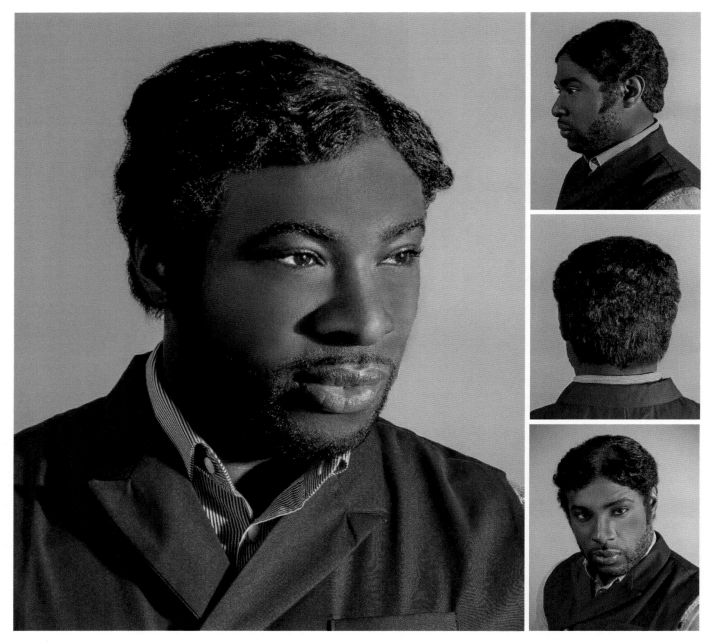

Figures 3.86–3.89   The completed mid-/late Victorian African-American man's style. Model: Eric J. Black.

four

THE GAY NINETIES

$\left(1885-1901\right)$

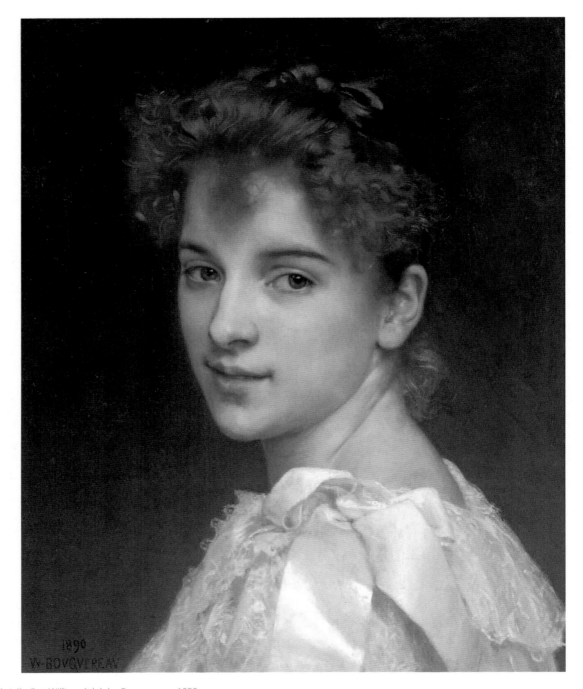

Figure 4.1   *Gabrielle Cot*, William-Adolphe Bouguereau, 1890.

Important Events

1886	The Statue of Liberty is constructed
1888	The Jack the Ripper murders occur in Whitechapel
1891	Sir Arthur Conan Doyle publishes the first Sherlock Holmes story
1892	Tchaikovsky's *Nutcracker Suite* premieres
1895	Oscar Wilde's *The Importance of Being Earnest* premieres
1898	The Spanish–American War is fought
1901	Death of Queen Victoria

Important Artists/Designers

Aubrey Beardsley, Paul Cezanne, Paul Gaugin, George Seurat, John Singer Sargent, Henri de Toulouse-Lautrec, John William Waterhouse, James McNeil Whistler

Important People/Style Icons

Princess Alexandra, Sarah Bernhardt, Mrs. Patrick Campbell, Annie Oakley, Ellen Terry, Oscar Wilde

1890s' Women

The "Gay Nineties" was a time of perceived prosperity and increased physical activity. These were the last years of Queen Victoria's reign, before the chaos of World War I would send the world into a tailspin. Clothing became simpler—the bustles and hoopskirts of the previous period had fallen out of fashion (corsets were still very much a part of a woman's daily wardrobe, however.) The idea of sportswear becomes important for one of the first times in history. Clothing became more tailored; likewise, hairstyles also became a bit simpler. Hair was still grown extremely long, and was considered to be a woman's crowning glory. Women were still wearing their hair piled high on their head, but unlike in the previous period, the shape was much more basic. Hair would often be waved, and then pulled up on top of the head in a French twist. Some women favored a simple topknot on the top of their head. Other women chose to coil their hair around on the top of the head, creating a large bun that was almost the same width as the head itself. Fashionable women's blouses were often high necked at this time, so women's hair was usually pulled up off the neck.

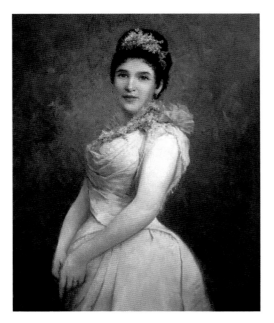

Figure 4.2   Detail from *Lady in a Yellow Dress with Lilacs in Her Hair*, Adolf Echtler, 1894. This painting shows a woman with the typical frizzled bangs and high wide bun of the 1890s.

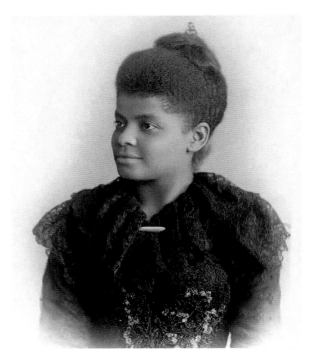

Figure 4.3   Photograph of Ida B. Wells Barnett, by Mary Garrity, circa 1893, Google Art Project. Restored by Adam Cuerden.

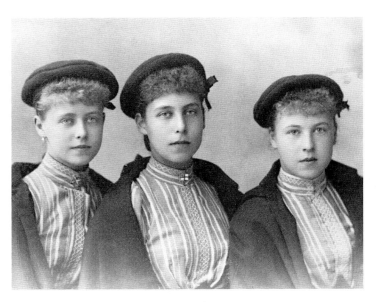

Figure 4.4   Photograph of Princess Marie, Princess Victoria Melita, and Princess Alexandra, circa 1891, Royal Collection of the United Kingdom. All three ladies wear a version of the bangs so popular in this era.

Gray hair was, perhaps surprisingly, very much in vogue at this time. Many women were using hair powders (used to absorb grease and create a soft look), which likely contributed to the trend of fashionable gray (or dusty) hair. The practice of curling hair with hot Marcel irons was still all the rage at this time. As a result, many women had damaged hair from the high temperatures of the curling irons. Photographs of women at this time often show the hair looking slight fuzzy and flyaway. Tightly curled or "frizzled" bangs were extremely popular at this time. Women would use the curling irons to painstaking curl a fringe of bangs. Examples of these bangs can be seen in Figures 4.1, 4.2, and 4.4. In fact, bangs were so popular that bang hairpieces (one example of which is the Lillie Langtry inspired "Skeleton Bangs") were available for purchase so every woman could wear the bangs of her dreams.

Evening hairstyles for women were often more elaborate and complicated. The twists and curls on top of the head would be more elaborate, and hairpieces might be used to add volume or interest. These hairstyles might incorporate jewels, fancy combs, or plumes.

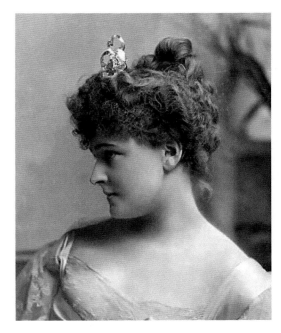

Figure 4.5   Photograph of Frances Evelyn Maynard "Daisy Greville", Countess of Warwick, by Lafayette Ltd, 1897.

1890s' Men

Men in the 1890s were quite dapper. They were still wearing their hair cut short and close to the head. It was often styled with a very clean part (either in the center or on the side), held in place with hair grease or pomade. Facial hair in this period was very dramatic. Men often grew large, elaborate mustaches that became a focal point of their look.

This mustache might be styled in a walrus shape, or it might be waxed into a handlebar. Small pointy beards or goatees were also fashionable for men.

The Aesthetic Dress movement influenced fashions for both men and women. The emphasis in clothing was on simple lines and luxurious fabrics. Hairstyles favored by Aesthetics were also more simple and flowing; they rejected the tightly bound updos and severe men's short haircuts of the time.

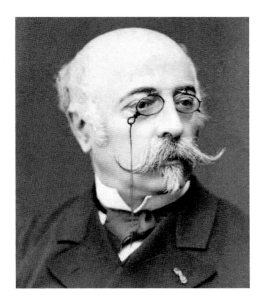

Figure 4.7 Photograph of French painter Paul Alexandre Protais, by Ferdinand Mulnier, 1890. This photograph shows an elaborate mustache and small goatee.

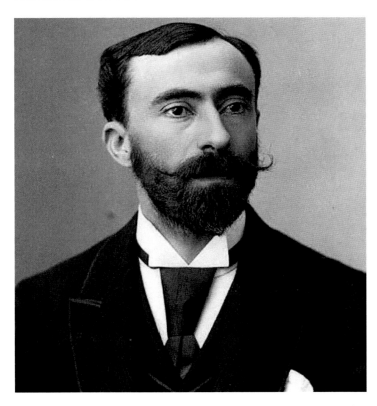

Figure 4.6 Photograph of Paul Bernard, by Marmand, circa 1893–1898. Bernard wears the deeply side parted hair, full mustache, and neat pointed beard that was fashionable in the 1890s.

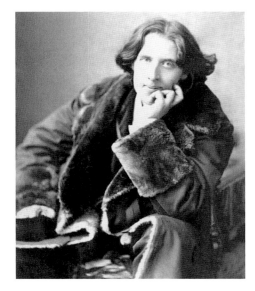

Figure 4.8 Photograph of Oscar Wilde in his favorite coat, by Napoleon Sarony, 1882. Note how Wilde's hair is much longer and looser than the styles worn by other men in this era.

1890s' Woman's Styling—Step by Step

This hairstyle is modeled after the ones in Figures 4.1 and 4.5.

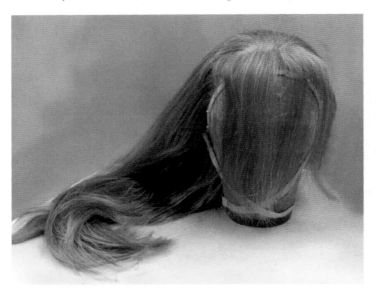

Figure 4.9   Step 1. Begin with a long wig (at least 16 inches at the nape of the neck) that has a section of shorter hair or bangs (three to five inches long) in the front. I used a long synthetic lace front wig for this style.

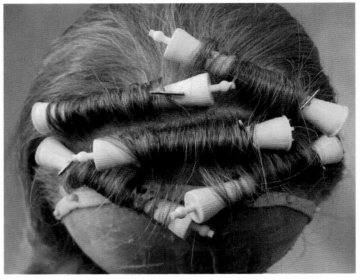

Figure 4.10   Step 2. Set the bangs on small perm rods, rolling towards the face.

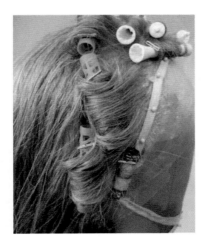

Figure 4.11   Step 3. Set several small pencil rollers along the hairline and behind the section of bangs. This will help add the frizzy texture commonly seen in hairstyles of this time period.

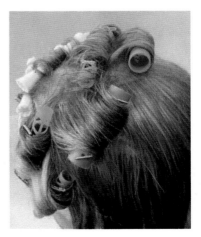

Figure 4.12   Step 4. Behind the pencil rollers, set a row of dime sized rollers, still setting the rollers away from the face.

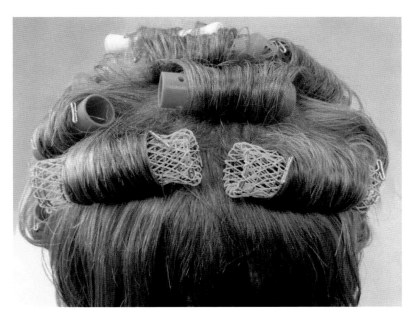 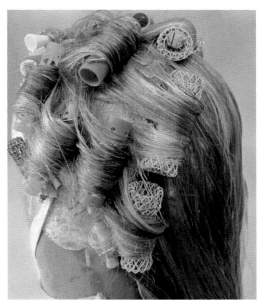

Figure 4.13 and 4.14 Step 5. You are now going to begin setting the hair on quarter sized rollers. Make sure to set your rollers in a brick pattern—this will keep you from having large gaps in your hairstyle.

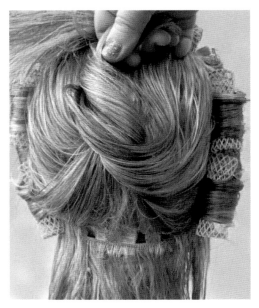 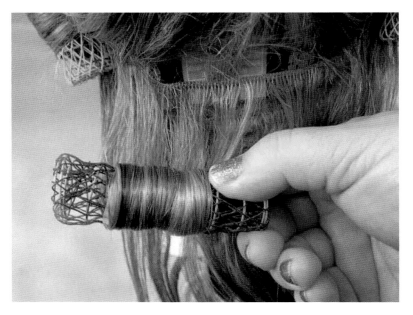

Figure 4.15 Step 6. Pull most of the hair in the back of the wig up out of the way in a twist. Make sure to leave a section of hair hanging down at the nape of the neck.

Figure 4.16 Step 7. Roll the hair at the nape of the neck on quarter sized rollers, rolling the hair up towards the crown of the head.

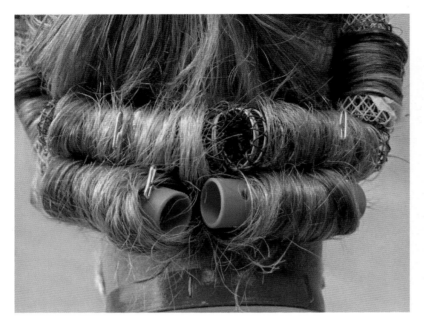

Figure 4.17 Step 8. Roll the bottom section of hair on dime sized rollers, again rolling upwards toward the crown of the head.

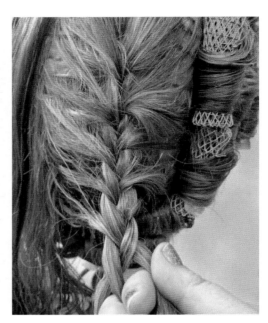

Figure 4.18 Step 9. Braid the hair in the back of the wig into two French braids. This will allow you to create texture in the hair without creating a lot of unnecessary volume.

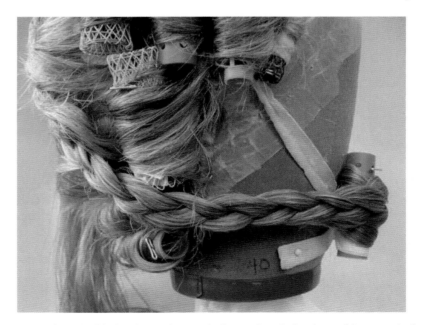

Figure 4.19 Step 10. Roll the ends of the braids onto dime sized rollers, and pin the braids out of the way at the front of the head.

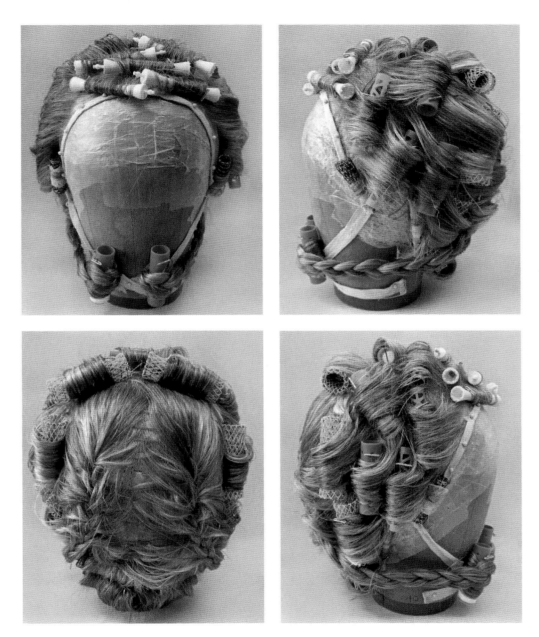

Figures 4.20–4.23 The finished 1890s' woman's style set.

Once you have finished setting the wig, steam each roller thoroughly if the wig is made of synthetic hair. If the wig is human hair, soak each roller with water sprayed from a spray bottle. After steaming or wetting, place the wig in a wig dryer for 75 minutes.

To style:

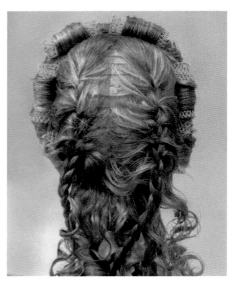

Figure 4.24 Step 11. Begin removing all the rollers, starting at the nape of the wig. Unbraid the braided section of hair. For now, leave the bang section of hair set on perm rods in the rollers.

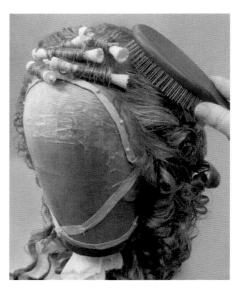

Figure 4.25 Step 12. Brush through all the hair with a large hairbrush.

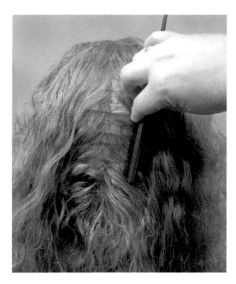

Figure 4.26 Step 13. Use a rattail comb to make a center part in the back of the wig.

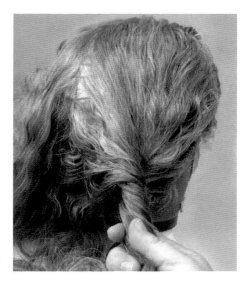

Figure 4.27 Step 14. Take half of the hair in your hand and twist the entire section of hair. Once twisted, twist the hair up the center back in order to create half of a French twist, leaving the ends loose. Make sure not to pull the twist so tight that you lose all the texture in the hair. Pin the twist securely up the center back with bobby pins.

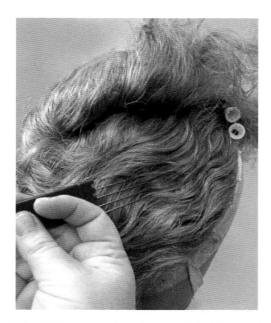

Figure 4.28   Step 15. Use a wire pick comb to smooth the hairs going into the twist. Once the hairs are in place, mist them in place with hairspray.

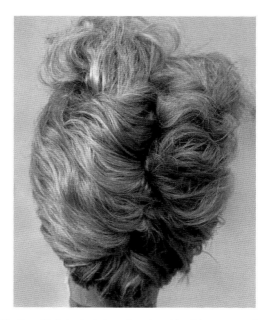

Figure 4.29   Step 16. Twist the hair on the other side of the wig to make a second French twist. The two twists should meet up in the center back of the wig.

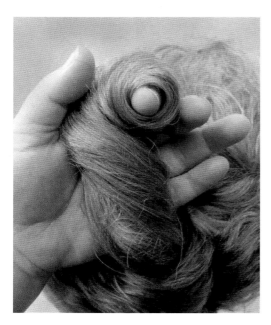

Figure 4.30   Step 17. Divide the loose hair at the top of the twists into three sections. Brush one section of the hair around two fingers to form a large curl.

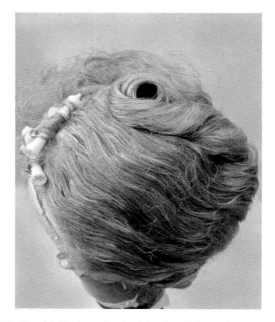

Figure 4.31   Step 18. Pin the curl so that it is relatively flat on the very top of the head.

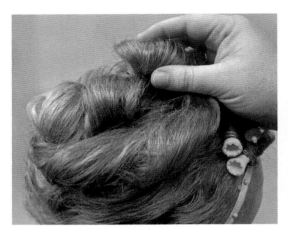

Figure 4.32 Step 19. Form the other two sections of hair into curls, and pin them into place.

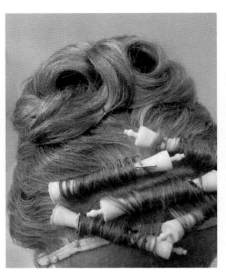

Figure 4.33 Step 20. Check your hairstyle from the front to make sure that it is symmetrical and that you are happy with the appearance of the curls.

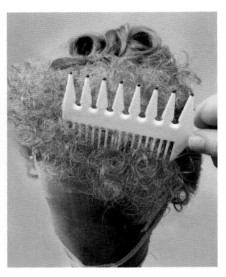

Figure 4.34 Step 21. Remove the rollers from the bangs. Use a pick to separate the curls.

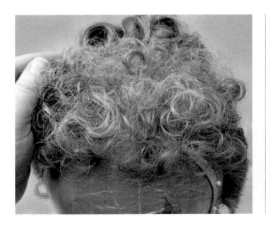

Figure 4.35 Step 22. Leave the curls a little bit frizzy. Use your fingers to arrange the curls in place. Pin them with bobby pins if necessary, making sure to hide the bobby pins.

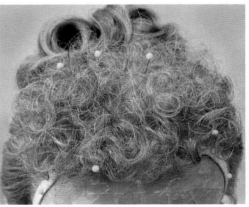

Figure 4.36 Step 23. Use round head pins to arrange the curls. Mist with hairspray and let them sit overnight.

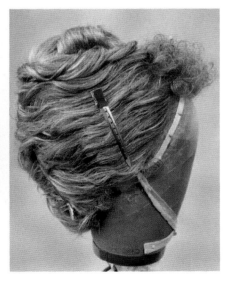

Figure 4.37 Step 24. To make the wig extra flat on the sides, use duckbill clips pinned into the waves. Again, mist the section with hairspray and let it sit overnight.

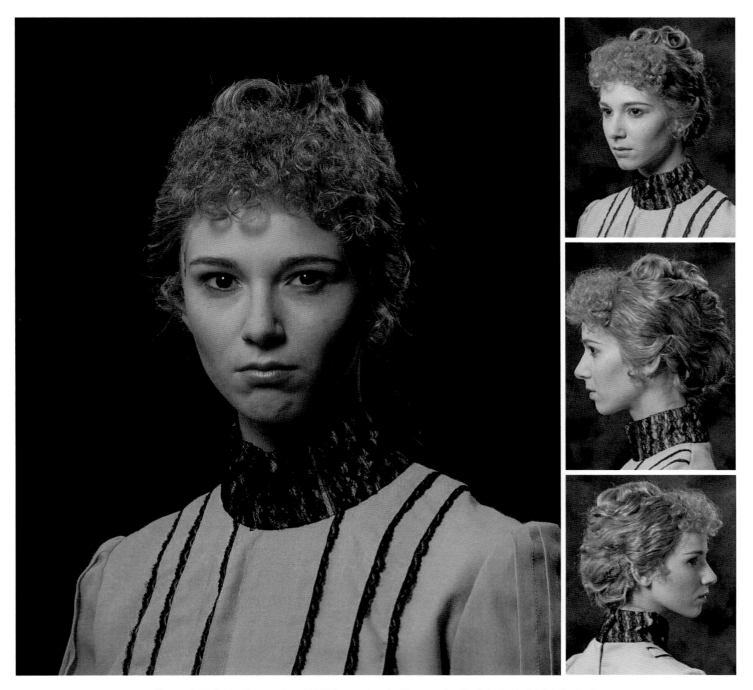

Figures 4.38–4.41   The completed 1890s' woman's style. Photography: Tim Babiak. Model: Sabrina Lotfi.

Variations

You can create variety in your 1890s' hairstyles by making use of different textures of hair. While many women's hair had the frizzy textures caused by hot curling irons, other women still used pomades and oils to create very slick looking hair.

You can also create variety by playing around with the bang section. Besides the frizzy curled bangs, you can also find example of bangs with a center part and bangs with sculpted spit curls. Other women still held onto a simple center part with no bangs at all. Many of the buns in these hairstyles are placed very high on the top of the head, but you can also place the bun lower to create variety.

Later in this period, the hairstyles begin to gain the volume that will define the next period. You can make use of this volume to create more fashion forward character looks.

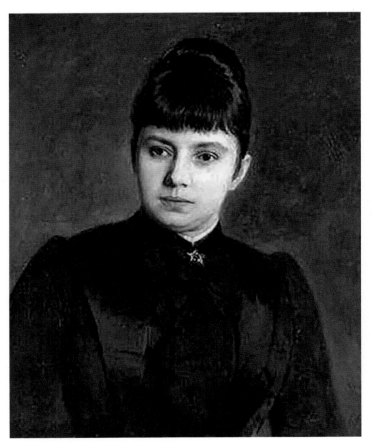

Figure 4.42 *Portrait of Lady Wearing a Black Gown*, Hans Kundmuller, 1890. The woman in this portrait wears a sleeker shiny style complemented by straight bangs.

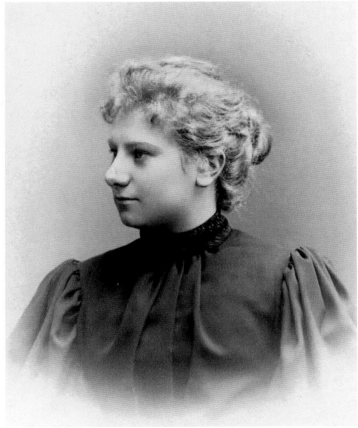

Figure 4.43 Photograph of Anna Greta Adamsen, pupil at Dramatiska Teatern, 1895. Notice how the hairstyle in this portrait is fuller on the sides than many styles from this period. This indicates that the hairstyle is from the later years of the 1890s.

1890s' Makeup

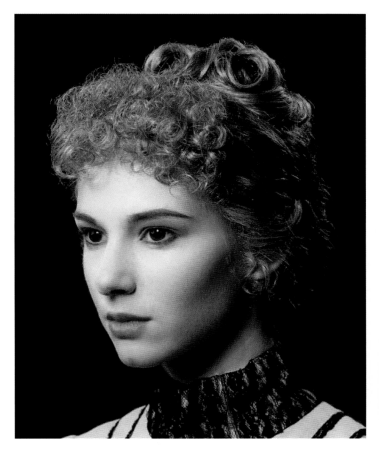

Figure 4.44   An example of this simple makeup look of the 1890s. Model: Sabrina Lotfi.

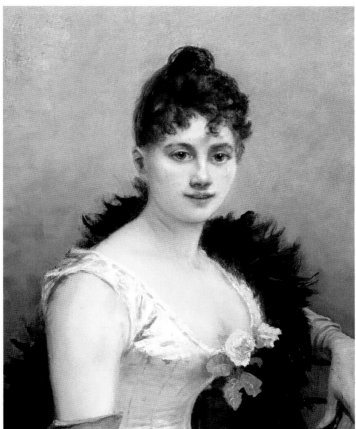

Figure 4.45   Detail from *Society Lady with Feather Boa*, Gustav Wertheimer, 1891. This lady is an example of the simple makeup look of the Gay Nineties.

Just as the clothing became simpler in this decade, so, too, did the makeup looks. People were beginning to become more active and spend more time outdoors, and their looks reflected this need for practicality. Pale skin remained de rigueur, however. Women at this time could use face powder (often patted on with a rabbit's foot), a little bit of rouge on her cheeks, castor oil rubbed into her eyelashes, and a bit of tinted lip salve and she would be ready for any activity that might come her way.

five

EDWARDIAN ERA/ GIBSON GIRL

(1901–1910)

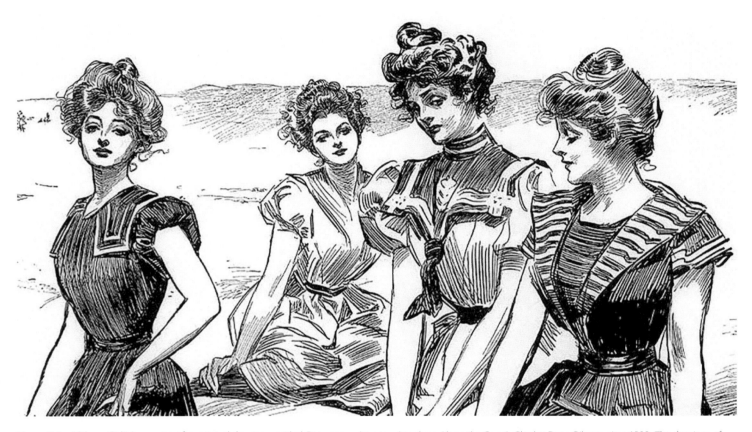

Figure 5.1   "Gibson Girl" (engraving after original drawing, entitled *Picturesque America, Anywhere Along the Coast*), Charles Dana Gibson, circa 1900. The drawings of women, like this one by artist Charles Dana Gibson, helped define the feminine ideal of the Edwardian era.

Important Events

1901   Edward VII becomes King of England
1903   First airplane flight by the Wright Brothers
1904   The New York subway opens
1904   Anton Chekhov's *The Cherry Orchard* premieres
1906   Harry Thaw murders architect Stanford White
1908   Ford introduces the Model T automobile
1909   W.E.B. DuBois helps found the NAACP

Important Artists/Designers

Thomas Eakins, Charles Dana Gibson, Gustav Klimt, Alphonse Mucha, Paul Poiret, John Singer Sargent, Louis Comfort Tiffany, Frank Lloyd Wright

Important People/Style Icons

Nancy Astor, John Barrymore, Camille Clifford, Lillie Langtry, Evelyn Nesbit, Theodore Roosevelt

Edwardian Women

The shape of fashion was changing greatly at the turn of the century, and this created what many referred to as the "New Woman." In Europe, this period of technological advancement and growing popularity of high fashion caused this era to be referred to as the "Belle Époque" ("Beautiful Era"). Art Nouveau was also extremely influential during this era. Art Nouveau's emphasis on natural forms and structures and curved lines had an echoing effect in women's fashion. Heavily upholstered bustles fell out fashion in favor of clothing that exaggerated the feminine contours of women's bodies. In much the same way, women's hairstyles transformed from rigid, constrained buns to casually tousled upswept hair.

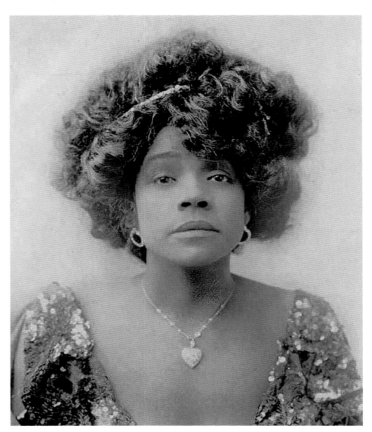

Figure 5.2 Photograph of Aida Overton Walker, by White, 1546 Broadway, 1261 Broadway, New York, 1907, Beinecke Rare Book and Manuscript Library. This is an example of a loosely tousled updo from this period.

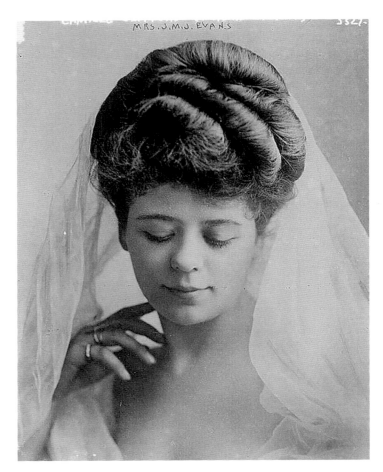

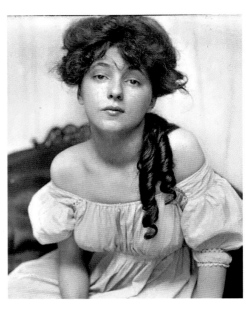

Figures 5.4   Photograph of Evelyn Nesbit when she was brought to the studio by Stanford White, circa 1900, Library of Congress Prints and Photographs Division.

Figure 5.3   Photograph of Camille Clifford (Mrs. H.L. Bruce) (Mrs. J.M.J. Evans), 1910, Library of Congress.

The idea was that this hair looked as though it had been carelessly pinned up by its wearer, and might come tumbling down at any second. Of course, a great deal of work went into styling these "natural" hairstyles. Artist Charles Dana Gibson was especially influential in creating the popularity of these large full hairstyles. These drawings became known as "Gibson Girls."

One popular Gibson Girl was Camille Clifford (Figure 5.3). Her towering updo of a high pompadour of curls in the front with the rest of her hair piled on top of her head was imitated by many women of the day. Another was artists' model Evelyn Nesbit (Figure 5.4), whose chestnut hair was her crowning glory.

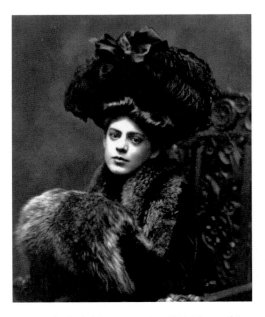

Figure 5.5   Photograph of Ethel Barrymore, circa 1901, Library of Congress Prints and Photographs Division. Barrymore models a typical Edwardian hat design that required voluminous hair for support.

To achieve these full hairstyles, women often needed to add pads, or "rats" to their hairstyles. Items known as "hair collectors" would sit on a woman's vanity. She would remove the loose hair from her hairbrush and insert it into the hole at the top of the hair collector. When the collector was full, the woman would remove the collected hair and use it to create stuffing that would add fullness to her hairstyle. In addition to being fashionable, hairstyles of this era also needed to be wide in order to support the large picture hats that were being worn. A popular hat design was the "Merry Widow" hat, which had piles of netting, feathers, and flowers.

In the majority of Edwardian hairstyles, the hair was pulled into a knot directly on the top of the head. Sometimes, however, a knot or coil of hair accentuated the nape of the neck (as in Figure 5.6). Still other women adopted the fashion of wearing part of their hair down, trailing over their shoulders (as in Figure 5.4).

Wavy textured hair was the most sought after during this period. Permanent waving machines were just being developed during this era—the early technology was a little terrifying! Women also explored some unusual hair products at this time to keep their crowning glories healthy and lustrous. Brilliantine, a hair oil, was used for shine, and some women even used a mercury ointment to keep their scalp healthy and to prevent dandruff! Many miracle cures, guaranteed to cure anything from gray hair to baldness, could be found in the advertisements of the era (see Figure 5.8).

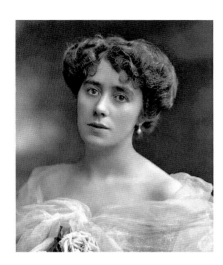

Figure 5.7 Photograph of Mrs. Alfred Charles William Harmsworth, by Lafayette Studio, London, 9 May 1902, Victoria and Albert Museum, Lafayette Archive. Mrs. Harmsworth has the coveted wavy hair texture from this time period.

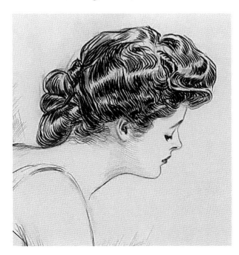

Figure 5.6 Left: Detail from "The Weaker Sex", by Charles Dana Gibson, 1903, Library of Congress. A coil of hair is visible at the nape of this woman's neck.

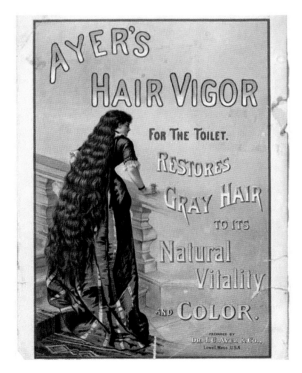

Figure 5.8 Advertisement for "Ayer's hair vigor for the toilet. Restores gray hair to its natural vitality and color", by Dr. J.C Ayer and Co., 1886, Library of Congress.

Edwardian Men

Men's hair in the Edwardian era was most often worn short, neat, and cleanly parted. Both side parts and center parts enjoyed popularity.

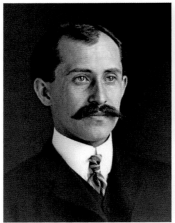 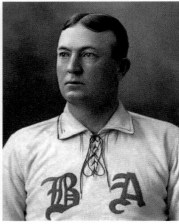

Figures 5.9 and 5.10   Left: Photographic portrait of Orville Wright, then aged 34, Library of Congress, 1905. Wright wears his hair slicked in place and neatly parted on the side and has a prominent mustache. Right: Denton True "Cy" Young, head and shoulders portrait, facing left, wearing a Boston Americans baseball team uniform, Library of Congress Prints and Photographs Division, 1902. Young wore his hair neatly combed into a center part.

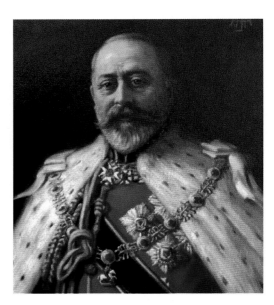

Figure 5.11   Portrait of H.M. King Edward VII, by Henry John Hudson, 1902.

Men, like women of the era, often used brilliantine to give their hair shine and hold it neatly in place. Macassar oil, an oil that was often made from coconut or palm oil, was also used during this era as a grooming and conditioning product. Because the oil had a tendency to travel from a man's hair onto the furniture he was resting his head against, people developed the antimacassar. This was a small crocheted cloth that was placed on the back of chairs to prevent the hair oil from sinking into the fabric of the furniture.

While there was not a huge variety in men's hairstyles, men could still express their individuality through their facial hair. Well trained handlebar mustaches were quite popular, as seen on Orville Wright in Figure 5.9. Edward VII (Figure 5.11) and W.E.B. Du Bois (Figure 5.12) both pair their handlebar mustache with a sharp, pointed trimmed goatee and beard.

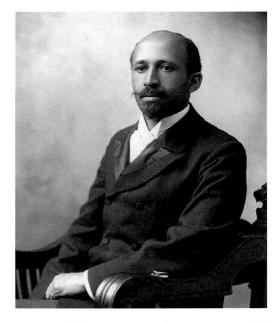

Figure 5.12   Photograph of W.E.B. Du Bois, taken in connection with the annual Niagara Movement meeting, summer 1907.

Gibson Girl Styling— Step by Step

This hairstyle is based on the Gibson Girl looks seen in Figure 5.1.

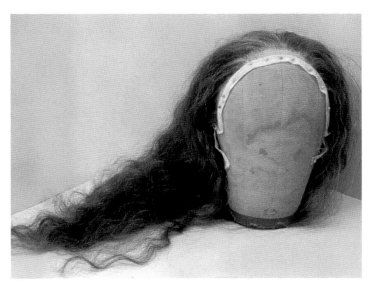

Figure 5.13 Step 1. Begin with a wig that is long (at least 14 inches long at the nape) and mostly one length. The wig in this picture is made of waved human hair, and the wig is fully ventilated.

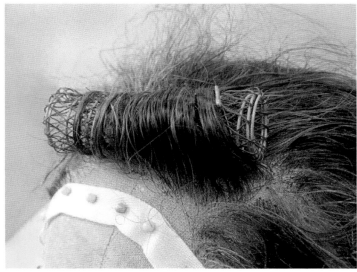

Figure 5.14 Step 2. Begin rolling the wig at the center front, using a nickel sized roller. Set the roller forward of the base, and at an angle to the hairline.

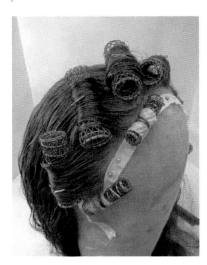

Figure 5.15 Step 3. Continue using nickel sized rollers set an angle down the front and one side of the wig. There is also a small tendril rolled in front of each ear.

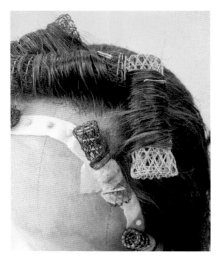

Figure 5.16 Step 4. Set another roller at the opposite angle of the first roller you placed at the center front hairline.

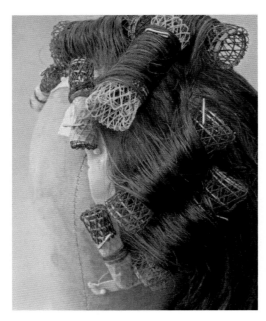

Figure 5.17   Step 5. Continue setting rollers at that angle down the other side of the hairline. A small tendril has been set in front of this ear as well.

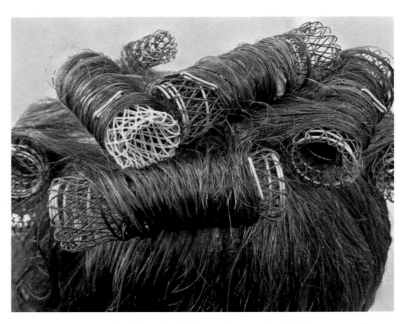

Figure 5.18   Step 6. Behind the angled rollers at the center front hairline, set two rollers going back towards the crown.

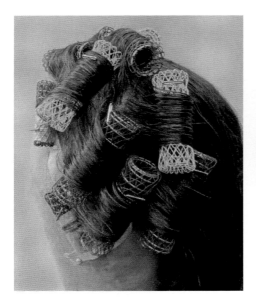

Figure 5.19   Step 7. Work your way down and around the side of the wig, setting rollers going away from the hairline.

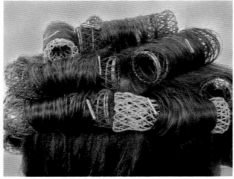

Figure 5.20   Step 8. Next, set a second row of rollers going down from the crown.

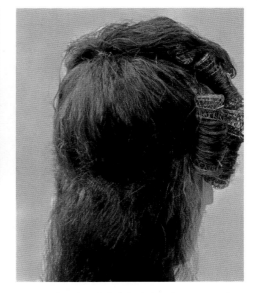

Figure 5.21   Step 9. Pull the hair at the crown and back of the head into a high ponytail. Make sure to leave at least two inches of hair around the back edges of the wig that is not pulled into the ponytail.

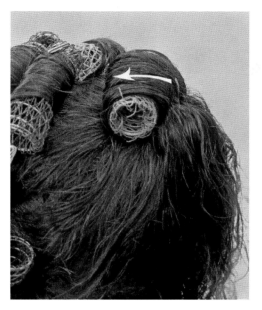

Figure 5.22 Step 10. Set the ponytail on nickel sized rollers, in a circular pattern.

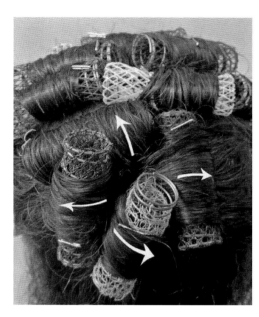

Figure 5.23 Step 11. Finish setting the hair in the ponytail—all the rollers should be rolled away from the center of the ponytail.

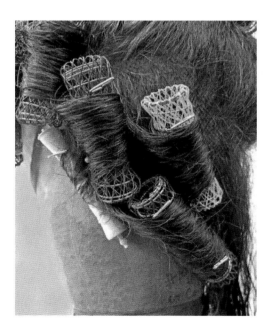

Figure 5.24 Step 12. Roll all remaining hair in the wig up towards the crown. If there are short tendrils of hair around the back, set them on medium sized perm rods, such as the yellow perm rod used here.

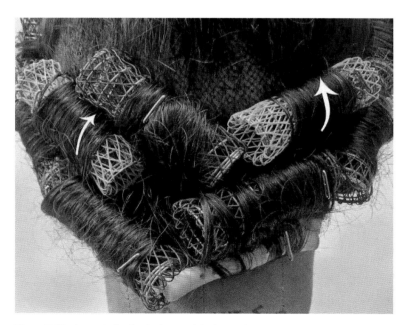

Figure 5.25 Step 13. The finished view of the hair at the nape of the neck, rolled towards the crown of the head.

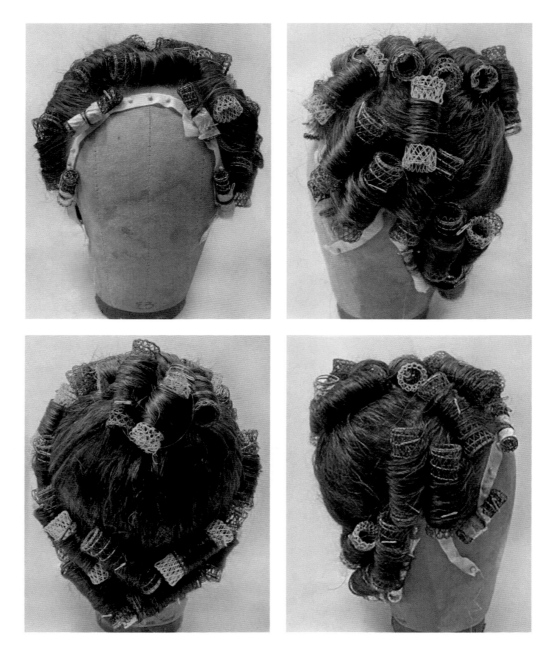

Figures 5.26–5.29   The finished Gibson Girl style set, viewed from all angles.

Once you have finished setting the wig, steam it if it is synthetic. If it is human hair, spray the hair through with water. Put the wig in the wig dryer after you have finished steaming and/or spraying, and dry it for 75 minutes.

To style:

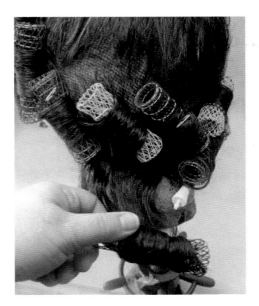

Figure 5.30 Step 14. Remove all the rollers beginning at the nape of the wig.

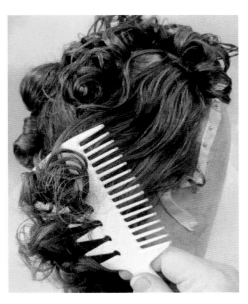

Figure 5.31 Step 15. Use a wide toothed comb to comb through all the curls of the wig.

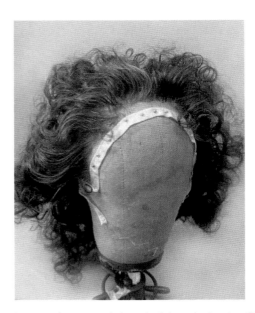

Figure 5.32 Step 16. After you comb through all the curls, the wig will have a lot of volume.

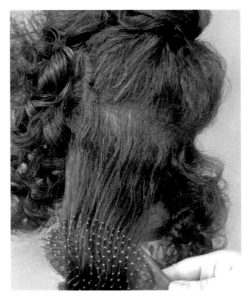

Figure 5.33 Step 17. Use a large brush to brush through the hair at the nape of the wig. Use a duckbill clip to pin the hair in the ponytail out of your way.

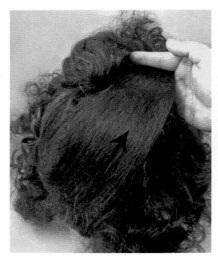

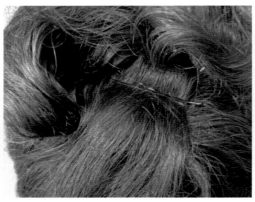

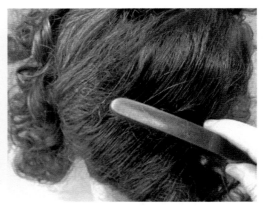

Figure 5.35   Step 19. Secure the section of hair with crossed bobby pins next to the base of the ponytail.

Figure 5.36   Step 20. Spritz the section of hair you just pinned with hairspray and smooth any flyways with your teasing/smoothing brush.

Figure 5.34   Step 18. Divide the hair at the nape in half. Smooth half of the hair diagonally up the back of the wig.

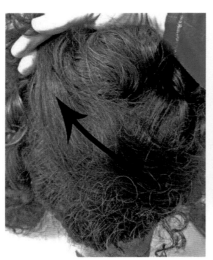

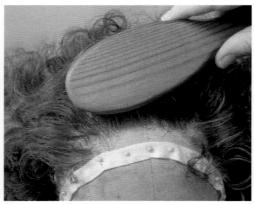

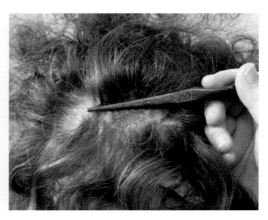

Figure 5.37   Step 21. Smooth the other half of the hair at the nape of the neck diagonally up and over the other side of the wig. Secure with bobby pins next to the base of the ponytail. Spritz with hairspray and smooth down the stray hairs.

Figure 5.38   Step 22. Now turn to the front of the wig. Use the large brush to brush through all the hair in the front section of the wig.

Figure 5.39   Step 23. Use the end of your teasing brush to separate out a small section of hair at the center front.

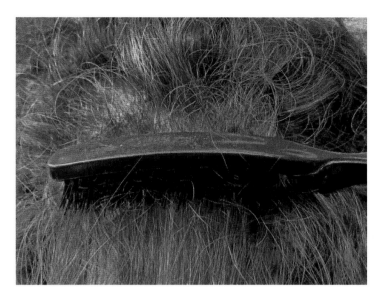

Figure 5.40 Step 24. Tease the hair to add volume and fullness at the front of the wig. Spray the hair lightly with hair spray after you finish teasing each section.

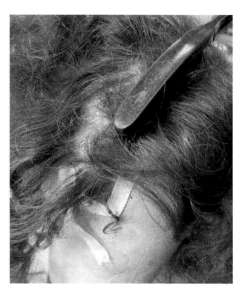

Figure 5.41 Step 25. Continue working your way down along the hairline towards the ear, teasing and spraying the hair as you go.

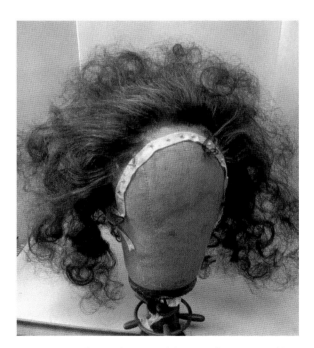

Figure 5.42 Step 26. After you have teased the entire front section of the wig, flip the hair back in the right direction and smooth the hair back. Spray with hairspray.

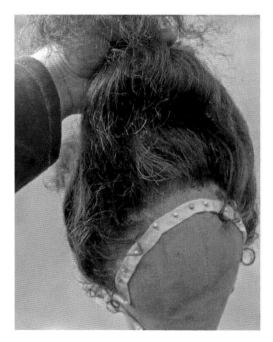

Figure 5.43 Step 27. Gather all the front section of hair together in your hand. You may need to use a smoothing brush to help the hair sweep up in the right direction.

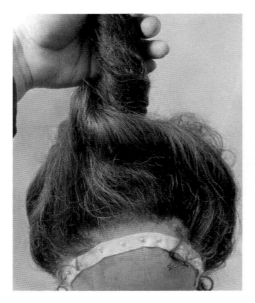

Figure 5.44 Step 28. Gently twist the hair into a loose coil.

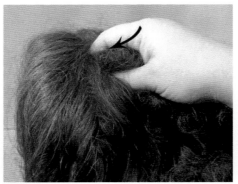

Figure 5.45 Step 29. Push the coiled hair down and forward. This will cause the hair to pouf out and form different shapes of wave in the front, depending on which direction you push in.

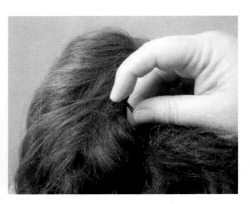

Figure 5.46 Step 30. When you are satisfied with the way the volume and waves look in the front, pin the coil of hair in place.

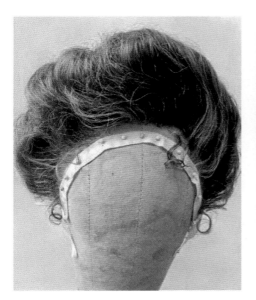

Figure 5.47 Step 31. Front view of the wig after the front section has been pinned in place.

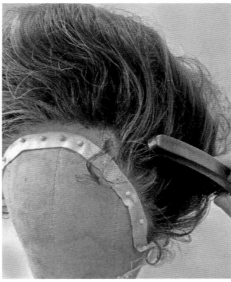

Figure 5.48 Step 32. Use hairspray and a smoothing brush to tidy up and sections of flyaway hairs.

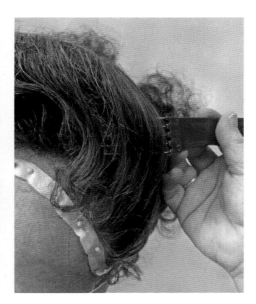

Figure 5.49 Step 33. You can adjust the volume or shape of the front by gently lifting sections with a teasing comb.

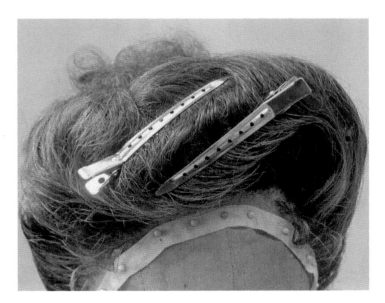

Figure 5.50 Step 34. I wanted to accentuate the wave in the front of this wig, so I used two duckbill clips to press the waves in place.

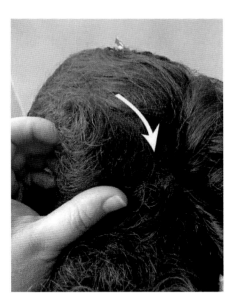

Figure 5.51 Step 35. Wind the end of the coiled hair into a cone shape. This will serve as the base for the high bun on your wig.

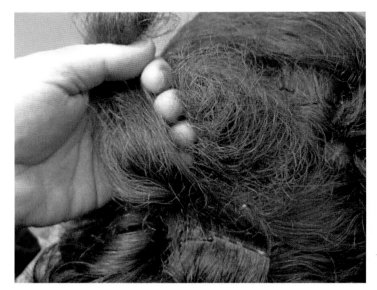

Figure 5.52 Step 36. Use a smoothing brush to smooth the pinned sections of hair from the nape of the wig around two fingers.

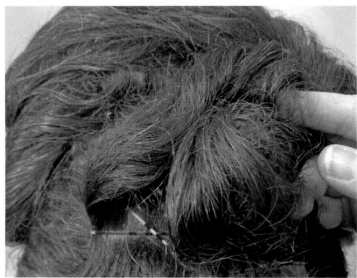

Figure 5.53 Step 37. Pin these curls you formed in place, continuing to create the bun of the wig.

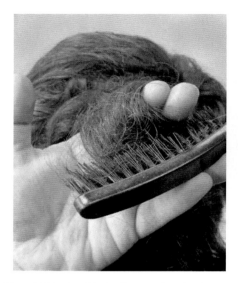

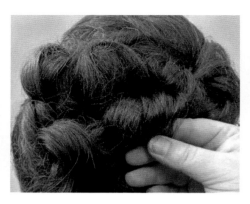

Figure 5.55   Step 39. Continue pinning the curls of hair from the ponytail to finish off the bun of the hairstyle.

Figure 5.54   Step 38. Use the smoothing brush to comb sections of hair from the ponytail around two fingers.

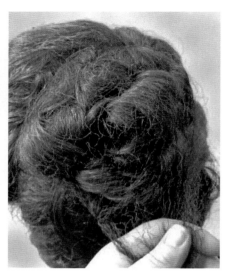

Figure 5.56   Step 40. Use a hairnet in a color that matches your wig. Pull the hairnet over the bun only. Hairnets come in a variety of sizes and colors. For this style, I used a bun sized hairnet, also sometimes called a chignon net.

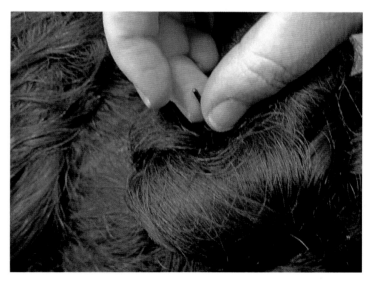

Figure 5.57   Step 41. Pin the hairnet both around and within the curls of the bun so that it is completely hidden.

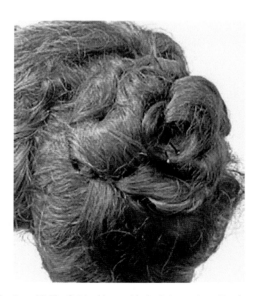

Figure 5.58   Step 42. The finished bun, with the hairnet pinned in place.

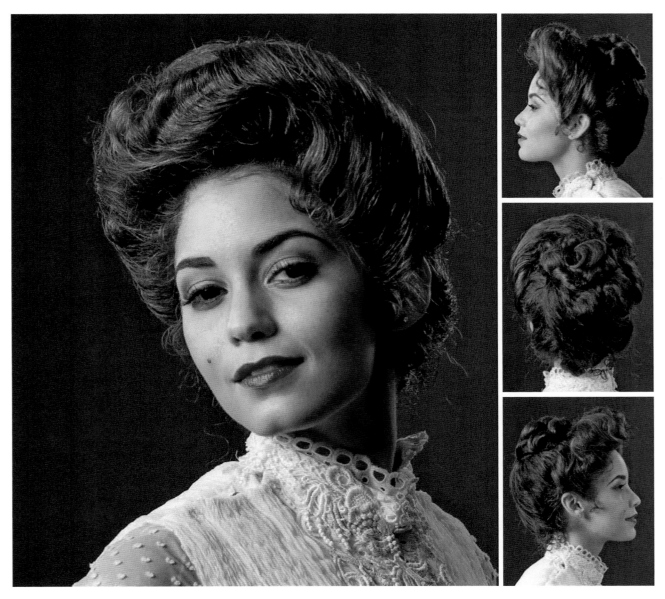

Figures 5.59–5.62   The completed Gibson Girl style. Photography: Tim Babiak. Model: Ivy Negron.

Variations

There are several ways to achieve great variety in your Gibson Girl looks. The Gibson Girls display many differences in hair texture, bun placement, and the arrangement of the waves around the face.

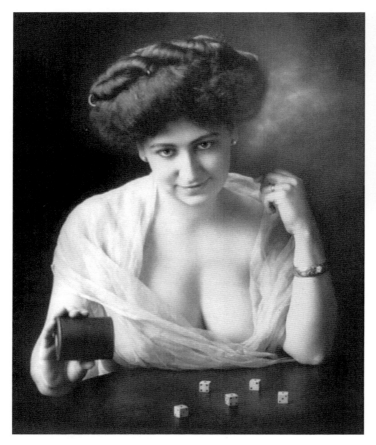

Figure 5.63   Photographic print "A Winning Miss", Library of Congress, Prints and Photographs Division, 1911. This lady wears a high wide hairstyle with very defined rolls on top.

Varying the shape of the silhouette of the hair from wider hairstyles to hairstyles that are more vertical can also help you to produce a diverse looking production.

The most fashionable hair color of the era was a reddish chestnut brown (such as the hair color of Evelyn Nesbit), but all hair colors and textures can be used successfully in this period.

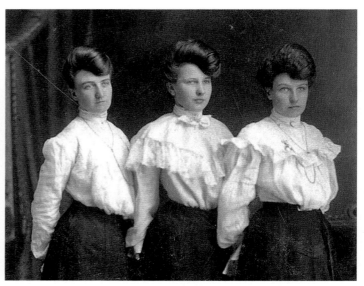

Figure 5.64   Portrait of three sisters from the Spencer family, private collection of David Ball, circa 1902. These ladies wear a version of Edwardian hairstyles that are more vertical in silhouette.

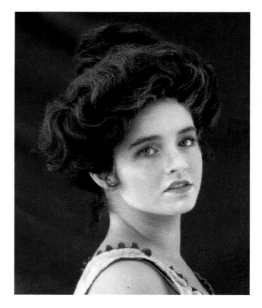

Figure 5.65   This wig, styled by Maur Sela, shows the rich, red-brown color so popular in the early 1900s.

Edwardian/Gibson Girl Makeup

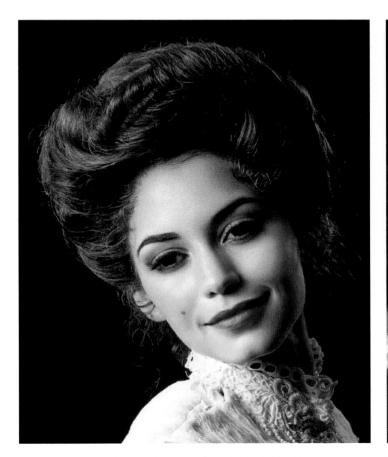

Figure 5.66 The ideal makeup look of a Gibson Girl. Model: Ivy Negron.

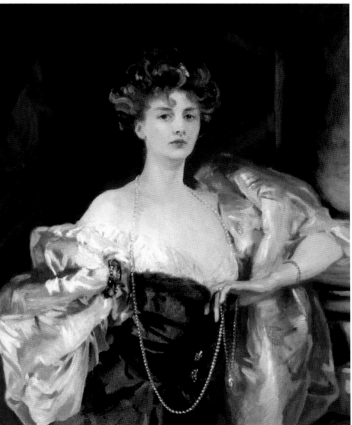

Figure 5.67 Detail from *Portrait of Helen Vincent, Viscountess d'Abernon*, John Singer Sargent, 1904, Birmingham Museum of Art.

Edwardian women were still seeking that perfectly pale smooth complexion. They tried to get rid of freckles using concoctions made of buttermilk or lemon juice. Tinted face powders were commonly used to perfect the skin. Blotting papers, made of tissue pressed with powder, were also used. Rouge made of carmine or safflower was commonly used to bring color to the cheeks and lips. Rosy pink lips were a fashion trend, achieved by staining the lips with geranium or poppy petals. In 1909, Gordon Selfridge began to place cosmetics on open counters in his store on Oxford Street in London. This began to change the idea of cosmetics from something that was purchased secretly to something that was more openly bought and used. Eyebrows were often focus of the Edwardian face, and thus eyebrow pencils became very popular. The ideal shape was for an eyebrow that was lifted in the center and curved downward towards the outer corner of the eye.

six

THE TEENS

$\left(\textit{1911–1920}\right)$

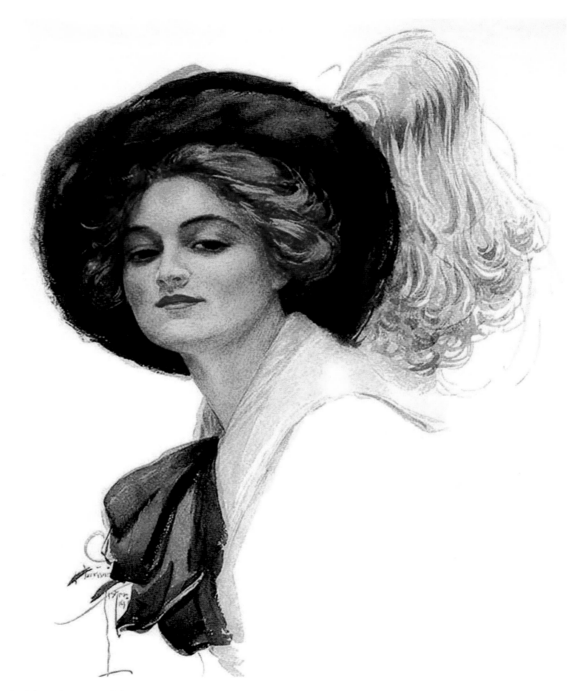

Figure 6.1   Dorothy Gibson, by Harrison Fisher, 1911.

Women in the Teens

In the "Teens," women were still expected to have great volumes of wavy hair that was then piled on their head. A permanent waving process was invented by Charles Nessler in 1905. He came to America in 1915 and opened a shop for waving hair. The hair was wrapped around brass rollers and hooked up to an electrical heating device. The process took six hours. The Art Nouveau and Orientalism movements also contributed to the romantic, exotic styles for women's hair. The volume of the hairstyles move down the head so that the fullness was concentrated either down around the ears, as in Figure 6.2, or on the back/crown area of the head, as in Figure 6.3.

Coronets of braids were popular at this time, as were piled masses of hair. The hair was often draped quite low over the forehead, sometimes nearly touching the eyebrows.

The Orientalism trend (popularized by designers such as Paul Poiret) also led to a craze for turbans. These turbans sometimes made

Important Events

1910	Ballet Russe performs *Scheherazade*, setting off a craze for Orientalism
1911	Triangle Shirtwaist Factory fire
1912	The *Titanic* strikes an iceberg and sinks on its maiden voyage
1914	Charlie Chaplin makes his first appearance as the Little Tramp character
1914–1919	World War I
1915	D.W. Griffith releases the film *Birth of a Nation*
1916	Norman Rockwell paints his first cover for the *Saturday Evening Post*
1917	Russian Revolution
1918	Czar Nicholas and his family are assassinated

Important Artists/Designers

Georges Braque, Marcel Duchamp, Wassily Kandinsky, Alphonse Mucha, Georgia O'Keefe, Paul Poiret, Norman Rockwell, Hans Unger

Important People/Style Icons

Irene Castle, Coco Chanel, Charlie Chaplin, Isadora Duncan, Eleanora Duse, Douglas Fairbanks, Mary Pickford

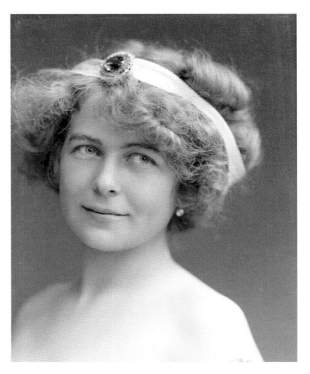

Figure 6.2 Gerda Andre, actor and singer, by Atelier Jaeger, Stockholm, undated, circa 1910, Swedish Performing Arts Agency.

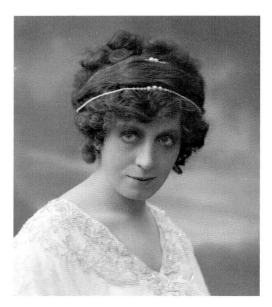

Figure 6.3 Pauline Brunius in *Gardesofficeren* at Svenska Teatern, by Atelier Jaeger, Stockholm, 1911, Swedish Performing Arts Agency.

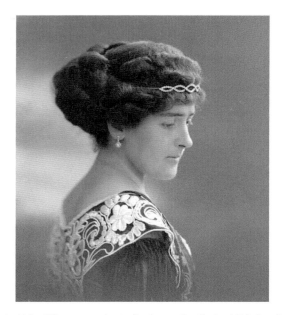

Figure 6.4 Helga Ekberg, actor, by Atelier Jaeger, Stockholm, 1912, Swedish Performing Arts Agency. In this picture, notice that the ears are mostly covered, the wavy hair is draped low across the forehead, and the bulk of the hair has been piled on the back of the head. The style is accented with a small jeweled band.

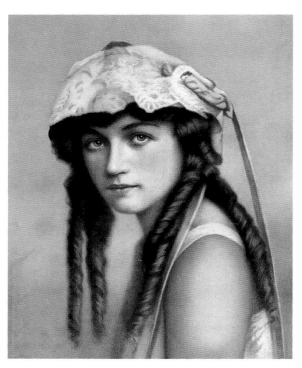

Figure 6.5 Detail of a movie poster for the American film *The Cinema Murder*, featuring Marion Davies, 1919, Paramount-Artcraft Pictures.

a narrower hairstyle necessary, so that the hair would fit inside. The large picture hats that were still in fashion required the support of a larger, wider hairstyle. Your fashion preferences would definitely have influenced your hairstyle during this era! In addition to turbans, fabric bandeaus and jeweled headpieces were often worn in this period, giving the hairstyles a vaguely Grecian look. Examples of this trend can be seen in Figures 6.2 and 6.4. There was also a trend of taking portrait of women where their long curls and ringlets were worn down around the shoulders (Figure 6.5). These looks were thought to be quite romantic and bohemian.

At this time in history, Madame C.J. Walker (Figure 6.6) was pioneering the development of haircare products for African Americans. Suffragettes begin to make simpler hairstyle choices to compliment more masculinely tailored clothes. Movies also begin to influence fashion. Late in the decade, dancer Irene Castle begins to make short hair popular, a trend that would explode in popularity in the 1920s.

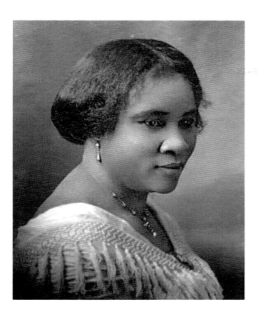

Figure 6.6 Madam C. J. Walker, the first self-made U.S. woman millionaire of any race, by Scurlock Studios, Washington DC, between 1905 and 1919, Smithsonian Institution.

Men in the Teens

Men's hair in the teens continued to be simple, short, and neat. The hair was often slicked straight back off the head, although styles with a part could still be found.

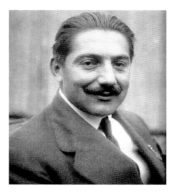

Figure 6.8 Georges Boillot at the Indianapolis 500, 1914, National Library of France. This is an example of a typical slicked back hairstyle.

The hair was often cropped so short that the skin was visible through the hair over the ears. The Arrow Collar Company produced an advertising campaign that was popular enough to set the ideal look for many men during this period.

The occasional neatly groomed mustache could still be found during this period, but the trend was generally toward being clean shaven.

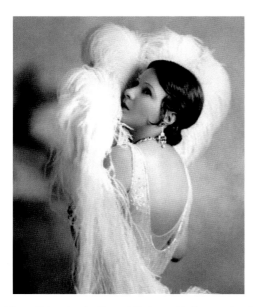

Figure 6.7 Norma Talmedge, by General Photographic Agency, circa 1919. This hairstyle is a precursor to the shorter styles that would explode in popularity in the 1920s.

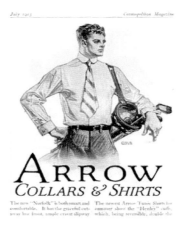

Figure 6.9 Arrow Collar Ad, 1913, *Cosmopolitan* magazine.

Teens' High Crown Woman's Styling— Step by Step

This hairstyle was inspired by Figure 6.3, but with a narrower silhouette.

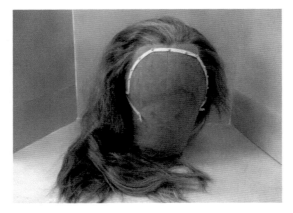

Figure 6.10   Step 1. Begin with a wig that is very long (at least 16 inches at the nape of the neck) and mostly one length. You may also need to incorporate a matching color switch in the final hairstyle. For this style, I used a synthetic lace front wig and a matching switch.

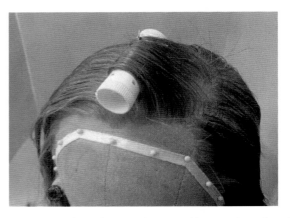

Figure 6.11   Step 2. Make a side part in the wig, and begin setting a dime sized roller to one side of the part.

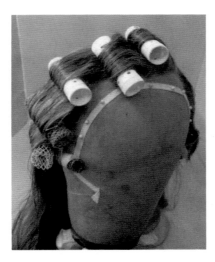

Figure 6.12   Step 3. Continue setting the rollers horizontally down the side of the head. Increase to quarter sized rollers once you get to the temple area. As you set the rollers, pull the hair slightly down onto the forehead.

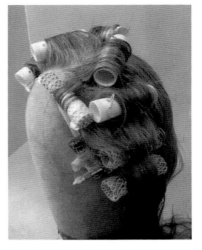

Figure 6.13   Step 4. On the other side of the part, you can set a tendril of hair on a dime sized roller if there happens to be short layers in your wig. Set a row of horizontal rollers going down the side of the head, just as you did on the opposite side. The first roller beside the part should be angled slightly so that it forms a "V" shape with the roller on the other side of the part. Again, move from dime sized rollers to quarter sized rollers.

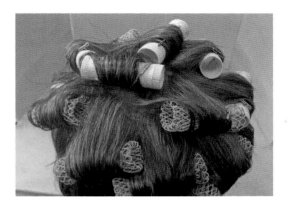

Figure 6.14 Step 5. Set a dime sized roller directly behind the "V" of the rollers at the part. Use quarter sized rollers to set alternating diagonal rows back to the crown of the head.

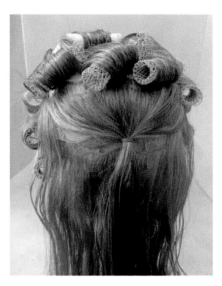

Figure 6.15 Step 6. Just below the crown of the head, pull a section of hair into a small ponytail.

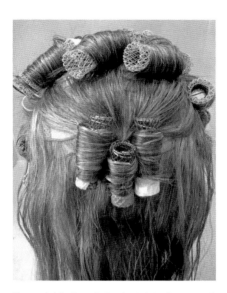

Figure 6.16 Step 7. Set the hair in the ponytail onto several dime sized rollers.

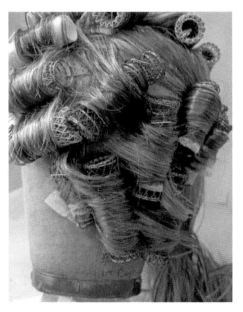

Figure 6.17 Step 8. Use quarter sized rollers to set the hair below the ponytail rolling towards the ponytail. If there are any shorter tendrils of hair behind the ears, set them on pencil sized rollers.

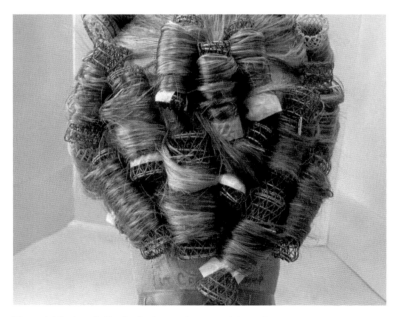

Figure 6.18 Step 9. The finished set at the nape of the neck.

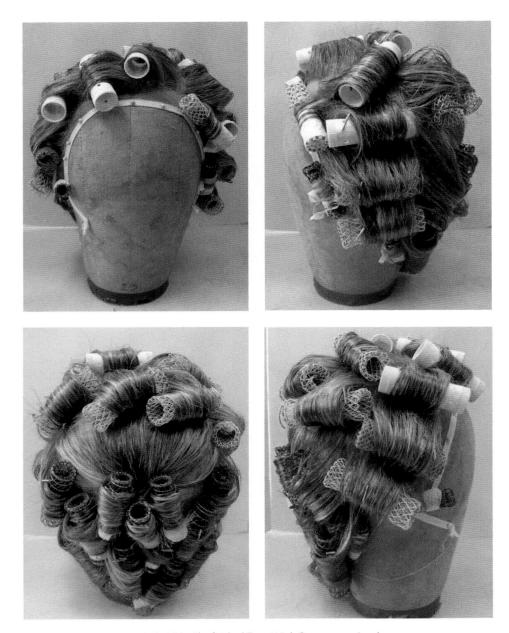

Figures 6.19–6.22   The finished Teens' High Crown woman's style set.

Once you have finished setting the wig, steam each roller thoroughly if the wig is made of synthetic hair. If the wig is human hair, soak each roller with water sprayed from a spray bottle. After steaming or wetting, place the wig in a wig dryer for 75 minutes.

To style:

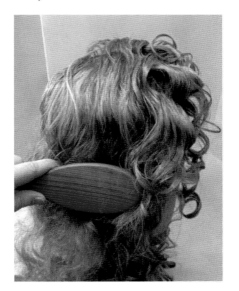

Figure 6.23 Step 10. Remove all the rollers from the wig, beginning at the nape of the neck. Brush through the entire wig with a large brush.

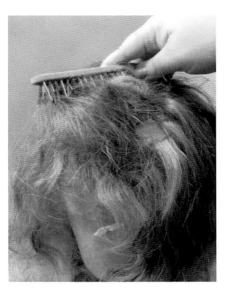

Figure 6.24 Step 11. Lightly tease the hair all around the hairline.

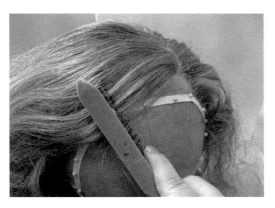

Figure 6.25 Step 12. Use a teasing/smoothing brush to smooth the teased hair down and away from the part. Make sure to brush the hair down onto the forehead.

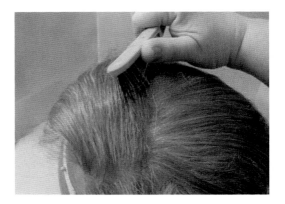

Figure 6.26 Step 13. Use the brush to make sure that there is a clear divide between the front section that is smoothed towards the ears, and the back section that is smoothed towards the crown of the head.

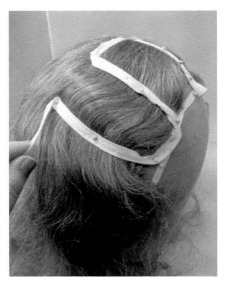

Figure 6.27 Step 14. Use a piece of blocking tape to shape the hair in the front section into large waves.

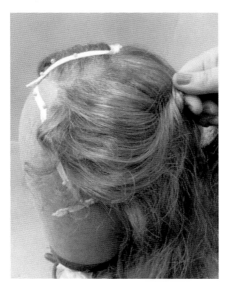

Figure 6.28 Step 15. On the other side of the head, pull the front section back over the ear and twist it a little bit. Pin the twist in place.

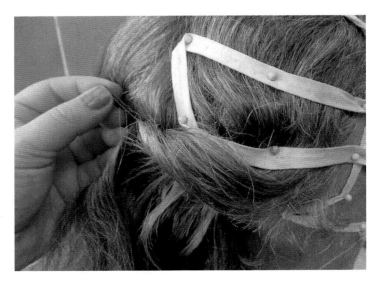

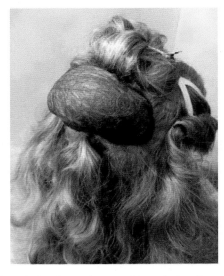

Figure 6.29 Step 16. Pull the hair at the bottom of the waved section up and twist it and pin it like you did on the first side.

Figure 6.30 Step 17. Pin a hair pad in a matching color just above the small ponytail you created earlier. Notice how the remaining hair in the front section has been pinned up out of the way with a duckbill clip.

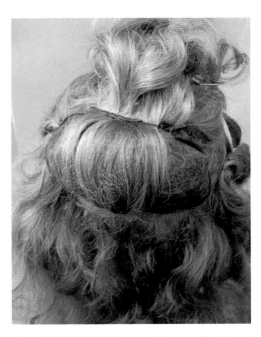

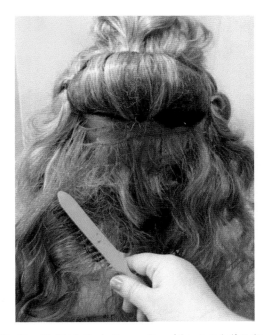

Figure 6.31 Step 18. Pull the hair in the ponytail up over the hair pad and anchor it with crossed bobby pins. It is not necessary for the entire hair pad to be covered at this time, as you are going to dress more hair over it in later steps.

Figure 6.32 Step 19. Divide the bottom section of the wig in half. Lightly tease the left side of the wig and mist it with hairspray.

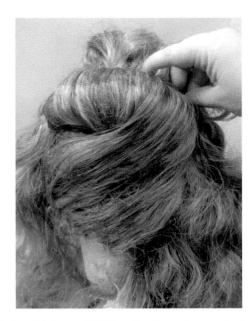

Figure 6.33 Step 20. Smooth this left section diagonally up the back of the wig and pin it so that the section covers the outside part of the hair pad.

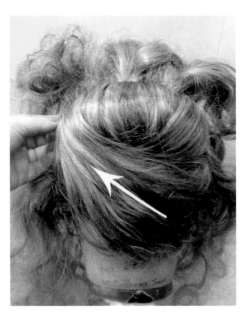

Figure 6.34 Step 21. Tease and smooth the right side of the wig diagonally up and over towards the left side of the hair pad (it should overlap the first section you did.) Pin this section in place.

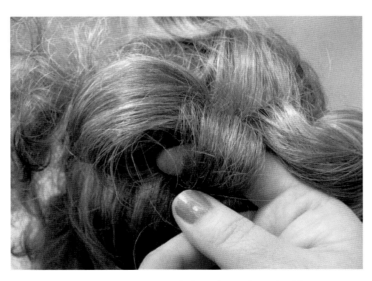

Figure 6.35 Step 22. Begin arranging the loose hair at the ends of the sections into curls and rolls by brushing sections of hair around your finger with a smoothing brush.

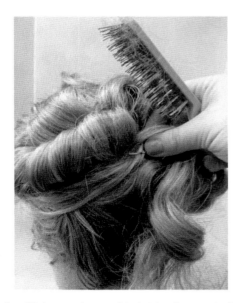

Figure 6.36 Step 23. Arrange the rest of the hair into loops and rolls around the hair pad. You may need to move and pin sections of hair around in order to create a balanced final product.

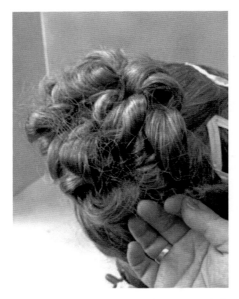

Figure 6.37 Step 24. Once you have arranged all the hair, cover it with a matching color hairnet and pin so that the hairnet does not show.

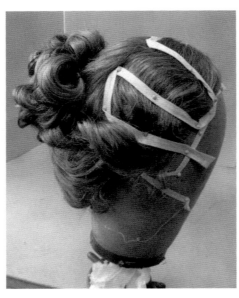

Figure 6.38 Step 25. You could finish the hairstyle at this point, and dress it with a bandeau or headband.

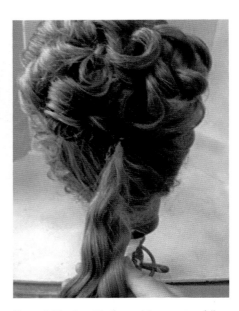

Figure 6.39 Step 26. If you wish to create a fuller, more elaborate hairstyle, pin a matching switch underneath the center of the finished curl cluster.

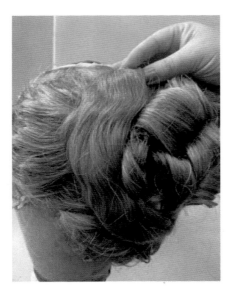

Figure 6.40 Step 27. I created the texture in this switch by simply braiding it and setting it. Once dry, I unbraided the switch and used the wavy texture as part of the finished look. Wrap the switch up and around the cluster of curls. Pin the hair in place with hairpins as you move around the head.

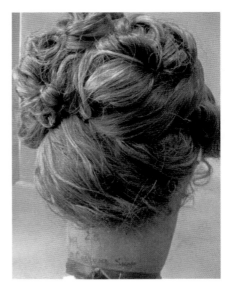

Figure 6.41 Step 28. Hide the tail end of your switch under the bottom of your curl cluster. Pin it in place with bobby pins.

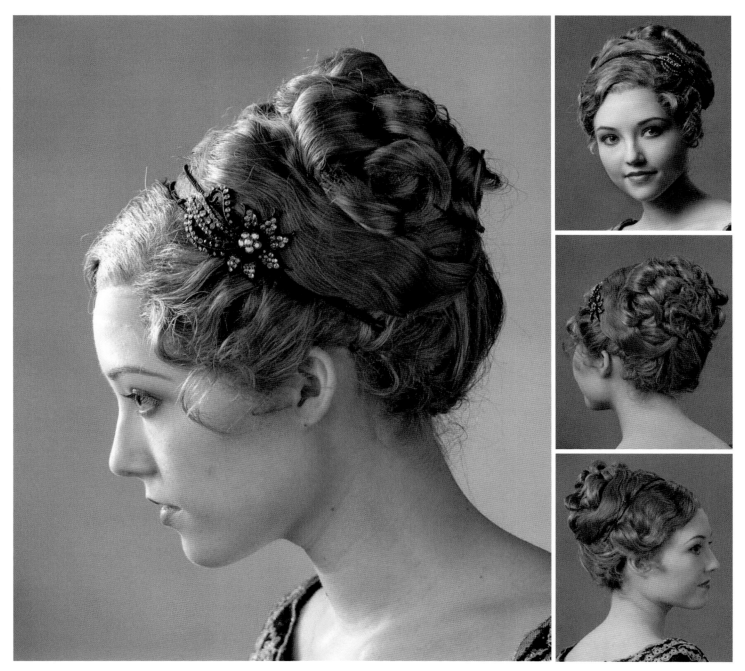

Figures 6.42–6.45   The completed Teens', High Crown woman's style. Photography: Tim Babiak. Model: Josephine McAdam.

Teens' Full Width Woman's Styling—Step by Step

This hairstyle is based on Figure 6.2.

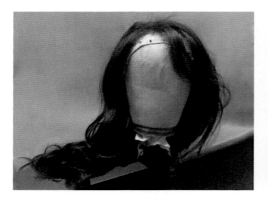

Figure 6.46 Step 1. Begin with a wig that has a lot of long length and some shorter sections around the face (or full bangs).

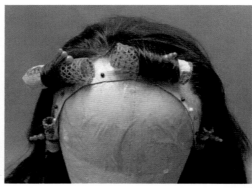

Figure 6.47 Step 2. Use quarter sized rollers to set the bangs low over the forehead. Also set small tendrils of hair in front of the ears.

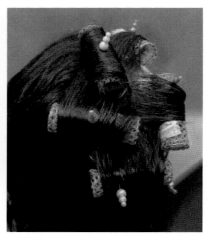

Figure 6.48 Step 3. Set a quarter sized roller rolling back off the face behind the bangs. Continuing working down the side of the head, angling the roller a little more each time. The bottom rollers should end up horizontal.

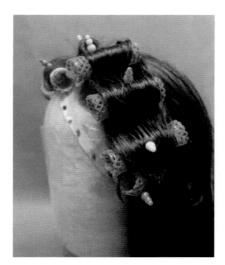

Figure 6.49 Step 4. Place horizontal rollers going down the opposite side.

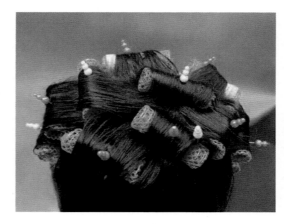

Figure 6.50 Step 5. Use rows of diagonal rollers to join each row of rollers on the back of the head.

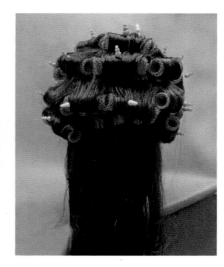

Figure 6.51 Step 6. Continue working your way down the back of the head, setting in horizontal rows.

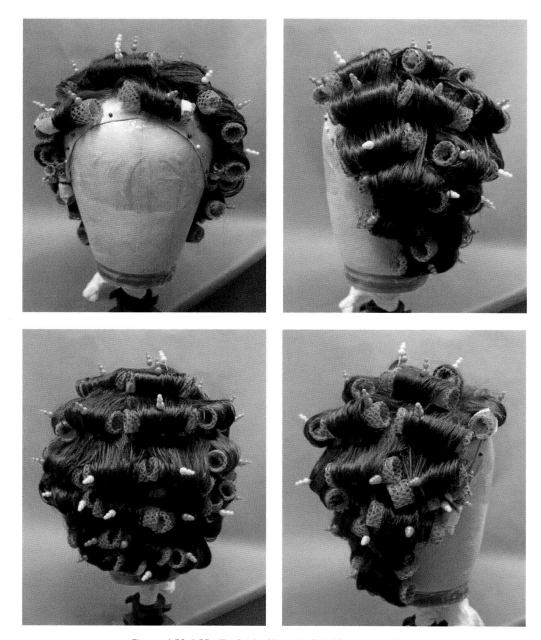

Figures 6.52–6.55   The finished Teens' Full Width woman's style set.

Once you have finished setting the wig, steam each roller thoroughly if the wig is made of synthetic hair. If the wig is human hair, soak each roller with water sprayed from a spray bottle. After steaming or wetting, place the wig in a wig dryer for 75 minutes.

To style:

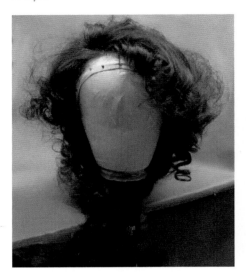

Figure 6.56   Step 7. Remove all the rollers and brush through the entire wig with a large brush.

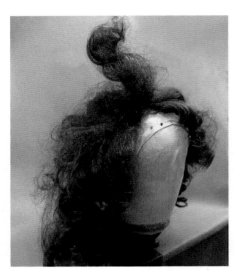

Figure 6.57   Step 8. Take sections of hair behind the bangs and gently tease them, applying light layers of hairspray as you go.

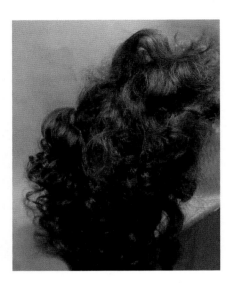

Figure 6.58   Step 9. Behind the teased sections, pull a section of the hair into a small ponytail just beneath the crown.

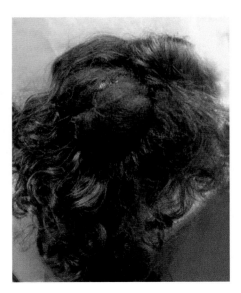

Figure 6.59   Step 10. Place a rat or hair pad just behind the teased sections of hair.

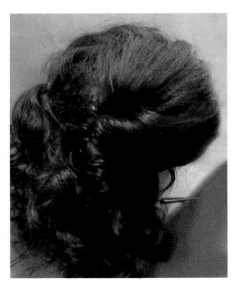

Figure 6.60   Step 11. Gather the front teased sections on the right side of the head into your hand. Smooth the top layer with a smoothing rush. Drape this section over the hair pad, twist, and pin in place next to the ponytail.

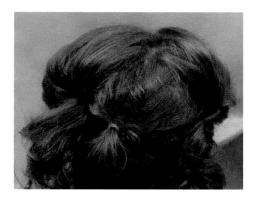

Figure 6.61 Step 12. Repeat the process on the opposite side of the wig.

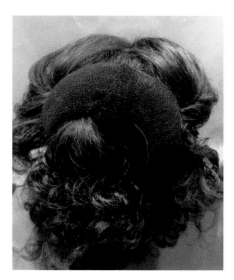

Figure 6.62 Step 13. Use another hair pad, this one "U" shaped, and pin it in an arc around the top of the ponytail.

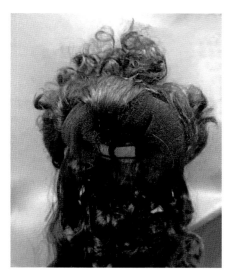

Figure 6.63 Step 14. Bring the hair in the ponytail up over the hair pad and begin to cover it, spreading the hair as you go. Leave the ends loose.

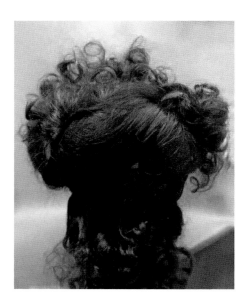

Figure 6.64 Step 15. Drape a section of hair from the left side of the wig, using it to continue covering the hair pad.

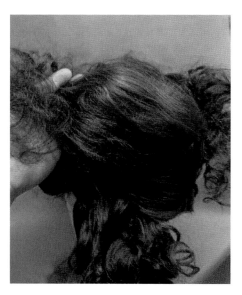

Figure 6.65 Step 16. Bring up a section from the right side of the wig and drape it to keep covering the hair pad. You may need to tease the underside of this section.

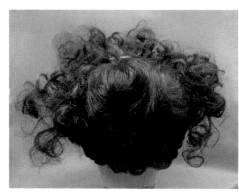

Figure 6.66 Step 17. Bring up the remaining length of hair and pin it so the hair pad is completely covered.

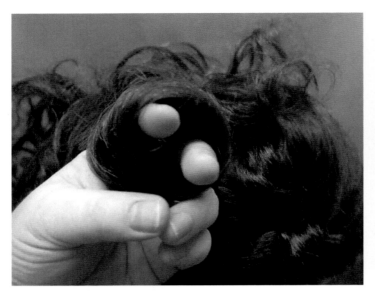 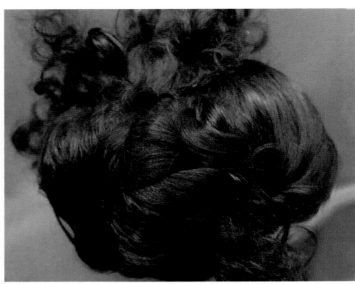

Figure 6.67 and 6.68   Step 18. Begin arranging the loose ends into large rolls by brushing a section around two fingers and then pinning it in place.

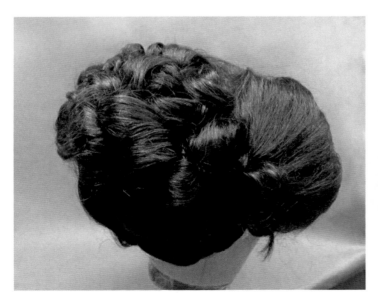

Figure 6.69   Step 19. The completed back of the wig.

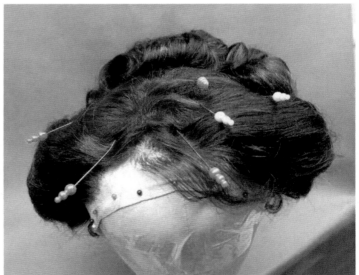

Figure 6.70   Step 20. Use large pins to accentuate the waves in the front of the hairstyle. Mist with hairspray and allow to set. You can also use a lifting comb to lift extra volume into the sides of the wig over the ears.

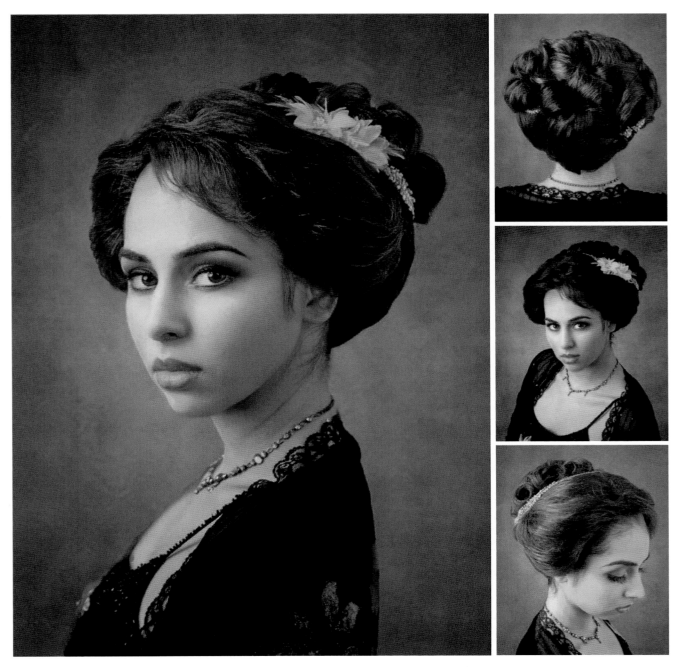

Figures 6.71–6.74   The completed Teens' Full Width woman's style. Model: Linette Zare.

Variations

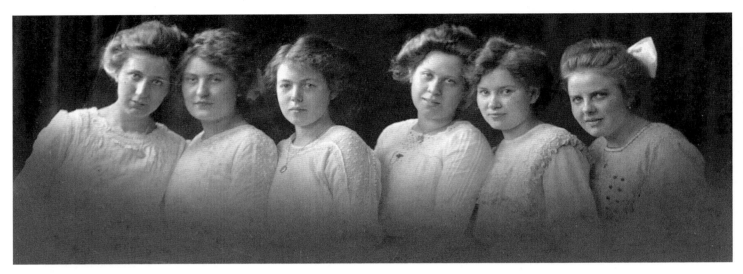

Figure 6.75   Professional photograph of a group from around the turn of the 19th/20th century, photographer unknown, 1912.

Varying the placement of the fullness in the hairstyle will allow you to create many different teens-appropriate looks (see Figure 6.75). You can also include the occasional shorter hairstyle, such as the one in Figure 6.76.

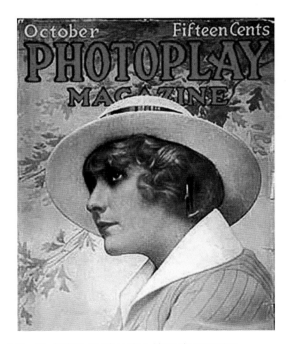

Figure 6.76   Pearl White, October 1914, *Photoplay* magazine.

Teens' Makeup

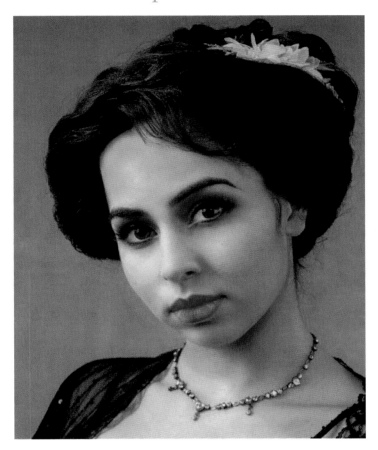

Figure 6.77 The healthy romantic blush of a typical woman of the Teens. Model: Linette Zare.

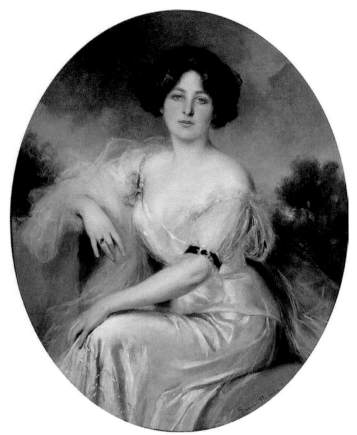

Figure 6.78 *Lady Elsie Duveen, nee Solomon,* Francois Flameng, 1910. Notice this lady's flushed rosy cheeks and stained lips.

Makeup in the teens focused on a more healthy, robust look for women. Women were becoming much more active, inspired by fads for sports like bicycle riding, golf, and badminton. They were still using things like powdered starch or oatmeal to powder their face. Pancake makeup began being manufactured in 1914, kicking off sales of commercial foundation products. Rouge for flushed rosy cheeks and stained lips was plentiful. Paste eye shadows in colors like gray, brown, and lemon also started to become popular.

seven

THE ROARING TWENTIES

(1920–1929)

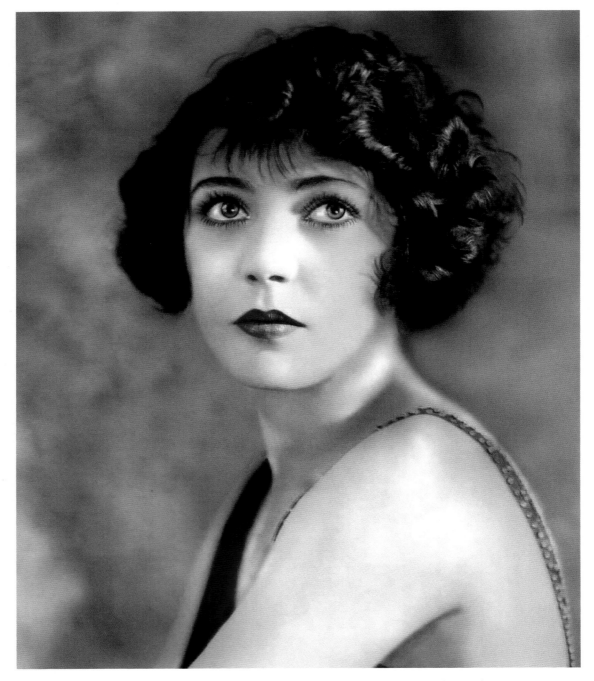

Figure 7.1   Renee Adoree (colorized), Goldwyn Pictures, circa 1922, Bain News Service; Library of Congress Prints and Photographs Division.

Important Events

1920   Prohibition of alcohol begins in the United States

1920   The Nineteenth Amendment, giving women the right to vote, is ratified in the United States

1922   The tomb of King Tut is discovered in Egypt

1927   *The Jazz Singer*, the first feature length movie with recorded dialogue, debuts

1928   Mickey Mouse debuts in the animated short *Steamboat Willie*

1929   Several gangsters are shot and killed in the St. Valentine's Day Massacre

1929   The stock market crashes, beginning the Great Depression

Important Artists/Designers

Coco Chanel, Erté, Max Factor, Salvatore Ferragamo, Jeanne Lanvin, Tamara de Lempicka, Maxfield Parrish, Jean Patou, Man Ray, Elsa Schiaparelli

Important People/Style Icons

Josephine Baker, Theda Bara, John Barrymore, Clara Bow, Louise Brooks, Al Capone, Charlie Chaplin, F. Scott and Zelda Fitzgerald, Ernest Hemingway, Al Jolson, Buster Keaton, Charles Lindbergh, Gloria Swanson, Rudolph Valentino

1920s' Women

Fashion changed dramatically for women in the 1920s. After hundreds of years of being confined in corsets and having long hair put up into elaborate hairstyles, woman gained new freedom from their clothes and heavy hair. Beginning in World War I, nearly all women who drove ambulances had their hair cut for reasons of sanitation and ease. In popular culture, a ballroom dancer by the name of Irene Castle cut off her long hair for reasons of convenience. The trend spread rapidly, and women everywhere began bobbing their hair.

In May of 1920, the *Saturday Evening Post* published F. Scott Fitzgerald's short story "Bernice Bobs Her Hair." This story of a small-town girl who is tricked by her cousin into chopping off her hair and subsequently becomes a femme fatale further served to give this haircut a special place in history. Fashion was also undergoing a revolution—women's clothes were less confining, and more masculine shapes and clean lines were very much in vogue. The close fitting cloche hats of the era also required short simple haircuts to fit underneath.

There were many variations of the bob haircut. The Shingle involved cutting the hair close to the scalp at the nape of the neck and leaving the hair gradually longer as the barber went higher, without showing a definite line. This haircut was very easy to style in a number of ways. The Eton Crop was a very short haircut, named after the

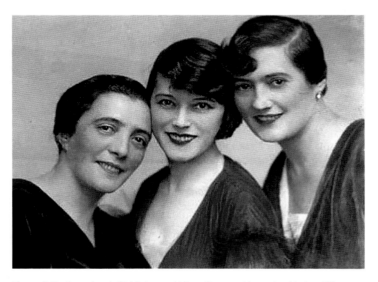

Figure 7.2   Ilona Aczel, Gizi Bajor, and Vilma Gomory, Hungarian National Theatre, 1927. These women model typical bobbed haircuts of the 1920s.

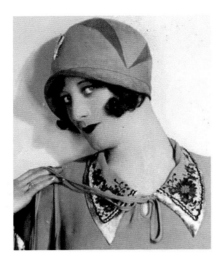

Figure 7.3 Joan Crawford, April 29, 1927, Library of Congress Prints and Photographs Division. Crawford models a close-fitting cloche hat that covers nearly all her short bobbed haircut.

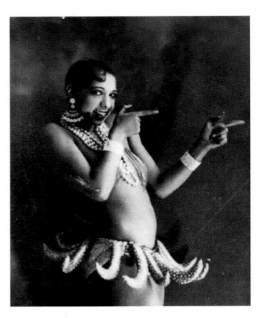

Figure 7.4 Josephine Baker in Banana Skirt from Folies Bergere production *Un Vent de Folie*, by Lucien Walery, 1927. Josephine Baker shows off her short, pomaded hairstyle.

English boy's prep school, that left both the ears and neck exposed. This haircut was made popular by Josephine Baker (Figure 7.4), the famous African American entertainer who rose to fame performing in France.

The Dutch Boy Bob was made famous by movie stars Louise Brooks and Colleen Moore (Figure 7.5). This haircut was usually worn straight to just above the jaw line, with blunt cut bangs helping to frame the face.

Another film star who set trends in the 1920s was Clara Bow. Her tousled curls, sad, down turned eyes, and well defined Cupid's bow lip earned her the name of the "It Girl."

In the earlier part of the 1920s, hair was often shorter, smoother, and sleeker, such as we see in Figures 7.2 and 7.5. This texture was often achieved by water waving or finger waving, a method of hair dressing that involved wetting the hair with curling lotion, combing it into waves with your fingers, and letting it dry.

Later in the decade, hairstyles had more texture—either like the messy curls of Clara Bow, or the more rigidly defined waves seen in Figure 7.7. The more rigid styles were likely created with a Marcel curling iron, an iron that created a three dimensional wave when pressed into the hair (Figure 7.8).

Despite the prevalence of the bob, some women refused to believe the trend would last. They feared cutting their hair, only to literally come up short when long hair came back into fashion. Many of these

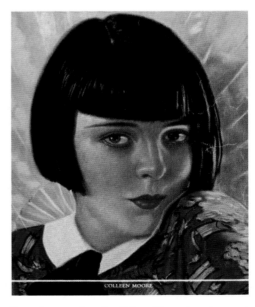

Figure 7.5 *Photoplay* cover, featuring Colleen Moore, based on a painting by Livingston Greer, January 1926.

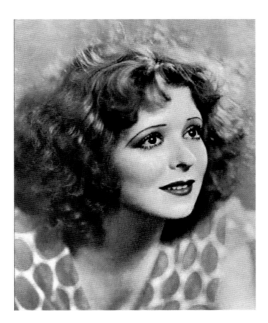

Figure 7.6 Clara Bow, *Photoplay*, 1932. Bow's curls are an example of a 1920s' hairstyle with a lot of texture.

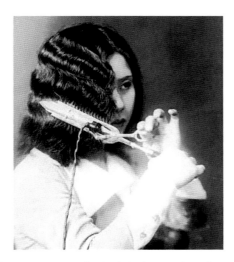

Figure 7.8 Japanese woman curling her hair, photographer unknown, 1920s. This woman is using a waving iron to achieve perfect waves in her hair.

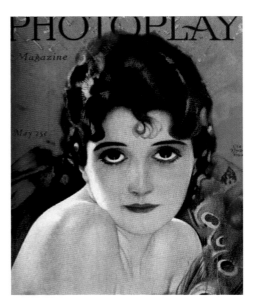

Figure 7.7 American actress Clara Kimball Young on the cover of *Photoplay*, reproduced as an ad on page 3809 of the May 1, 1920 *Motion Picture News*, by Rolf Armstrong, May 1920. A short, waved hairstyle, typical of the early part of the 1920s.

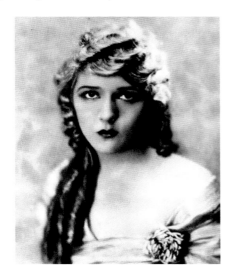

Figure 7.9 American actress Mary Pickford on the cover of the *Photoplay*, by Nelson Evans, October 1921.

women secured their hair in a tight low bun that mimicked the close fitting silhouette of the bob. Other women chose to wear a romantic style of hair with long ringlets, made popular by silent actress Mary Pickford, who was famous for playing plucky young ingénues. Whether women's hair was long or bobbed, the silhouette was very close to the head, and the hair was usually dressed low on the forehead.

1920s' Men

Men in the 1920s often had haircuts where the hair was longer on the top and sides, but quite short and neatly trimmed in the back. Like the women of the period, men also had Marcel waves in their hair. Movie stars like Rudolph Valentino helped set the fashion of heavily slicked back hair.

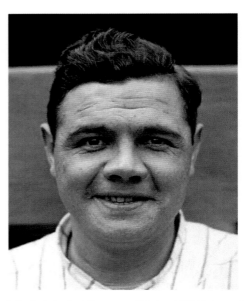

Figure 7.11   Babe Ruth, by Paul Thompson NY, circa 1920, Heritage Auction Gallery.

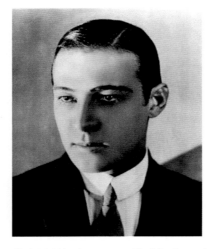

Figure 7.10   Actor Rudolph Valentino on page 15 of the September 1922 *Photoplay*, by Donald Biddle Keys. Valentino's slicked back hair and heavily made up face were a popular look in the 1920s.

Men following this fashion were often referred to as "sheiks"—this term came from the characters in all the Arabian/Middle Eastern film settings popular at the time. To achieve the desired slicked back, cleanly parted looks, men used hair products like brilliantine, an oily grooming liquid for hair that gave a highly glossy finish. Brylcreem also made its debut in this decade—it was invented as a pomade in England in 1928. Marcel waves were as popular for men as they were for ladies. However, not all men adopted the slicked back look. Some men wore their hair in a looser, more adventurous looking textured hairstyle, such as the look worn by Babe Ruth in Figure 7.11.

Stylish mustaches were very fashionable in the 1920s. Because women were enjoying freedoms through short boyish haircuts and more masculine clothing, men would grow mustaches to assert their masculinity. Popular styles of mustache included the very thin pencil mustache and the short toothbrush mustache popularized by Charlie Chaplin.

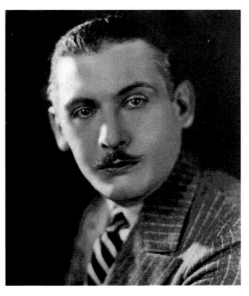

Figure 7.12   Lew Cody, star of *Photoplay*, 1924. Notice Cody's very neatly groomed mustache.

1920s' Flapper Styling—
Step by Step

This hairstyle was inspired by Figure 7.2, with a little more curl added for visual definition.

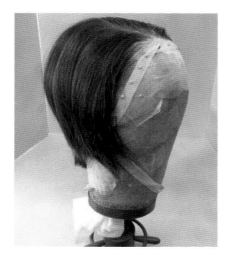

Figure 7.13 Step 1. Begin with a wig that is cut quite short in the back, with longer hair (at least four inches long) on the top, front, and sides. (This wig could actually be used without any additional styling as a simpler kind of boyish 1920s' look.) I used a fully ventilated lace front human hair wig for this styling project.

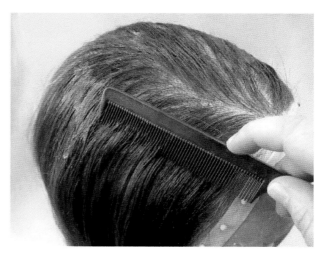

Figure 7.14 Step 2. Make a clean part in the wig. Comb setting lotion through the wig.

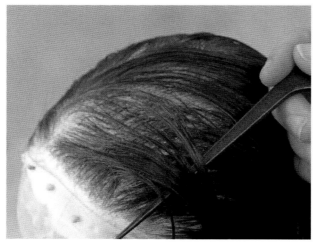

Figure 7.15 Step 3. Use a rattail comb to section out an area of hair that is approximately one inch by one inch square.

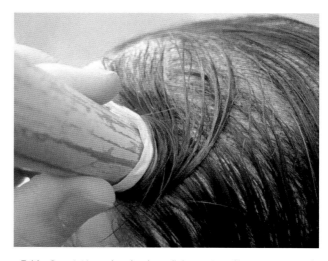

Figure 7.16 Step 4. Use a dowel rod to roll the section of hair into a pin curl.

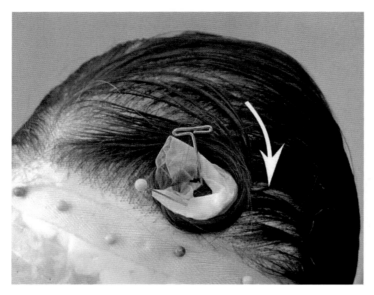

Figure 7.17 Step 5. This curl is rolled clockwise towards the face, coming forward of the hairline.

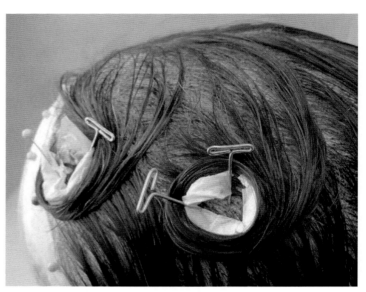

Figure 7.18 Step 6. Continue rolling pin curls in a horizontal row around the head. All the curls in this row should be rolled clockwise.

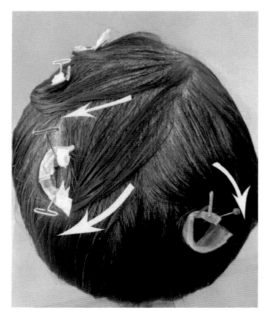

Figure 7.19 Step 7. As you come around the part, continue rolling the curls in a clockwise direction.

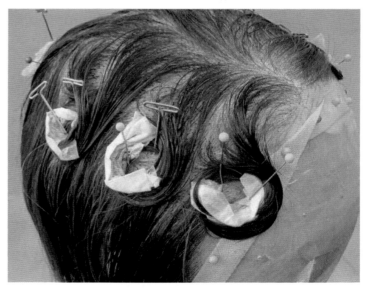

Figure 7.20 Step 8. The last pin curl in this row should also come forward of the hairline. Setting your curls in front of the hairline is especially helpful if you are styling a hard front wig—this will help the waves conceal the edge of the wig once the hair is styled.

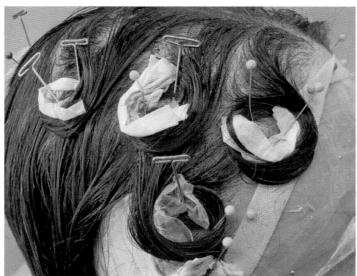

Figure 7.21 Step 9. The next row of pin curls should be rolled in a counterclockwise direction. Also make a tiny pin curl in front of the ear.

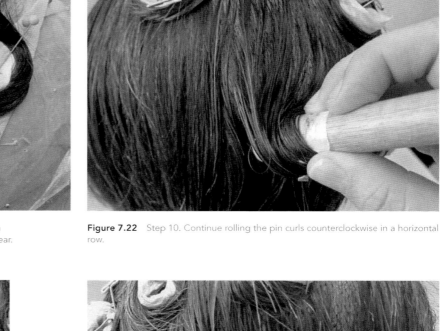

Figure 7.22 Step 10. Continue rolling the pin curls counterclockwise in a horizontal row.

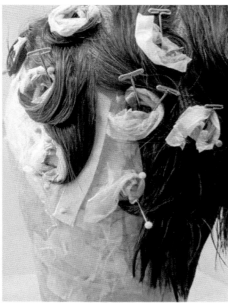

Figure 7.23 Step 11. Finish this row of pin curls with a curl that comes past the hairline onto the face. Make another small pin curl in front of the ear. If there is enough length in the hair, make small pin curl behind the ear.

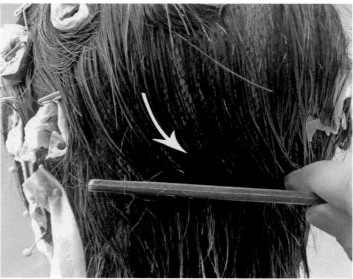

Figure 7.24 Step 12. The rest of the hair in this wig is too short to pin curl. (If the hair in your wig is long enough, continue pin curling the wig all the way down to the nape of the neck in alternating rows.) Instead, we are going to finger wave the back. Begin by combing all the hair to the right. You may need to add more setting lotion and water if the wig has become too dry.

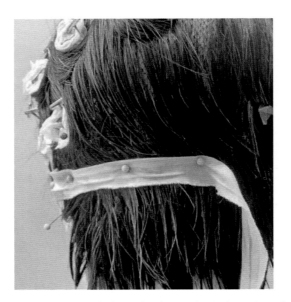

Figure 7.25 Step 13. Secure the hair in this direction by pinning a piece of blocking tape over it.

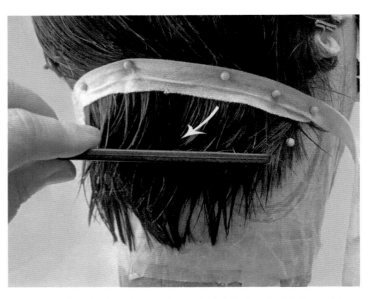

Figure 7.26 Step 14. Drop down and comb the hair back to the left. Secure it in place with the blocking tape.

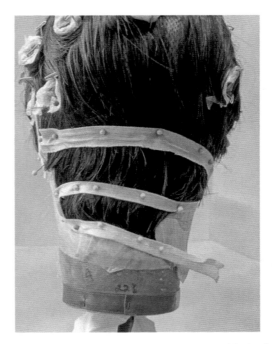

Figure 7.27 Step 15. Finish off the set by combing the ends of the hair back towards the right and securing them with the tape.

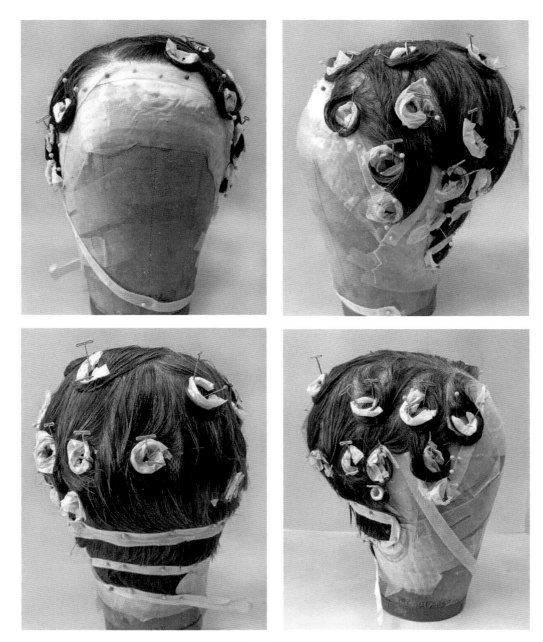

Figures 7.28–7.31   The finished 1920s' Flapper style set.

Once you have finished setting the wig, steam it if the wig is made of synthetic hair. If the wig is made of human hair (as this one is) spray it liberally with water. Put the wig in a wig dryer to dry for 75 minutes.

To style:

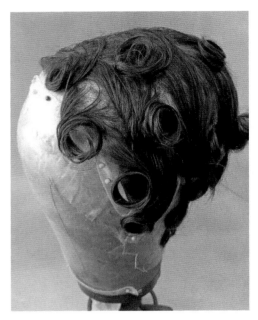

Figure 7.32 Step 16. Remove the blocking tape from the back of the wig and undo all the pin curls, removing the endpapers.

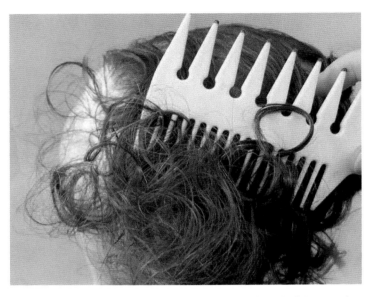

Figure 7.33 Step 17. Use a wide toothed comb to comb through all the pin curls.

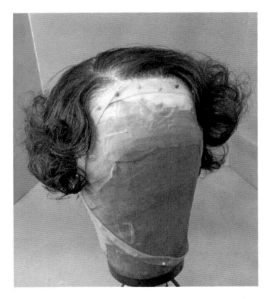

Figure 7.34 Step 18. The wig after it has been completely combed through.

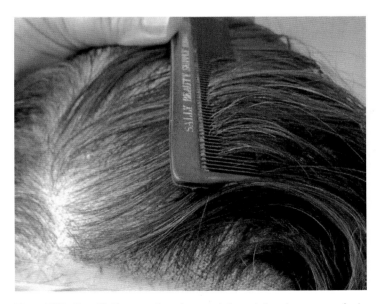

Figure 7.35 Step 19. Use a rattail comb to comb through the wig even more finely.

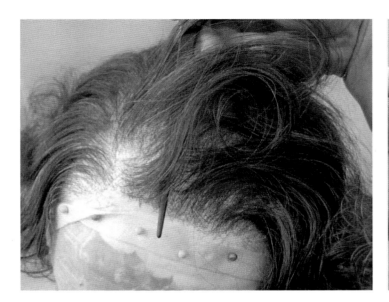

Figure 7.36 Step 20. Use the end of the rattail comb to section out the hair next to the part.

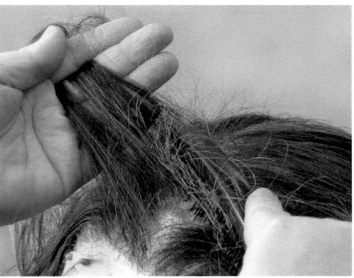

Figure 7.37 Step 21. Use a teasing/smoothing brush to lightly tease the underside of the hair in the section.

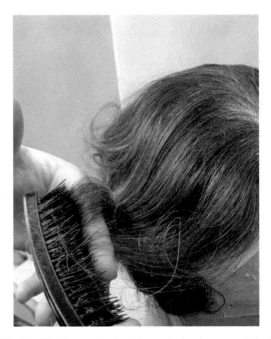

Figure 7.38 Step 22. After teasing the hair, use the brush to smooth the hair back down. Next, use the brush to brush the curls at the ends of the hair around your fingers to make them neat.

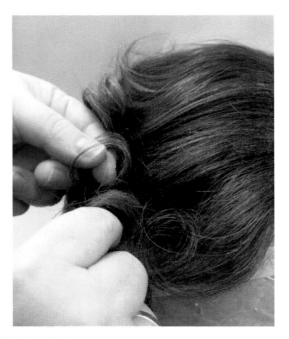

Figure 7.39 Step 23. After you have formed the curls around your finger, gently pull them apart and arrange them in an attractive way. Continue smoothing and arranging the curls, working your way around the entire head.

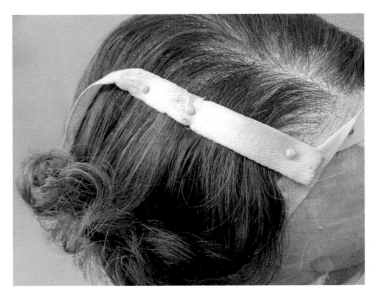
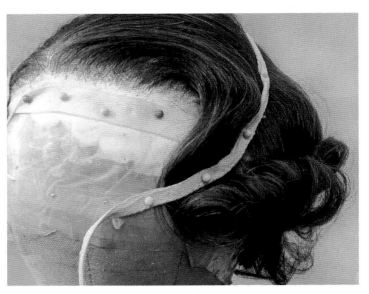

Figure 7.40 Step 24. Once you have finished the curls, use a piece of blocking tape to hold the waves in place.

Figure 7.41 Step 25. Use the tape to pull the wave onto the forehead.

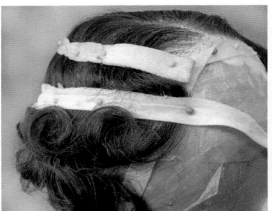
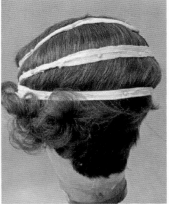
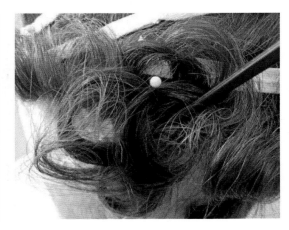

Figures 7.42 and 7.43 Step 26. Continue pinning the waves and curls in place with the blocking tape.

Figure 7.44 Step 27. You can also arrange the curls where you want them by holding them in place with pins. Once you have finished taping and pinning the hair, mist the wig with hairspray and let it set overnight. When you are ready to use the wig, carefully unpin and remove the blocking tape and pins.

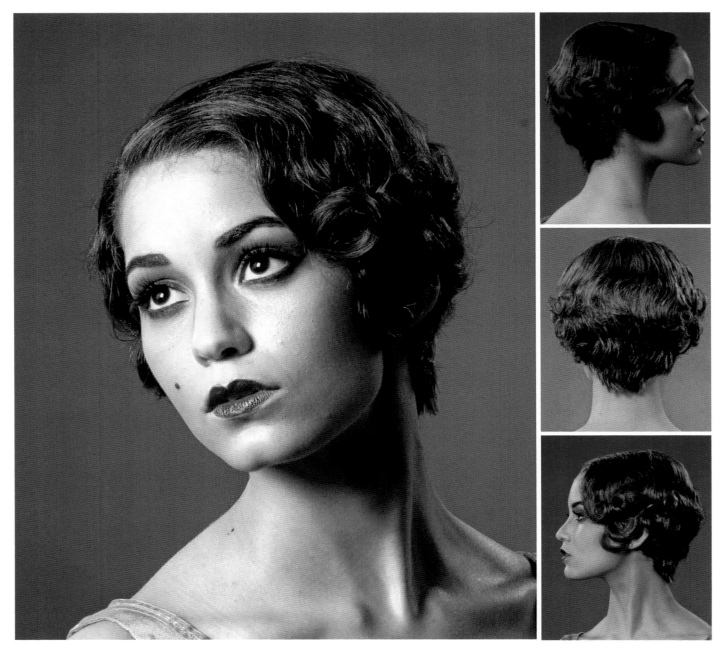

Figure 7.45–7.48   The completed 1920s' Flapper style. Photography: Tim Babiak. Model: Ivy Negron.

1920s' Finger Wave Styling— Step by Step

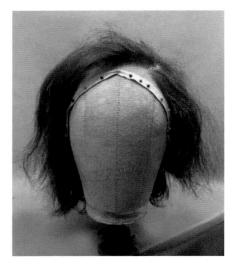

Figure 7.49   Step 1. Begin with a wig that mostly one length and hits just past the chin. I used a fully ventilated human hair wig for this style.

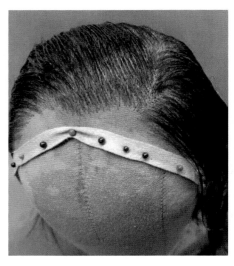

Figure 7.50   Step 2. Make a deep side part in the wig. Thoroughly saturate the wig with setting lotion. Comb the hair to the left of the part back off the face.

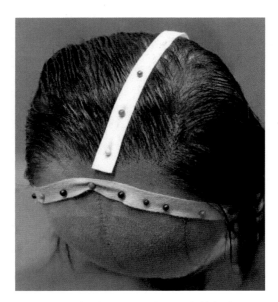

Figure 7.51   Step 3. Use a blocking tape and pins to hold this first section of the wave in place.

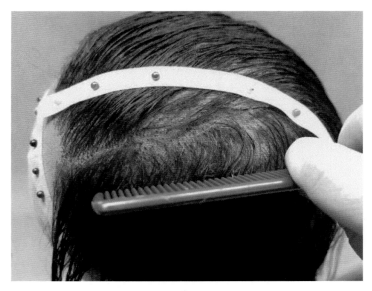

Figure 7.52   Step 4. Continue combing the wave around the end of the part. As you move around the end, you will now be combing the hair on the right side of the part towards the face.

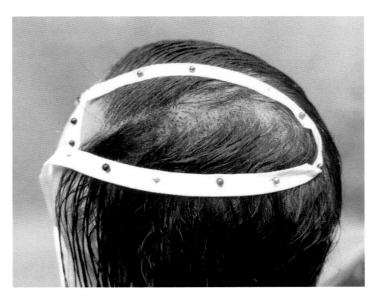

Figure 7.53 Step 5. Continue using the blocking tape and pins to secure the wave. Notice how the wave comes down in front of the front hairline.

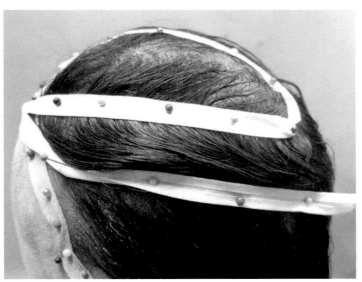

Figure 7.54 Step 6. Once the tape is secured, begin combing the hair back in the opposite direction. Pin as you go. If you slightly push up on the blocking tape, you can create a ridge in the wave.

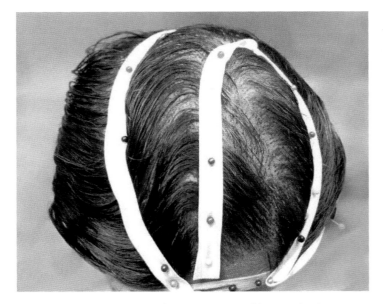

Figure 7.55 Step 7. Continue working your way around the entire head, alternating directions.

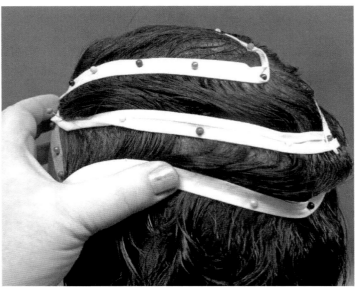

Figure 7.56 Step 8. You can also add ridges to the waves by pinching them with your fingers.

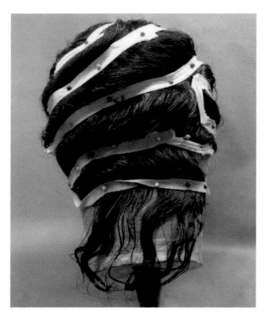

Figure 7.57 Step 9. Wave down the entire wig until you reach the edge of the wig base.

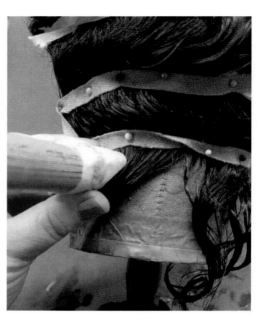

Figure 7.58 Step 10. Use a dowel rod to set the remaining length of hair into pin curls.

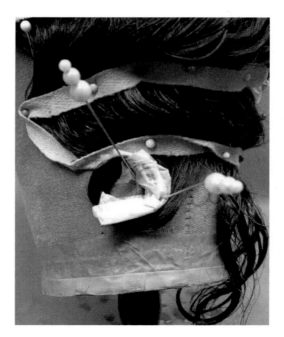

Figure 7.59 Step 11. Use pins to secure the pin curl in place.

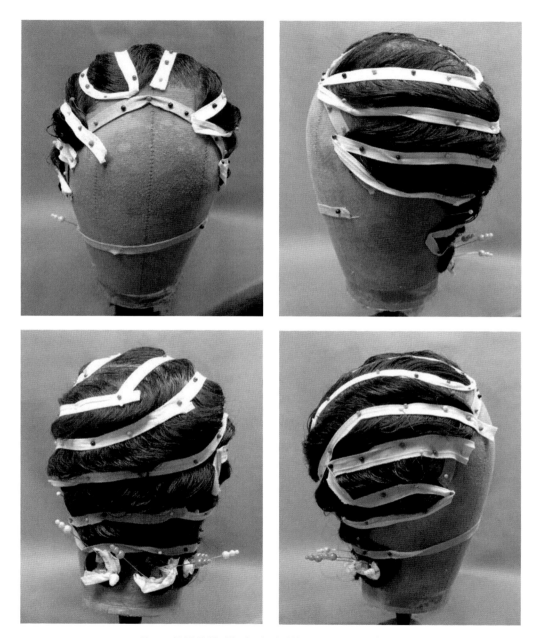

Figures 7.60–7.63   The finished 1920s' Finger Wave style set.

Once you have finished setting the wig, steam it if the wig is made of synthetic hair. If the wig is made of human hair (as this one is) spray it liberally with water. Put the wig in a wig dryer to dry for 75 minutes.

To style:

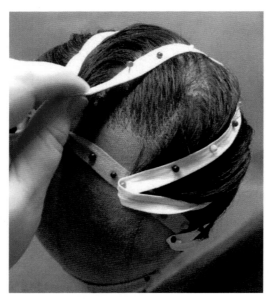

Figure 7.64   Step 12. To style, begin by removing the blocking tape. Begin the removal in the same place you started the set, at the front hairline (working from the bottom may pull the waves out of place). Also remove the pins in the pin curls.

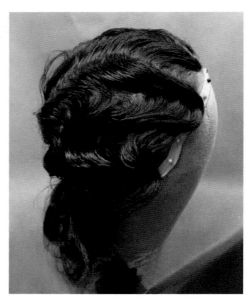

Figure 7.65   Step 13. Comb through the pin curls at the bottom. For a softer style, you could comb through the entire wig, but for this example, we will leave the majority of the wig slicked.

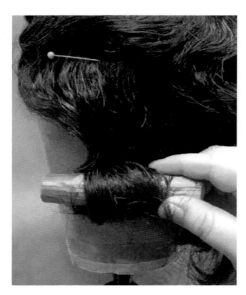

Figure 7.66   Step 14. Use a dowel rod to neatly roll the pin curls and bobby pin them at the nape.

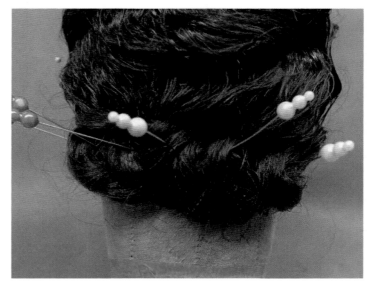

Figure 7.67   Step 15. To finish the styling, direct the pin curls flat to the side using pins. Mist with hairspray and allow to dry.

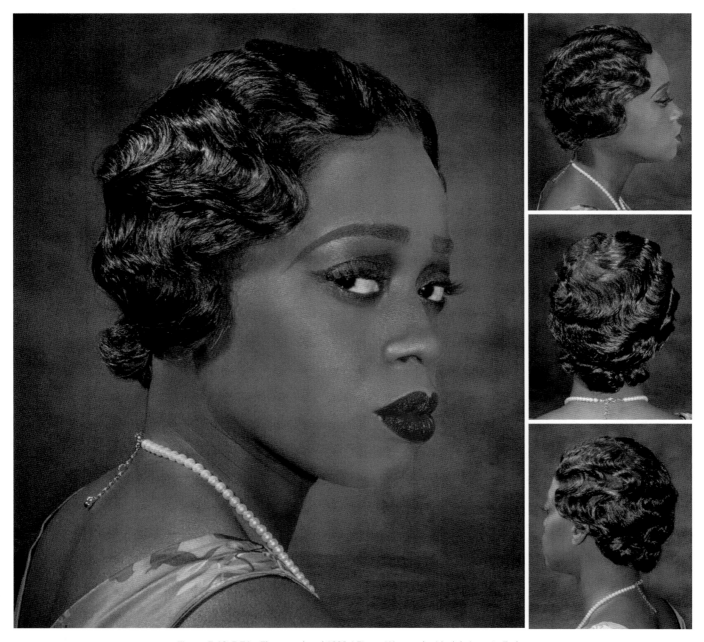

Figure 7.68–7.71   The completed 1920s' Finger Wave style. Model: Antonia Taylor.

Variations

1920s' looks were usually dark, dramatic, and exotic. You can vary the looks by mixing in a range of dark colors, from jet black to deep auburn. You can purchase Dutch Boy Bob wigs that are ready to go straight out of the box. You can also purchase short boyish straight wigs and short waved wigs that do not require much styling that are appropriate to this period.

1920s' Makeup

In addition to the freedom to have shorter hair and dresses, women now felt confident to openly wear cosmetics. Max Factor

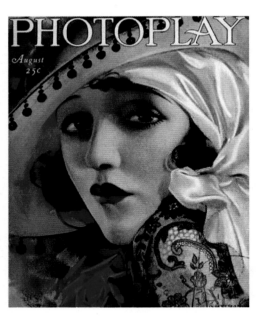

Figure 7.73 Bebe Daniels on the cover of *Photoplay* magazine, by Rolf Armstrong, August 1921.

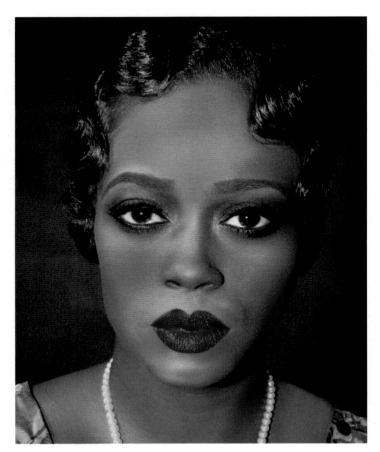

Figure 7.72 A vampy look inspired by the 1920s. Model: Antonia Taylor.

realized that many women desired to look like their favorite film star, and he was one of several who began marketing the cosmetics he used as a film makeup artist. It Girls and Vamps had a variety of products at their disposal to use. Pancake makeup, which gave a smooth matte look to the skin, was very popular. Eyebrows were thin, and penciled in a shape that extended down to the outside corner of the eye (see Figures 7.6 and 7.73 for examples). The eyebrows also often had a slight lift in the center by the nose, which gave the wearer a perpetually sad or vulnerable look. Eyes were accented with kohl and glossy shadows. Mascara came in cake form and was applied with a small comb to both top and bottom lashes, giving the lashes a clumpy, doll like look. Rouge was bright and was placed in circles in the center of the cheeks. Lips were drawn slightly inside the natural lip to give them a small shapely appearance. Special attention was paid to the upper lip and making it well defined. The Cupid's Bow shape with its very defined peaks was particularly coveted. Lip colors were usually quite dark red in this era. In fact, much of the makeup was a bit exaggerated in color and intensity, influenced by film looks and the need to exaggerate them so faces were clear through the grainy film quality of the time.

eight

THE 1930S

$$\left(\textit{1930–1939}\right)$$

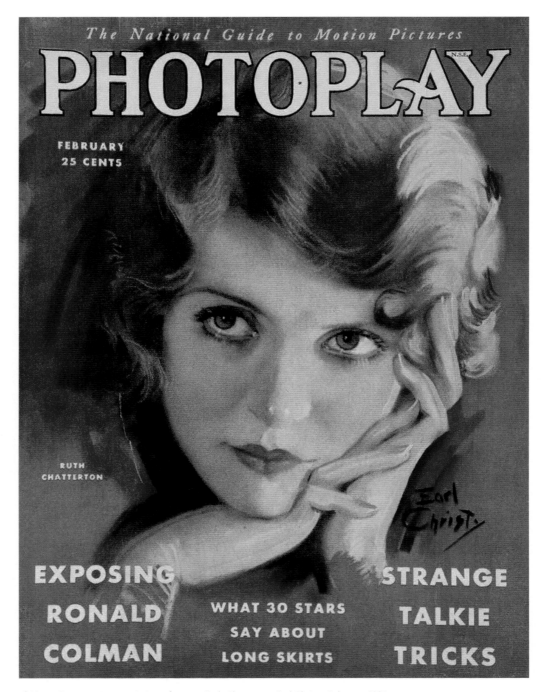

Figure 8.1   Front cover of *Photoplay* magazine, a painting of actress Ruth Chatterton, Earl Christy, February 1930.

Important Artists/Designers

Grant Wood, Mark Rothko, Salvador Dalí, Adrian,
Madame Grès, Madeline Vionnet

Important People/Style Icons

Joan Crawford, Bette Davis, Marlene Dietrich,
Douglas Fairbanks, Jr., Errol Flynn, Clark Gable,
Greta Garbo, Jean Harlow, Lana Turner, Mae West,
Anna Mae Wong

1930s' Women

The 1930s took the radical new looks of the 1920s and intensified them, making them even more glamorous and detailed. Hairstyles moved away from the simpler boyish looks of the 1920s towards a more voluptuous and feminine look. For example, in Figure 8.2, Joan Blondell's hairstyle displays the more exaggerated sculptural waves that define this period.

Hats also remained a hugely important fashion element in the 1930s. The hats of this era moved from the cloche hats of the 1920s that cover nearly the entire head to smaller hats that perched on the head like a plate, often at a jaunty angle. This led to many 1930s' hairstyles being rather smooth on top, such as in the style modeled with a hat in Figure 8.3.

Even if the hairstyle was smoother on top, there were usually still small curls framing the face. Hair during this period was often set using either pin curls, finger waves, or a combination of both. Setting lotions or curling fluid helped provide the sleek control often seen in styles

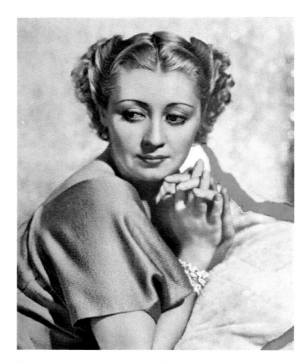

Figure 8.2   Colored photo of Joan Blondell from *Photoplay* magazine, August 1936.

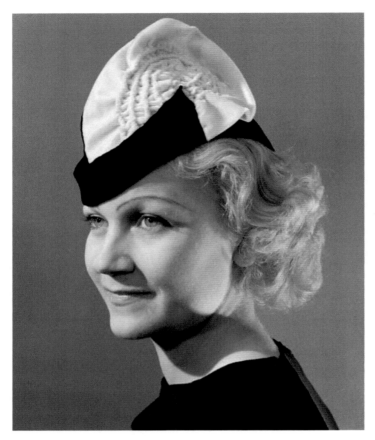

Figure 8.3   Model De Decker with hat, by Willem van de Poll, 1936, Dutch Collection/Archive, Van de Poll Reportage.

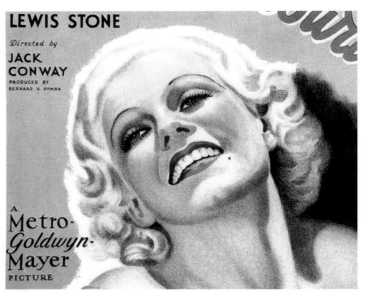

Figure 8.4   Detail from a poster from the 1934 film *The Girl from Missouri*, featuring Jean Harlow, the original 1930s' "blonde bombshell."

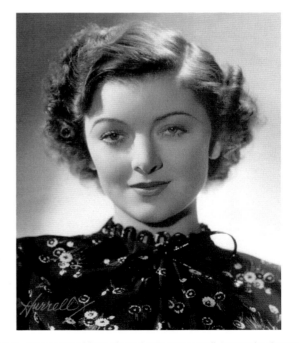

Figure 8.5   Myrna Loy publicity photo, by George Hurrell. Notice the deep wave coming down onto the left side of her forehead.

from this era. The 1930s was also the era of the peroxide blonde. Film star Jean Harlow (Figure 8.4) caused a stir when she bleached her hair to a platinum blonde color for the film *Platinum Blonde*.

Another movie star look that was popular in the 1930s was a deep side part with a wave that dipped down on the opposite side of the face, such as the one shown on Myrna Loy (Figure 8.5). This wave accentuated the mysterious beauty of stars such as Loy, Norma Shearer, and Greta Garbo. This wave would dip further and further down onto the face until it became the peek-a-boo look that was popular in the 1940s.

1930s' Men

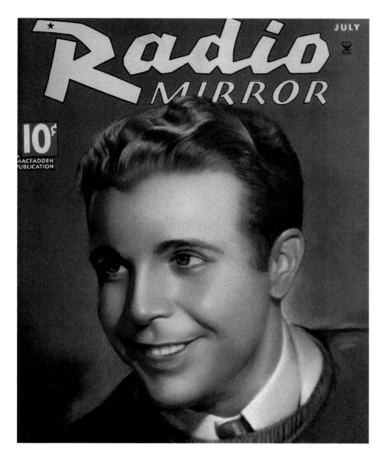

Figure 8.6   Dick Powell on *Radio Mirror* magazine, by A. Mozert, July 1935.

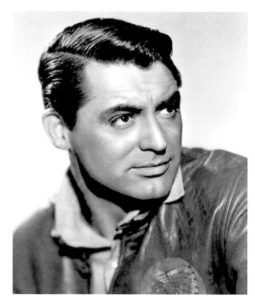

Figure 8.7   Cary Grant publicity photo for *Only Angels Have Wings*, 1939.

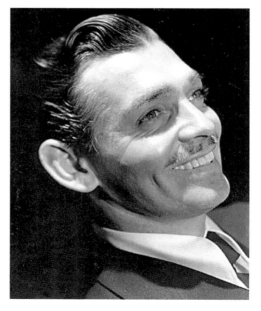

Figure 8.8   Publicity still of Clark Gable, 1938, MGM Studios.

The ideal gentleman in the 1930s was clean cut, with neatly trimmed, groomed, and pomaded hair, and a clean shaven face, such as in the magazine cover in Figure 8.6. Matinee idols, as in the 1920s, continued to set the trends for audiences everywhere. The exaggerated slicked back hair and heavily made up face of the 1920s gave way to a more realistic looking man in the 1930s. The hair was still controlled with pomades and other products, but the finish was not as glassy as the previous decade. No facial hair at all was the dominant trend, such as that illustrated by Cary Grant (Figure 8.7), but several prominent actors, including Clark Gable (Figure 8.8) and Errol Flynn sported neat, well-groomed pencil mustaches.

1930s' Blonde Bombshell Styling— Step by Step

This reference picture for this hairstyle is Figure 8.4, worn by Jean Harlow.

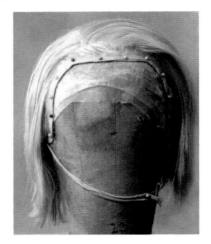

Figure 8.9 Step 1. Begin with a wig that is just below chin length, with layers of four to six inch long hair throughout the wig. I used a platinum blonde lace front wig made with synthetic hair.

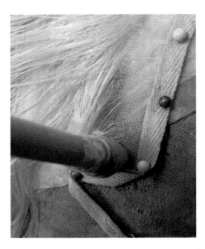

Figure 8.10 Step 2. Use a small dowel rod to set a tiny pin curl in front of each ear. Secure the pin curl with roundhead pins.

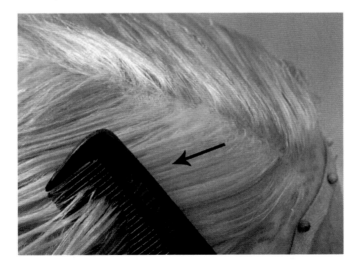

Figure 8.11 Step 3. Make a side part in the hair. I have chosen to place the part on the left side for this style. Comb a small amount of setting lotion mixed with water throughout the wig. Because the wig in the example is synthetic, large amounts of setting lotion are not needed to shape the style, because steaming the set will also help hold the set. Once you have distributed the product through the wig, comb the hair at the part away from the face.

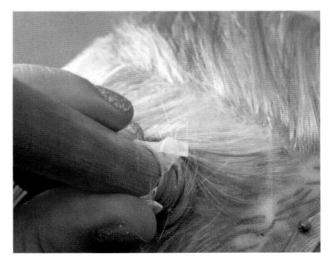

Figure 8.12 Step 4. Use a larger dowel rod (approximately the diameter of a quarter) to begin shaping your pin curls. This first row of pin curls should be rolled in a counterclockwise direction.

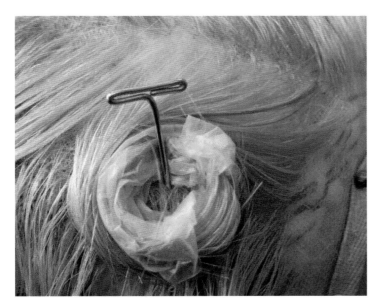

Figure 8.13   Step 5. Secure the finished pin curl with a curl clip, hairpin, or t-pin (shown here).

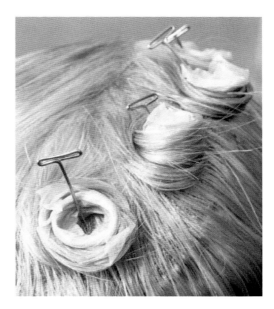

Figure 8.14   Step 6. Work your way along the part, rolling all your pin curls in the same direction (counterclockwise).

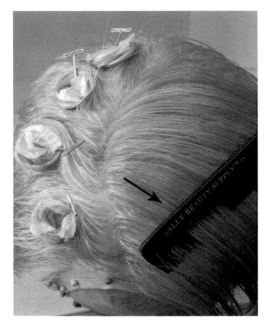

Figure 8.15   Step 7. Continue set the hair in counterclockwise pin curls as you circle around the part. Comb the hair on the other side of the part towards the face.

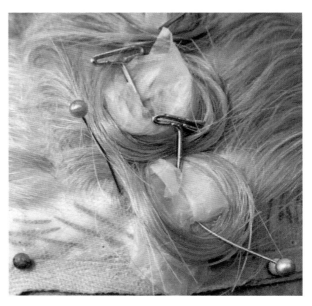

Figure 8.16   Step 8. Continue rolling the pin curls in a counter clockwise direction. As you get to the hairline of the wig, allow the pin curl to dip down onto the forehead. A small round head pin has been used here to provide a little lift to the hair right at the part.

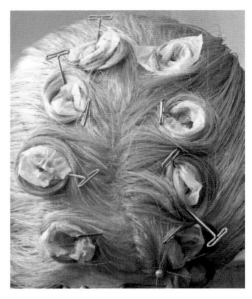

Figure 8.17 Step 9. The finished first row of pin curls, viewed from the top.

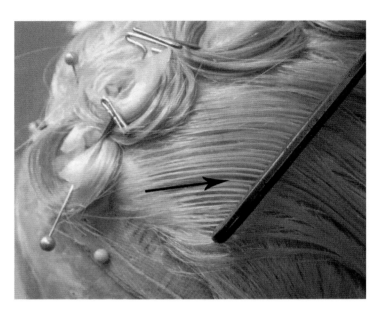

Figure 8.18 Step 10. The next row of pin curls will be rolled in a clockwise direction. Begin by combing the next section of hair away from the face.

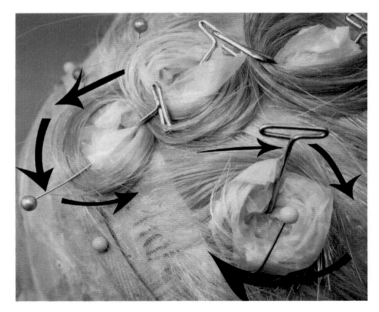

Figure 8.19 Step 11. Roll the first pin curl of the second curl so that it sits slightly behind the hairline. Continue rolling the pin curls in this row clockwise, working your way around the head.

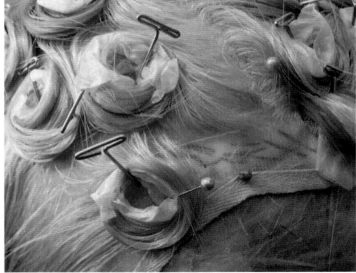

Figure 8.20 Step 12. When you get to the last pin curl of this row, set that curl so that it comes onto the face, past the hairline. Set curls in front of the hairline is very helpful when you are styling a hard front wig—it will help you conceal the front edge of the wig.

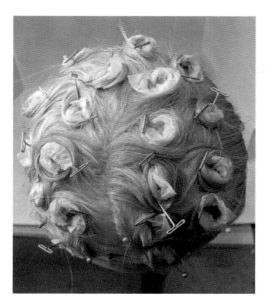

Figure 8.21 Step 13. The completed second row of pin curls, viewed from the top.

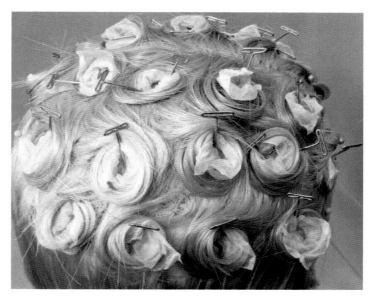

Figure 8.22 Step 14. The third row of pin curls should be rolled counter clockwise (in the same direction as the first row). However, because the hairstyle we are creating is asymmetrical, the third row of pin curls should only go about halfway around the head.

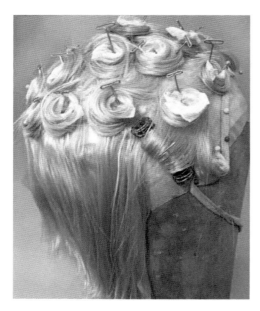

Figure 8.23 Step 15. The remaining hair on the left side of the wig should be set with a small roller.

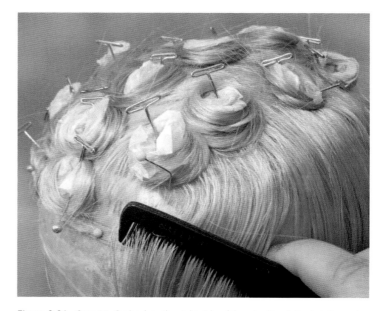

Figure 8.24 Step 16. Go back to the right side of the wig. Comb the hair towards the face.

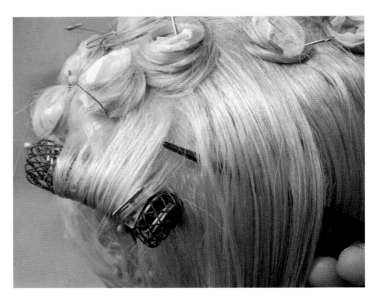

Figure 8.25   Step 17. Begin rolling the hair on dime sized rollers. The rollers should be rolled toward the face and be placed diagonally.

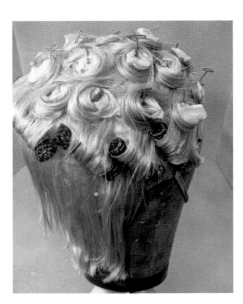

Figure 8.26   Step 18. Continue rolling diagonal sections of hair, working your way around the wig. The last roller should meet up with the first roller you placed on the left side of the wig.

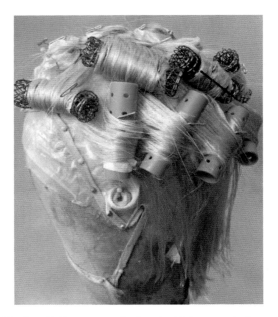

Figure 8.27   Step 19. The next row of rollers should also be set in diagonal sections, but this time, the diagonal is going away from the face on this side (when you reach the opposite side, it will be going away from the face).

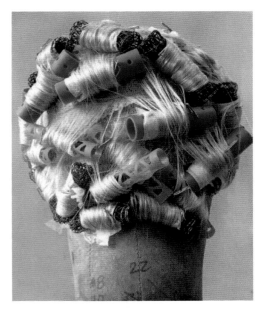

Figure 8.28   Step 20. As you work your way down the wig, keep alternating the direction of your diagonal sections. You will also likely need to use smaller rollers as you get to the shorter layers of hair at the bottom of the wig.

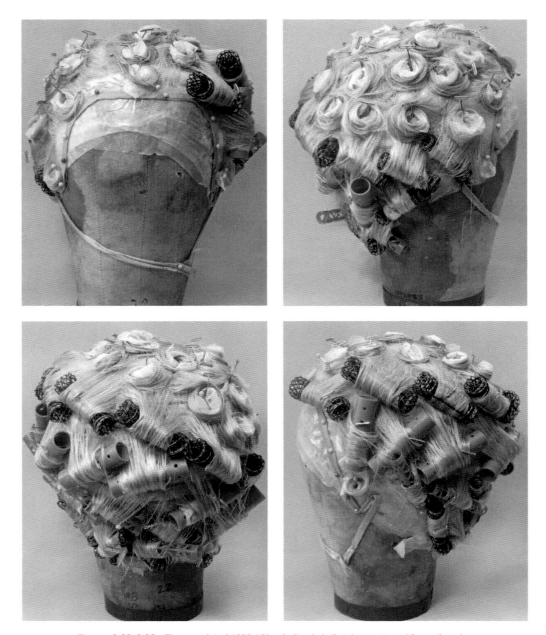

Figures 8.29–8.32　The completed 1930s' Blonde Bombshell style set, viewed from all angles.

The set is now complete. If the wig is synthetic hair, steam the roller set in place. If the wig is human hair, thoroughly wet the finished set. Place the wig in a wig dryer for 75 minutes until completely dry and then allow to cool fully.

To style:

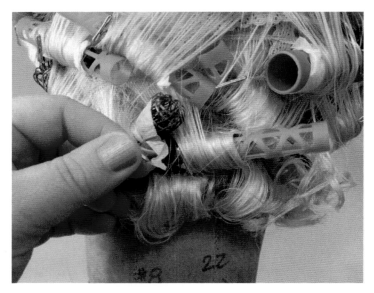

Figure 8.33 Step 21. Begin removing the rollers at the nape of the neck of the wig and work your way up until all the rollers have been removed. Do not undo the pin curls yet.

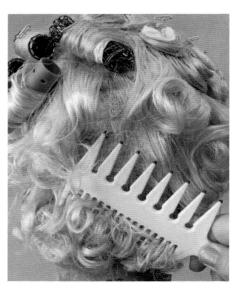

Figure 8.34 Step 22. As you unroll each row of rollers, use a wide toothed comb to gently pick through the curls.

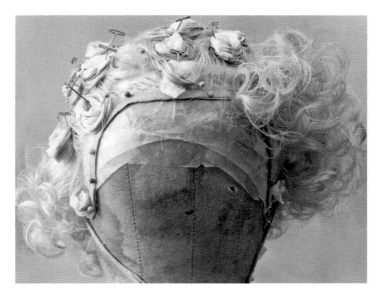

Figure 8.35 Step 23. Continue to use the pick to comb out all the unrolled hair. Once you have completed the combing, go ahead and undo the pin curls.

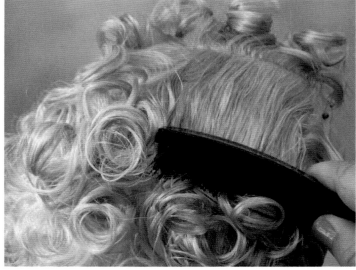

Figure 8.36 Step 24. Use a smoothing brush to thoroughly brush through the hair that was set in pin curls.

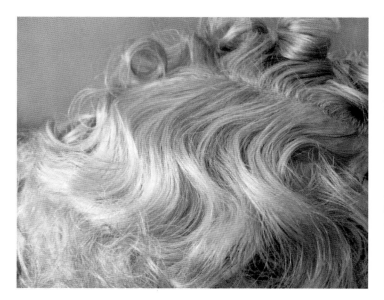

Figure 8.37 Step 25. After brushing through the section, use your hand to pat the hair towards the part until the waves begin falling into place.

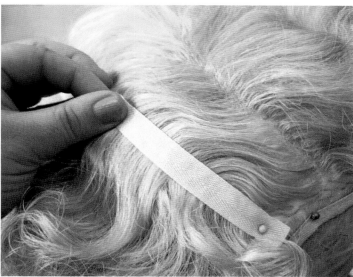

Figure 8.38 Step 26. Use a long piece of blocking tape to block the waves in place. Pin the blocking tape in the center of the crest of the first wave. Pin every inch or so to hold the wave in place. Make sure to close all gaps and breaks in the waves as you are pinning the blocking tape.

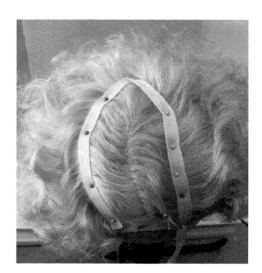

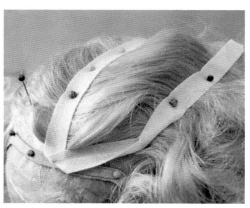

Figure 8.40 Step 28. Use the tape to push the ridges of the waves up so that they are more defined.

Figure 8.39 Step 27. Work your way, back and forth around the head, just as you did when you were setting the pin curls. Here is a top view of the blocking tape being pinned into place.

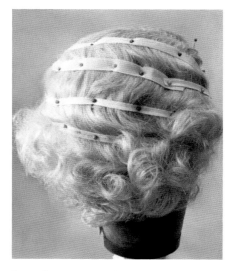

Figure 8.41 Step 29. All the wavy section has now been taped and pinned in place.

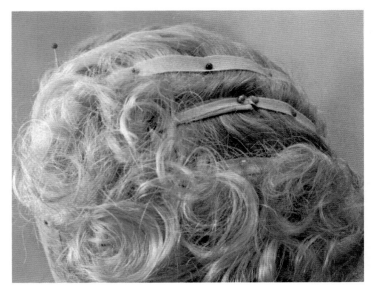

Figure 8.42 Step 30. Notice how the pinned waves do not go all the way around on the right side of the wig. This is because the hairstyle is asymmetrical.

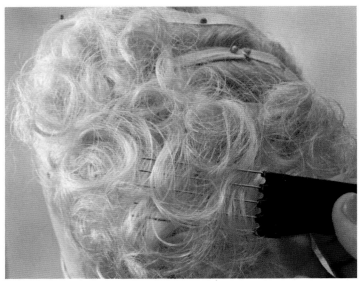

Figure 8.43 Step 31. Use a lifting comb to fluff out the curls on the rest of the wig.

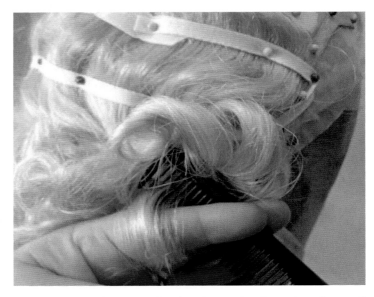

Figure 8.44 Step 32. Use a rattail comb to shape each curl around your finger until you are happy with the placement of each. Once you have made all the wig's curls neat, spray the wig with hairspray.

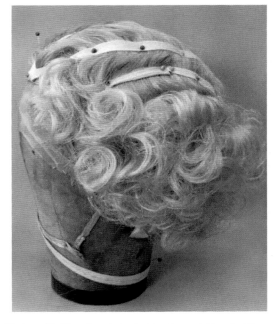

Figure 8.45 Step 33. Allow the wig to sit at least overnight so that the waves and curls may settle into place. Once you are ready to use the wig, remove the tapes and unpin the wig from the canvas block.

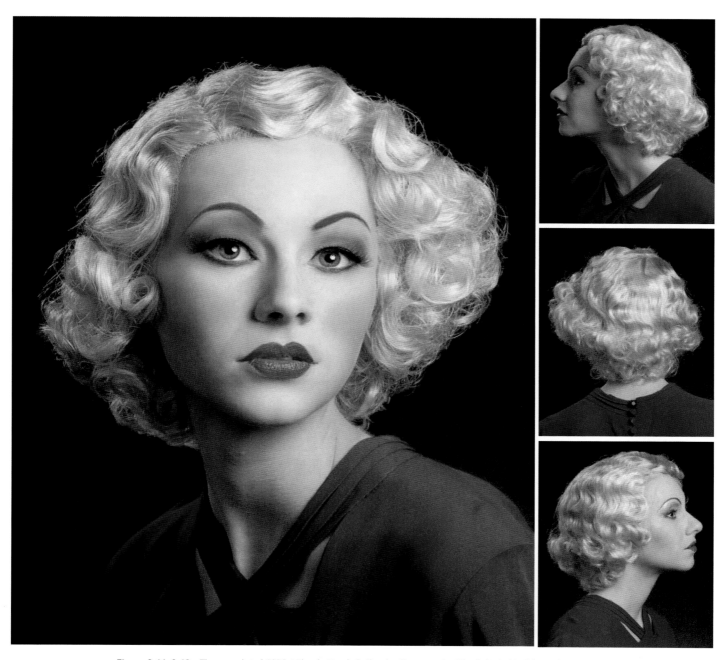

Figure 8.46–8.49 The completed 1930s' Blonde Bombshell style. Photography: Tim Babiak. Model: Ariel Livingston.

Variations

You can achieve variety in your 1930s' wig looks by changing the location of the part. You can also experiment with texture. Shaping each curl around your finger may create an elegant screen siren; picking out those curls so that they have a frizzy texture may look more like a ditzy showgirl. Some styles remained sleeker—you could use the blocking to tape to secure the waves all the way down and eliminate the curled section entirely. You could use a larger dowel rod to create bigger pin curls on the top section—this will make the top smoother, like the style seen in the photograph of the model seen in Figure 8.3. While the platinum blonde color dominated the trends, there were still darker mysterious beauties like Greta Garbo, so do not be afraid to use a variety of hair colors.

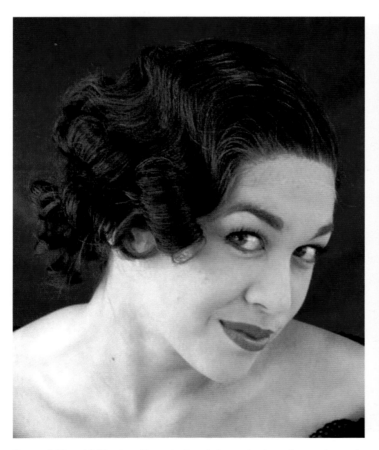 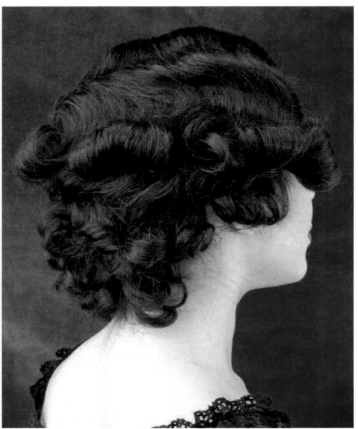

Figures 8.50 and 8.51   Anna Fugate's wig style is one that is much smoother on the top, with defined curls in the back.

1930s' Makeup

Makeup in the 1930s was more refined than it had been in the 1920s. Where the 1920s had a dramatic, glossy, and smudgy aspect, the 1930s featured brighter colors and cleaner lines. Pencil thin eyebrows were a very important part of this look. The preferred shape was a smooth arc, giving the wearer a bit of a surprised look. Some women even shaved off their eyebrows entirely and drew the new shape on! Top and bottom eyelashes were still accented with cake mascara. Cream eye shadows were available in colors like pink, spring green, powder blue, and lavender. Cheek colors moved from the brighter orangey red of the 20s to a softer rosy pink color. Raspberry red lips were the most fashionable color. Lip gloss was invented during the 1930s, so women were able to give their lips a shiny look.

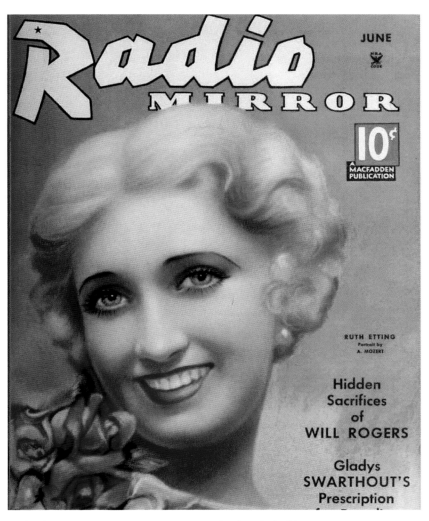

Figure 8.52   Ruth Etting on the cover of *Radio Mirror*, June 1935. Etting wears a typical makeup look of the 1930s.

nine

THE 1940S

(1940–1949)

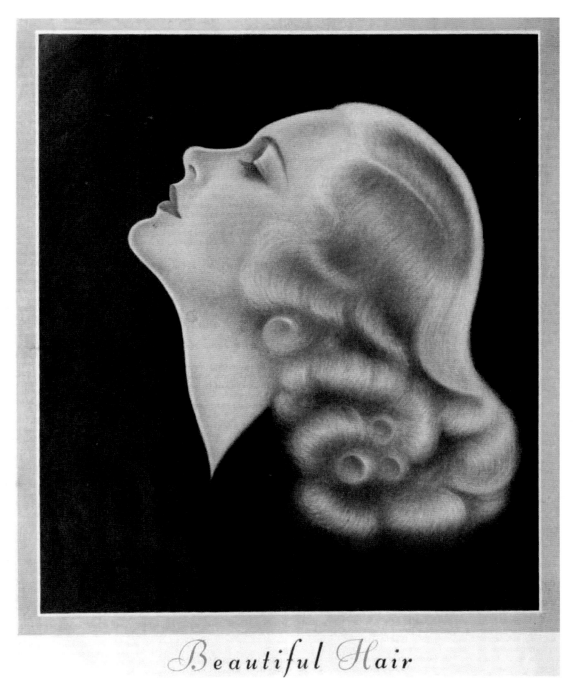

Beautiful Hair

Figure 9.1   Breck shampoo, hair lotion, and hair cream advertisement in *The Ladies Home Journal*, 1948.

Important Events

1941   The Japanese attack Pearl Harbor
1941   Orson Welles directs *Citizen Kane*
1943   Ayn Rand publishes *The Fountainhead*
1944   D-Day—Allied troops invade the beaches
         of Normandy
1944   Tennessee Williams' *The Glass Menagerie* is
         produced
1945   Adolf Hitler commits suicide; the United
         States bombs Hiroshima and Nagasaki
1945   VE Day—World War II formally ends.
1946   The bikini swimsuit is introduced

Important Artists/ Designers

Balenciaga, Gil Elvgren, Willem de Kooning,
Edward Hopper, Jeanne Lanvin, Jean Patou, Jackson
Pollock, Mark Rothko, Elsa Schiaparelli, Alberto
Vargas, Andrew Wyeth

Important People/Style Icons

Lauren Bacall, Humphrey Bogart, Ava Gardner,
Rita Hayworth, Lena Horne, Veronica Lake, Hedy
Lamarr, Carmen Miranda, Rosalind Russell, Lana
Turner, Esther Williams

1940s' Women

The 1940s was a decade of pinup models, sweater girls, and back home sweethearts. As World War II raged on in Europe, women back home often went to work and took on traditionally masculine jobs that were left empty when thousands of soldiers went to war. Ironically, although gender roles were changing, women's fashion was becoming extremely feminine. Hairstyles were growing longer—the 1920s bob became the 1930s shingle, which then became the 1940s pageboy.

This longer, more feminine haircut provided many style options, and popular movie actresses were still setting the trends in hair. Movies were thought to keep up spirits during wartime, and thus they dominated popular entertainment in the forties. Movie magazines and cosmetics ads made it even easier for the average women to access all the details of her favorite star's look.

Actress Veronica Lake was famous for her long blonde peek-a-boo hairstyle that mysteriously draped over one eye.

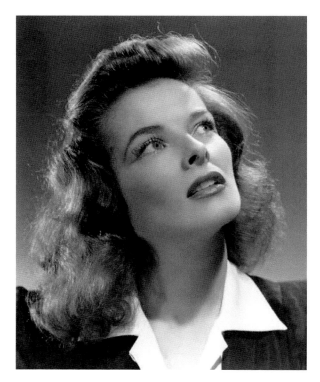

Figure 9.2 MGM studio photograph of Katherine Hepburn, *Photoplay* magazine, August 1942. Hepburn wears a typical version of the 1940s' pageboy hairstyle.

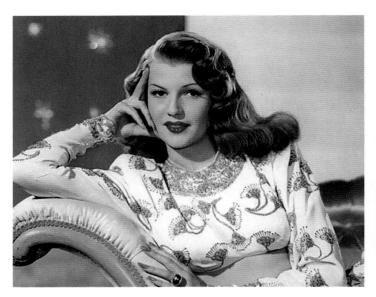

Figure 9.3   Promotional photograph of Rita Hayworth for the 1946 film *Gilda*, in *Screenland* magazine, June 1946.

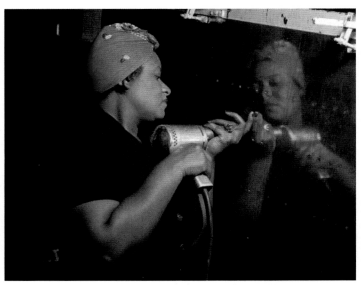

Figure 9.5   A real-life "Rosie the Riveter" operating a hand drill at Vultee-Nashville, Tennessee, working on an A-31 Vengeance dive bomber, by Alfred T. Palmer, February, 1943, U.S. Office of War.

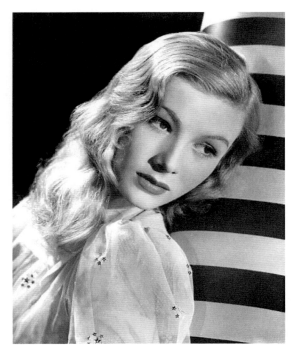

Figure 9.4   Paramount publicity headshot of Veronica Lake, 1943.

Rita Hayworth (Figure 9.3) wore a similar hairstyle dyed red. These long hairstyles were eventually thought to be a danger to women working in factories. Veronica Lake actually changed her widely imitated hairstyle to encourage factory safety. One method women used to keep their long hair from catching in machinery was putting it up in a snood, partly inspired by the 1939 film *Gone With the Wind*. This style soon took on such popularity the women began wearing it outside the factories. Head scarves and bandannas, like the one worn by Rosie the Riveter, were also used to tie hair up out of the way (figure 9.5).

Also gaining in fashion trends was the elaborate updo. These hairstyles took the trend of wearing hair neatly back in a snood and took it one step further. All of the hair was swept off of the neck and piled on top of the head in elaborate curls. Bangs helped to keep this style feminine. The bangs might be worn in a thick wave (figure 9.6) or in a cluster of curls (figure 9.7).

One extremely popular version of the updo was the Victory roll. These sculptural rolls of hair are what many people think of when they think of 1940s hair. True Victory rolls roll all the way down the head, forming a "V" shape in back. There is also a version of the hairstyle where just the hair around the face is rolled and the length of the hair is left loose in the back.

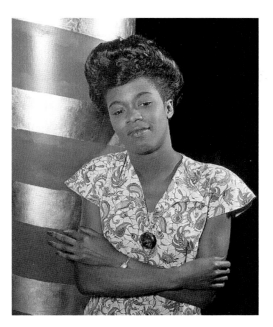

Figure 9.6 Sarah Vaughan at Café Society NYC, by William Gottlieb, circa September 1946.

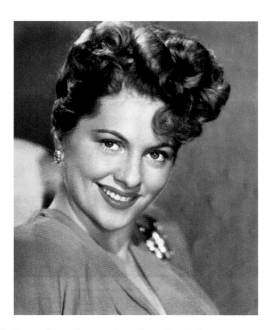

Figure 9.7 Photo of Joan Fontaine from *Photoplay*, 1943.

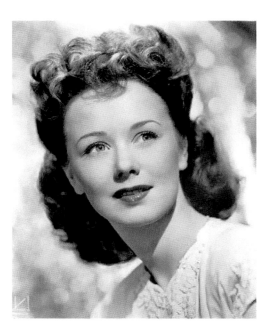

Figure 9.8 Photo of actress and vocalist Iva Withers, 1947. Withers wears a version of the half up/half down hairstyle with elaborately curled bangs.

1940s' Men

Men's hairstyle trends in the 1940s were usually determined by one of two things: movie stars or the military. Many men were forced to obey military regulations for their hair. These hairstyles were very short, buzzed almost to the skin in the back, and trimmed high over the ears (see figure 9.9). Some versions, like the high and tight haircut, left the hair slightly longer on top of the head. Crew cuts and flattops were also becoming popular haircuts at this time.

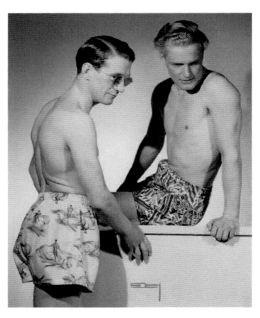

Figure 9.10   Two men in swimsuits from the Nordic Company's campaign with California clothing, by Erik Holmen, May 1947. These men wear two examples of 1940s' men's hairstyles.

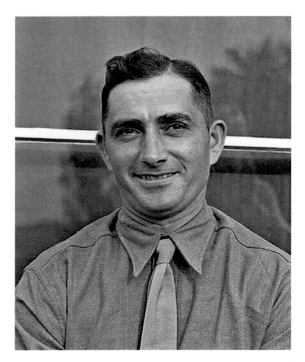

Figure 9.9   Portrait of a U.S military serviceman sitting on an exterior window sill of a house, by Tudor Washington Collins, circa 1940s, Auckland War Memorial Museum.

Civilian men, like military men, wore the back and sides of their haircuts very short and neat. The lines around the ears and neck were sharp and very precise. The hair on the top of the head was left longer. It might be parted on the side, or combed straight back—both ways used products like Brylcreem to hold the style in place. Natural wave to the hair was very fashionable, and the hairstyles were combed in such a way as to accentuate the waves of the hair in front.

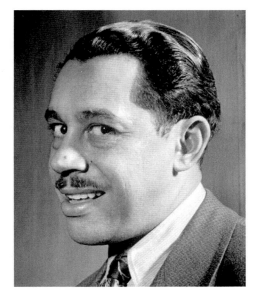

Figure 9.11   Portrait of Cab Calloway, by William P. Gottlieb, 1947, Columbia Studio, New York. Calloway's natural waves are accentuated by the use of hair products.

1940s' Glamour Girl/Peek-a-Boo Styling— Step by Step

This hairstyle was inspired by the photographs of Rita Hayworth and Veronica Lake, seen in Figures 9.3 and 9.4

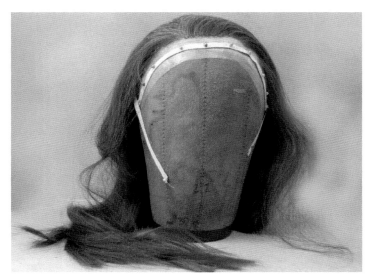

Figure 9.12 Step 1. Begin with a wig that is at least shoulder length (8 to 12 inches long at the nape of the neck is ideal). Long layers around the face are also helpful in creating this hairstyle. I used a fully ventilated lace front human hair wig that is in the longer range for this hairstyle.

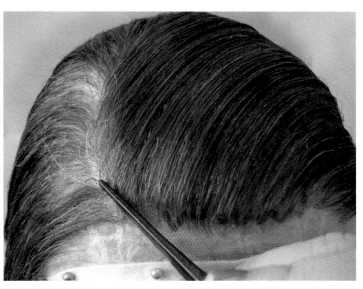

Figure 9.13 Step 2. Thoroughly wet the hair with water and setting lotion. Make a deep side part in the wig with the end of your rattail comb. Comb the hair above the part away from the face.

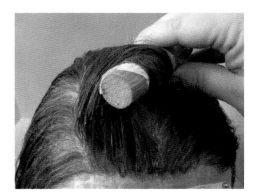

Figure 9.14 Step 3. Separate out a section of hair that is approximately one inch by one inch square. Use a dowel rod to make a pin curl in the wig, winding the hair clockwise towards the face.

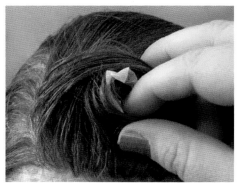

Figure 9.15 Step 4. After sliding the hair off of the dowel rod, give the pin curl a slight push towards the part. This will give lift to the root of the hair in the pin curl.

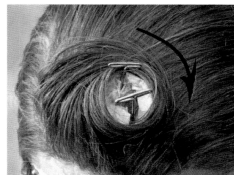

Figure 9.16 Step 5. Use t-pins, curl clips, or hair pins to secure the pin curl in place.

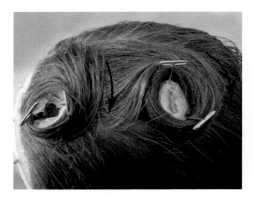

Figure 9.17   Step 6. Make a second pin curl behind the first one, still rolling the hair away from the face in a clockwise direction. Continue working your way around the part, setting pin curls.

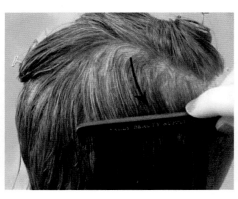

Figure 9.18   Step 7. As you come around the part, continue combing the hair in the same direction. The hair below the part will now be combed going towards the face.

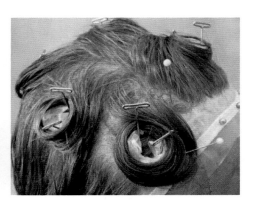

Figure 9.19   Step 8. The last pin curl should break the hairline and come forward onto the face.

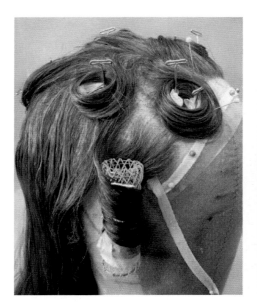

Figure 9.20   Step 9. For the next row, roll the hair going towards the face on a nickel sized roller. Pin the roller so that it sits vertically.

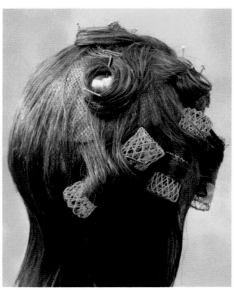

Figure 9.21   Step 10. Continue setting nickel sized rollers around the back of the head. These rollers should sit diagonally.

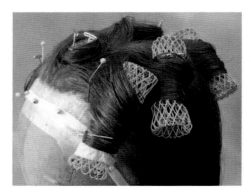

Figure 9.22   Step 11. As you work your way around the head, the rollers will sit higher up on the head. The last roller should sit just in front of the hairline. I have also placed a round headed pin in to give a bit of extra lift at the hairline.

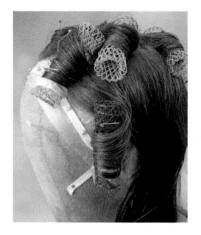

Figure 9.23 Step 12. Drop down another row and set this roller going towards the face.

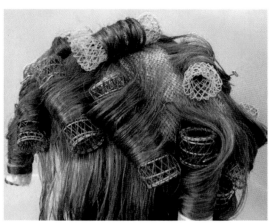

Figures 9.24 and 9.25 Step 13. This next row of rollers should be set in the opposite diagonal direction from the row above. Finish this row with a dime sized roller (the yellow roller in Figure 9.25).

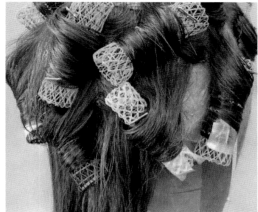

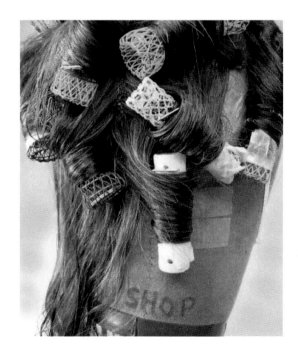

Figure 9.26 Step 14. The next row of rollers below should again change direction, beginning with a dime sized roller rolled towards the face.

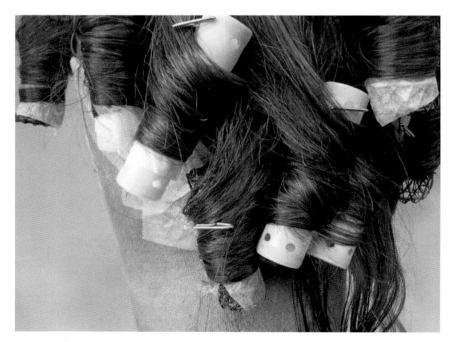

Figure 9.27 Step 15. Continue setting this row of rollers around the head. Alternate diagonal rows of rollers until you reach the bottom of the wig. I used pencil sized rollers at the bottom of the wig in order to get a tighter curl.

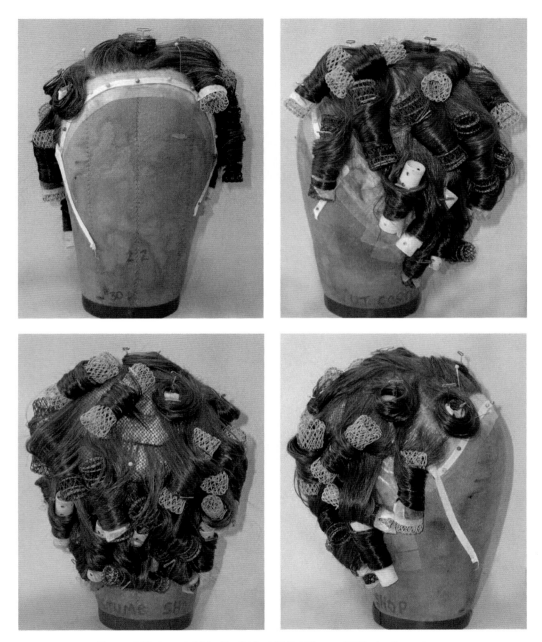

Figures 9.28 through 9.31   The finished 1940s' Glamour Girl/Peek-a Boo style set.

Once you have finished setting the wig, steam each roller thoroughly if the wig is made of synthetic hair. If the wig is human hair, soak each roller with water sprayed from a spray bottle. After steaming or wetting, place the wig in a wig dryer for seventy-five minutes.

To style:

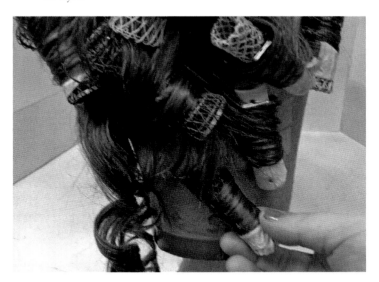

Figure 9.32   Step 16. Begin removing the rollers from the bottom of the wig, working your way up to the top.

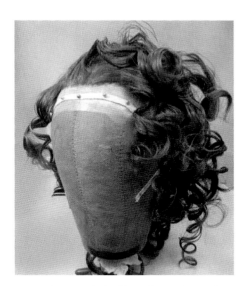

Figure 9.33   Step 17. The wig with all of the rollers and pin curls removed.

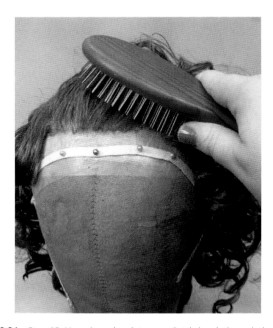

Figure 9.34   Step 18. Use a large brush to completely brush through the entire wig.

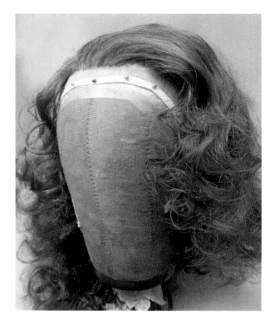

Figure 9.35   Step 19. Once the wig is brushed out, it will appear very soft. The shape of the waves should begin to be apparent.

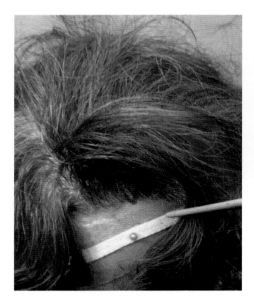

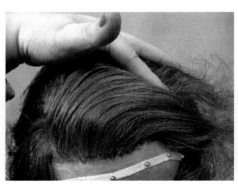

Figure 9.37   Step 21. Use your teasing/smoothing brush to smooth the hair in the top section back into place. Use your fingers to push the hair and help define the shape of the wave.

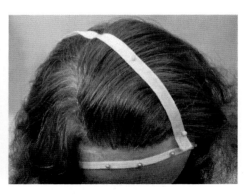

Figure 9.38   Step 22. Pin a piece of blocking tape in place and use it to hold and define the shape of the waves.

Figure 9.36   Step 20. Lightly tease the underside of the hair on the top of the wig. This will add a little volume to the wig and smooth out any roller breaks.

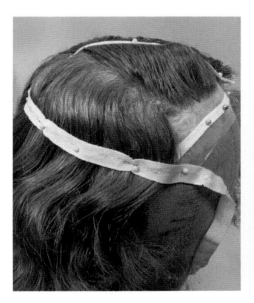

Figure 9.39   Step 23. Continue pinning the tape around the part until you come around the other side. Use the tape to shape the wave onto the face.

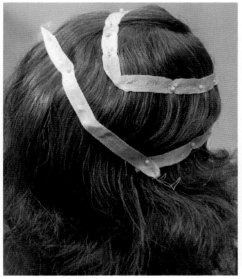

Figure 9.40   Step 24. Work your way back around the head, following the shape of the waves.

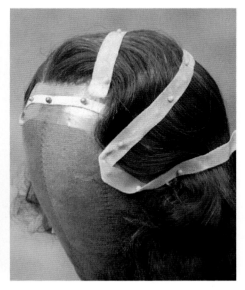

Figure 9.41   Step 25. The wave on the opposite side of the face should now also come forward of the hairline.

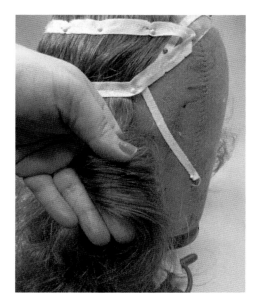

Figure 9.42 Step 26. Brush the hair below the part around your finger with your smoothing brush. This will create a nice sculpted curl that finishes off that side of the hairstyle.

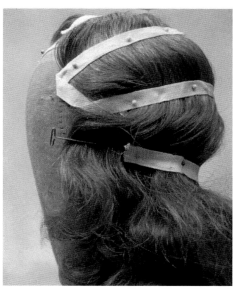

Figure 9.43 Step 27. Pin another piece of tape next to the curl you just created, and use it to define the waves under the curve of the head.

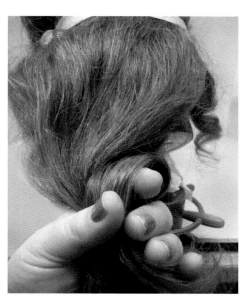

Figure 9.44 Step 28. Gather the remaining hair into your hand and brush it around a finger or two, shaping the hair into a large curl.

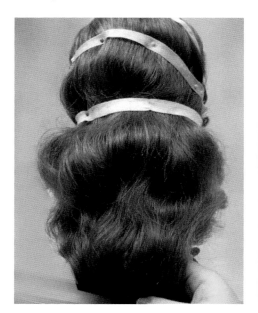

Figure 9.45 Step 29. Smoothly roll this curl underneath, shaping it with your fingers.

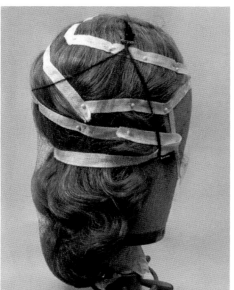

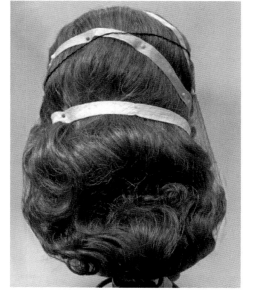

Figure 9.46 and 9.47 Step 30. Place a large hairnet over the back of the wig and use it to sculpt the hair into shape. Pin the hairnet until you are pleased with the way the hair is placed in the back. Mist the wig with hairspray and let it sit until the wig is ready to be worn.

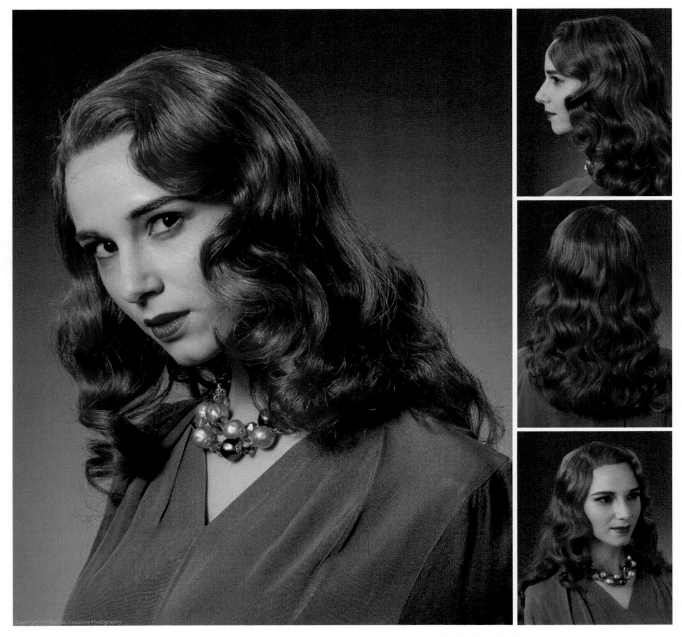

Figures 9.48–9.51   The completed 1940s' Glamour Girl/Peek-a-Boo style. Photography: Tim Babiak. Model: Sabrina Lotfi.

1940s' Victory Rolls/Pinup Girl Styling—Step by Step

This hairstyle uses elements of Figure 9.8, with more defined rolls at the front of the wig.

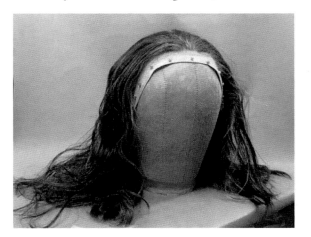

Figure 9.52 Step 1. Again, begin with a wig that at least comes to the shoulders (8 to 12 inches from the nape of the neck). I used a synthetic lace front wig.

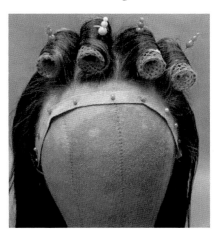

Figure 9.53 Step 2. Use your rattail comb to make a clean off-center part in the wig. Use quarter sized rollers to set the hair rolling away from either side of the part.

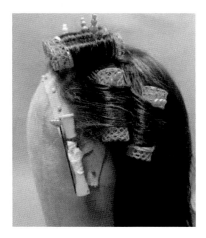

Figure 9.54 Step 3. Separate out the side sections and set them rolling back from the temple area. Repeat on the other side of the wig.

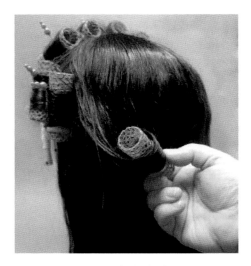

Figure 9.55 Step 4. At the back of the wig, use to the quarter sized rollers to roll diagonal sections of hair up towards the crown of the head. Rolling the rollers up instead of under will help you create a nice ridge in the back of the wig once the set is combed out.

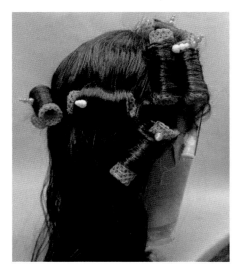

Figure 9.56 Step 5. Continue rolling the curlers up in diagonal rows that alternate angles.

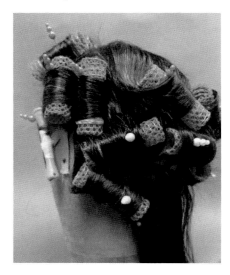

Figure 9.57 Step 6. Work your way all the way down the back of the wig in this manner.

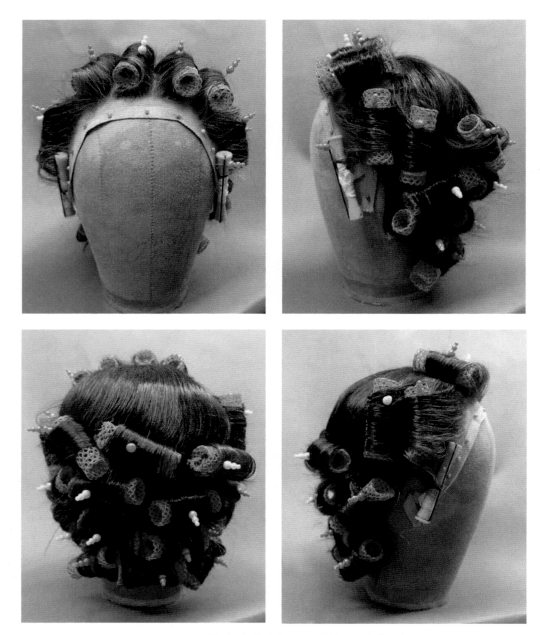

Figures 9.58–9.61   The finished 1940s' Pinup Girl/Victory Rolls style set.

Once you have finished setting the wig, steam each roller thoroughly if the wig is made of synthetic hair. If the wig is human hair, soak each roller with water sprayed from a spray bottle. After steaming or wetting, place the wig in a wig dryer for seventy-five minutes.

To style:

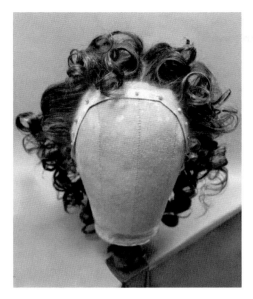

Figure 9.62 Step 7. Remove all the rollers from the wig, beginning at the nape of the neck.

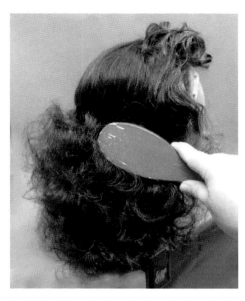

Figure 9.63 Step 8. Brush through the entire wig with a large brush.

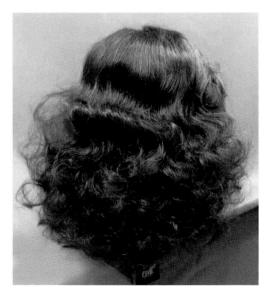

Figure 9.64 Step 9. The wig, after being entirely brushed out.

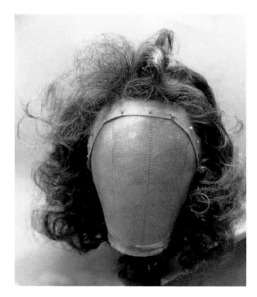

Figure 9.65 Step 10. Use the end of your teasing/smoothing brush to separate out a small section of hair in the front of the wig. Tease the underside of this section. Mist with hairspray.

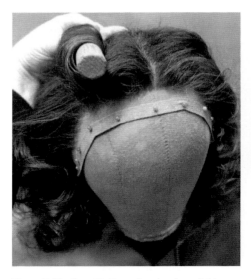

Figure 9.66 Step 11. Use a dowel rod to roll this section of hair into the first roll of the style. Secure with bobby pins.

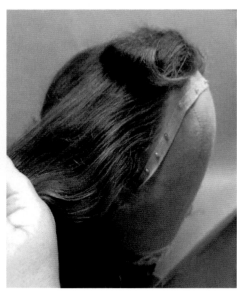

Figure 9.67 Step 12. Gather all the hair in the side section.

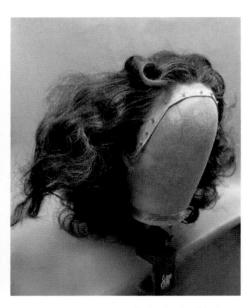

Figure 9.68 Step 13. Tease the back side of the hair in this section.

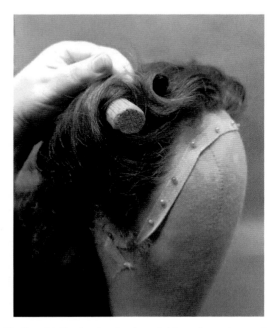

Figure 9.69 Step 14. Use the dowel rod to roll this section up into a roll that sits right beside the first one. Secure with bobby pins.

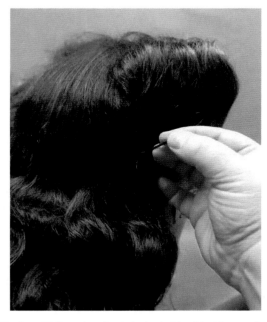

Figure 9.70 Step 15. Smooth and tuck the back side of the Victory roll, securing with bobby pins as needed.

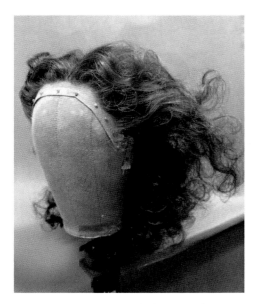

Figure 9.71 Step 16. Tease the back side of the hair on both the top and side of the other side of the wig.

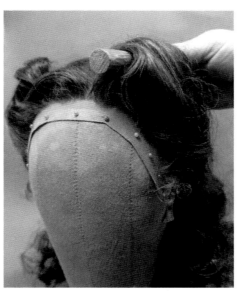

Figure 9.72 Step 17. Roll up all the hair on this side of the part into a single roll using the dowel rod.

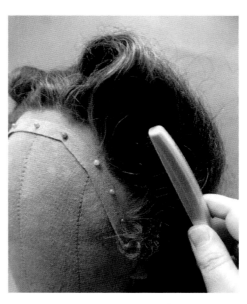

Figure 9.73 Step 18. To smooth any flyaways, mist the wig with hairspray and smooth with a smooth brush.

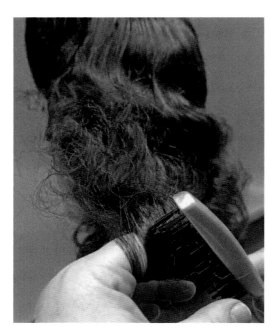

Figure 9.74 Step 19. Next, use the smoothing brush to neaten the back of the hairstyle. Brush sections of the hair around one or two fingers for shaping

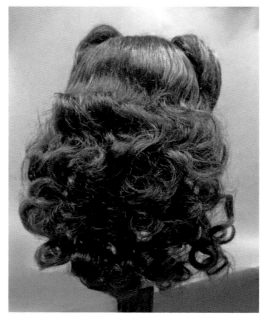

Figure 9.75 Step 20. The completed back of the wig. Notice the nice ridge naturally formed partway down by rolling the rollers upward.

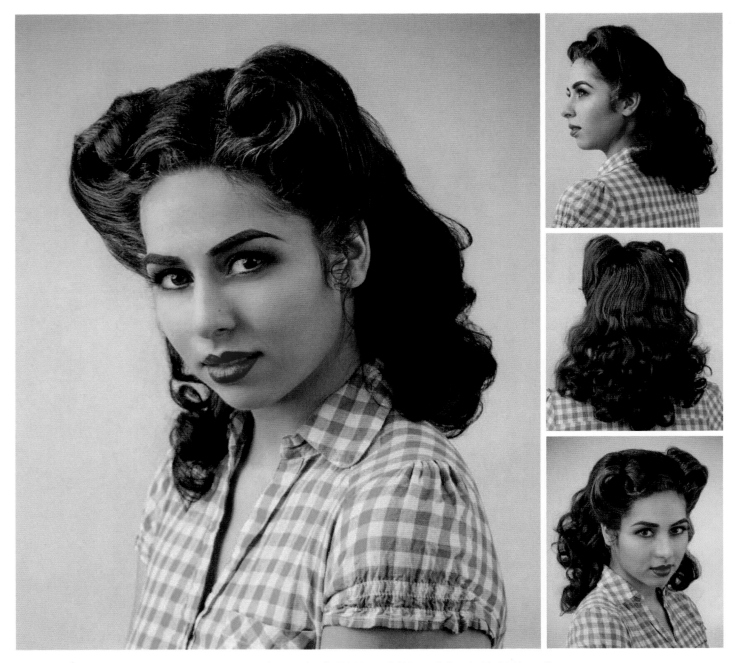

Figures 9.76–9.79   The Completed 1940s' Pinup Girl/Victory Rolls style. Model: Linette Zare.

Variations

Use scarves, snoods (Figures 9.80 and 9.81), and flowers to add variation and style to your 1940s' wigs. You can also do the rolls as a full updo that go all the way down the back to form the traditional "V" shape (Figure 9.82). Another way to vary the look is to place the Victory rolls asymmetrically. You can also create a wig with a strong wavy section in the front of the hair. This sculptural look is very typical of the 1940s. However you choose to vary your 1940s' styles, be sure that the end result is sculptural and feminine.

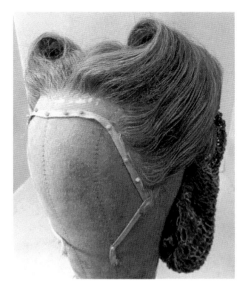
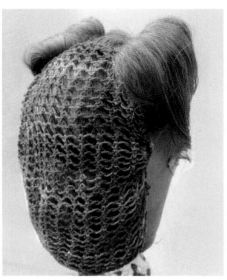

Figures 9.80 and 9.81 Front and back views of a Victory Roll hairstyle finished with a snood.

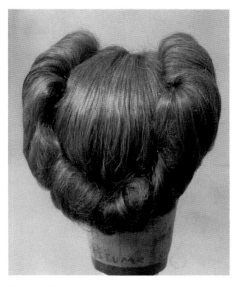

Figure 9.82 Back view of a wig styled with the traditional "V" shape.

1940s' Makeup

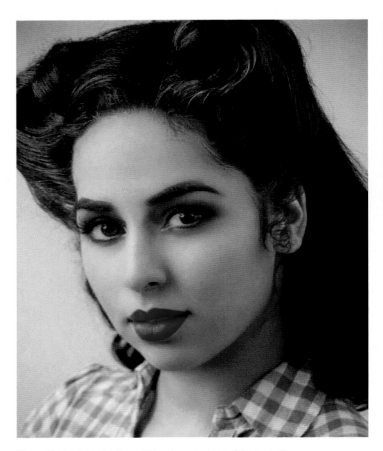

Figure 9.83   A 1940s' Pinup Girl makeup look. Model: Linette Zare.

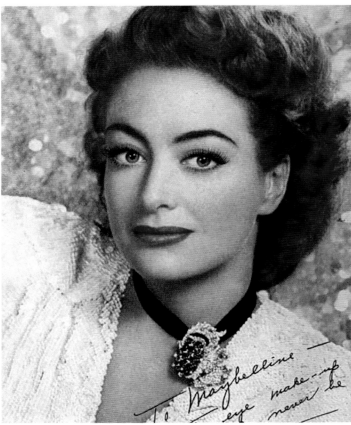

Figure 9.84   Photograph of Joan Crawford from a Maybelline advertisement in *Modern Screen*, by Paul Hesse, January 1946. Crawford's eyebrows and lip shape were the height of fashion in this era.

In the 1940s, just as women took on more masculine roles in the workplace, so too did the makeup fashions become more masculine. The dainty eyebrows of the 1930s became the much fuller, squared off brows of the 1940s. The tiny pinky red lips of the 30s became the overdrawn lips of the 1940s, and a new bolder warm based red became popular. Brick reds and orange based reds (see Figure 9.84) were especially fashionable shades of lipstick. The top lip in particular was flattened and overaccentuated. Creamy eye shadows, in many colors women could coordinate with their outfits, continued to be popular. Women could also buy leg makeup to mimic the look of stockings once nylon was rationed for World War II. They would even use an eyebrow pencil to imitate the look of a stocking seam running up the back of the calf.

ten

THE 1950S

$\left(1950-1959\right)$

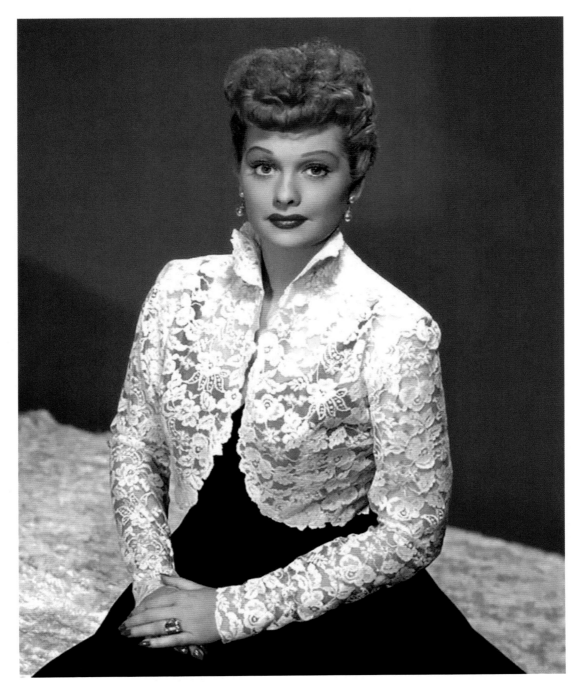

Figure 10.1   Lucille Ball in a 1950s' film still, 1950s, Flickr.

Important Events

1950–1953	The Korean War
1951	Color TV is introduced
1955	Disneyland opens
1955	Rosa Parks refuses to give up her seat on the bus, thus beginning the Civil Rights movement
1956	Elvis Presley appears on the Ed Sullivan show
1957	Grace Kelly marries Prince Rainier III of Monaco
1957	The Soviet Union launches Sputnik I
1959	Fidel Castro overthrows the regime of Fulgencio Batista in Cuba, establishing a communist government
1959	The airplane carrying singers Buddy Holly, Richie Valens, and J.P. "The Big Bopper" Richardson crashes, killing all three

Important Artists/Designers

Christian Dior, Hubert de Givenchy, Willem de Kooning, Charles James, Guy Laroche, Jackson Pollock, Mark Rothko

Important People/Style Icons

Lucille Ball, James Dean, Sandra Dee, Audrey Hepburn, Grace Kelly, Eartha Kitt, Marilyn Monroe, Bettie Page, Babe Paley, Elvis Presley, Elizabeth Taylor

1950s' Women

In the 1950s, women were now leaving the factories they had been urged to work in during World War II and were returning to domestic life. They were expected to look perfect for their husbands returning from the war, and they were expected to keep a perfect house without a hair coming out of place. Women usually wore their hair short and curly. Hats were very popular in the 1950s, so the hair underneath often needed to be short and neat. If they kept their hair long, it was usually put up neatly. Fashions, such as the "New Look" by Christian Dior, accentuated a woman's proportions of a small head, large bust, small waist, and full hips—very much an hourglass shape.

The Poodle Cut, made popular by Lucille Ball (Figure 10.1), was an especially popular hairstyle at the time.

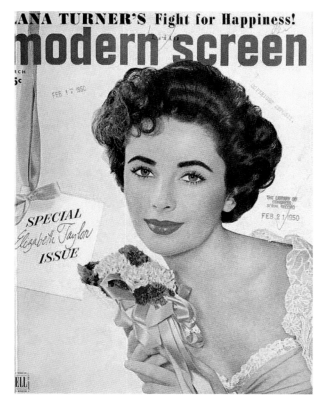

Figure 10.2 Photograph of Elizabeth Taylor on the cover of *Modern Screen*, by Nickolas Muray, 1950. This illustration shows a short hairstyle typical of the 1950s.

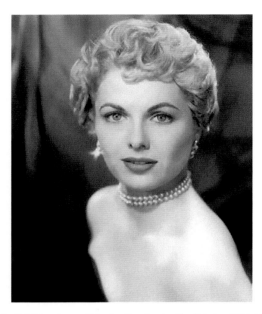

Figure 10.3   Publicity photo of Martha Hyer for the film *Sabrina*, 1954. Hyer wears the Poodle Cut hairstyle.

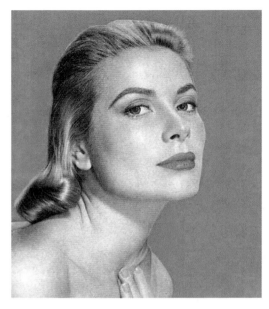

Figure 10.4   Photograph of Grace Kelly on the cover of *Modern Screen*, 1955, Dell Publications. Kelly personifies the look of the "Hitchcock Blonde."

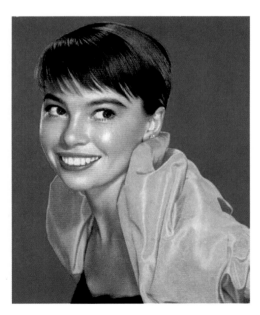

Figure 10.5   Photograph of Leslie Caron on the cover of *Eiga no Tomo*, 1953. This look is an example of the Gamine hairstyle.

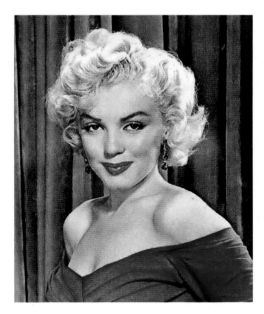

Figure 10.6   Photograph of Marilyn Monroe from the cover of the *New York Sunday News* magazine, 1952. Monroe wears a softly curled, curvy blonde hairstyle.

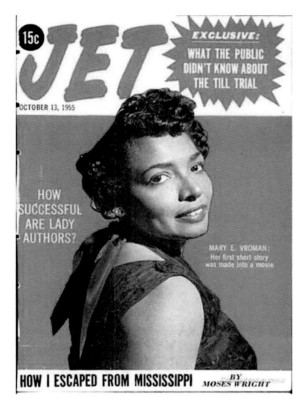

Figure 10.7   Photograph of Mary Elizabeth Vroman on the cover of *JET* magazine, October 1955. Vroman wears the tightly curled bangs and short hair typical of the 1950s.

1950s' Men

Many men in the 1950s were still wearing the extremely short haircuts held over from military days. The flattop, a version of the crewcut that had a very square shape on top, was especially popular with young men.

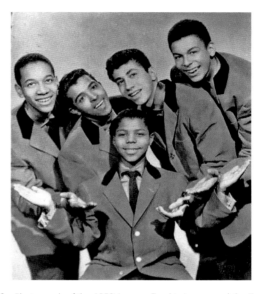

Figure 10.8   Photograph of the 1950s' group Frankie Lymon and the Teenagers, Gee records, *Billboard* magazine, March 1956. A variety of hairstyles and shapes can be seen in this photograph.

Film director Alfred Hitchcock had a reputation for putting icy cool blondes in his films. These actresses, including Grace Kelly, Kim Novak, and Janet Leigh, became known as "Hitchcock Blondes."

Teenage girls in this period, inspired by the film *Gidget*, began wearing their hair pulled back in a ponytail, often accented by a chiffon scarf. These girls were called "bobbysoxers," so called for the short socks they often wore with penny loafers. Beatnik girls, late in the 1950s, began ironing their hair straight. Audrey Hepburn and Leslie Caron, with their short bangs accentuating enormous eyes, helped to make the gamine look popular.

Bombshells such as Elizabeth Taylor and Marilyn Monroe wore more sensual, full, wavy hairstyles. Pinup queen Bettie Page made the heavy bangs that formed a slight curve on the forehead popular.

Nonconformist young men began growing their hair longer and styling it into elaborate pompadours. They used oils and hair grease to sculpt their hairstyles, giving them the nickname "greasers."

These hairstyles were made mainstream by performers such as Elvis Presley. The backs of these hairstyles were often combed straight back on the sides with a part down the center back. This hairstyle was called the "duck tail," "duck's ass," or "D.A." hairstyle because of its resemblance to the tail feathers of a duck.

Teddy boys in England wore fashions that mimicked those of the 1890s. Their hairstyles were often the ducktail or the quiff, a hairstyle with a lock of hair elaborately dressed over the forehead. Men's hair in the 1950s was also often wet looking, made so with the use of Brylcreem and pomade.

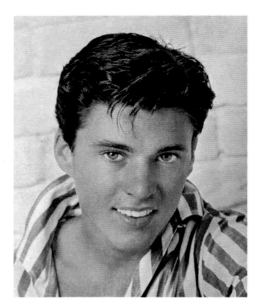

Figure 10.9   Photograph accompanying an article about Ricky Nelson in *Modern Screen* magazine, 1958. Teen idol Nelson wears an example of greased hair with a front curl.

1950s' Woman's Styling— Step by Step

This hairstyle is a combination of the short curly styles seen in Figures 10.2 and 10.6.

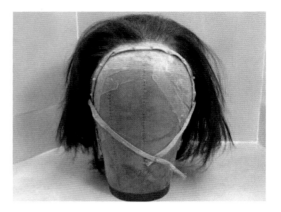

Figure 10.11   Step 1. Begin with a wig that is just below chin length, with some layers. The hair should be at least five inches long on top—it can be shorter in the back. This style works especially well with fully ventilated lace wigs, because they are less dense than hard front wigs, making it easier to keep the style trim and close to the head. Here, I used a fully ventilated human hair lace front wig.

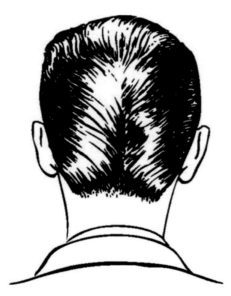

Figure 10.10   The Duck's Ass (or, in the, UK Duck's Arse) is a haircut style that was popular during the 1950s. It is also called the Duck's Tail, the Ducktail, or simply a DA.

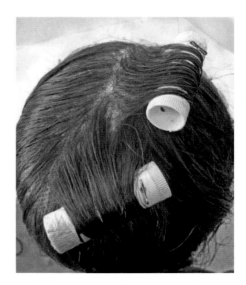

Figure 10.12   Step 2. Saturate the wig with water and setting lotion, and make a side part on a slight diagonal in the wig. Use nickel sized rollers to set two rollers with some drag at the roots on the larger side of the parted hair.

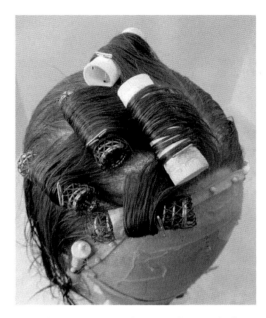

Figure 10.13   Step 3. Continue setting the wig on dime sized rollers, working down the side of the head. Include one roller that is set going down over the hairline,

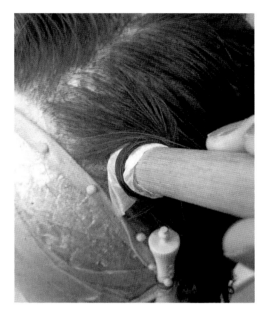

Figure 10.14   Step 4. Move to the other side of the part. Use a dowel rod to form the hair into pin curls. Setting this side on pin curls instead of rollers will ensure that there is less volume on this side of the wig.

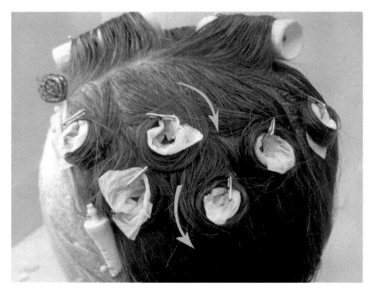

Figure 10.15   Step 5. The first row of pin curls should be set clockwise, rolling towards the face. The second row of pin curls should be set in the opposite direction, counterclockwise, rolling away from the face.

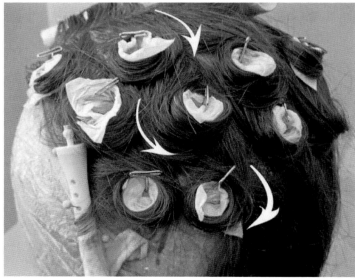

Figure 10.16   Step 6. Set three total rows of pin curls, alternating between clockwise and counterclockwise rows.

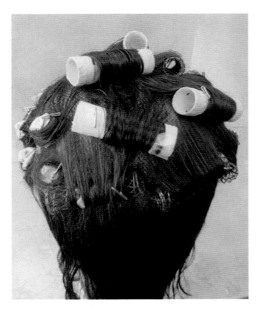

Figure 10.17 Step 7. Next, use rollers to set the rest of the wig. Begin with quarter size rollers on top of the head. Below the three quarter sized rollers, drop down to nickel sized rollers and continue setting the wig in alternating diagonal rows.

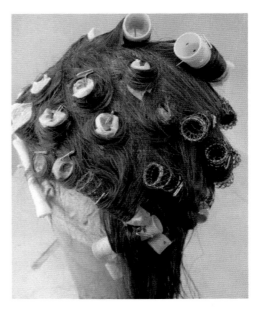

Figure 10.18 Step 8. Continue to decrease the roller size you are using as you work your way down the back of the wig. Below the row of nickel rollers, set a row of dime sized rollers, still setting in a diagonal direction. Notice how the rollers are used to fill in underneath where the pin curls have been set.

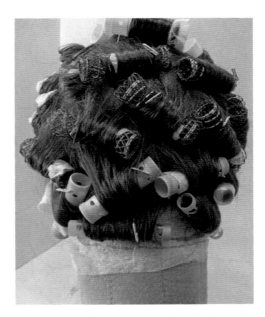

Figure 10.19 Step 9. Finish the set by setting a row of pencil rollers at the nape of the wig.

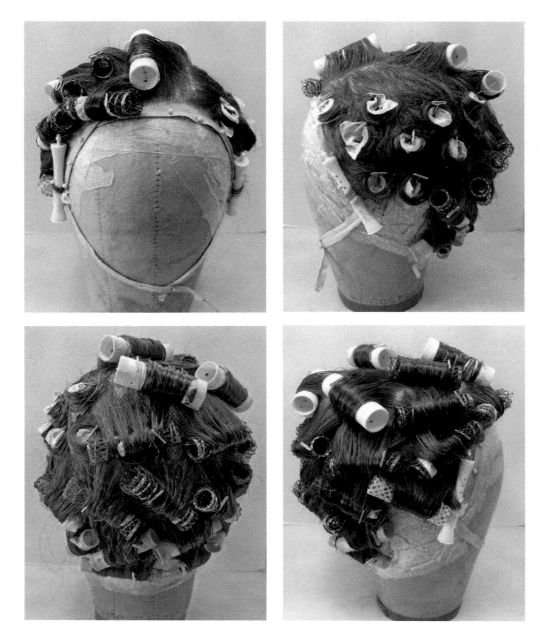

Figures 10.20–10.23 The finished 1950s' woman's style set.

Once you have finished setting the wig, steam each roller thoroughly if the wig is made of synthetic hair. If the wig is human hair, soak each roller with water sprayed from a spray bottle. After steaming or wetting, place the wig in a wig dryer for 75 minutes.

To style:

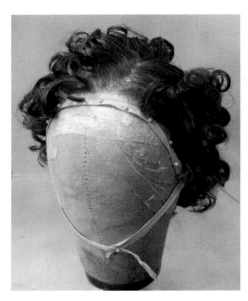

Figure 10.24 Step 10. Remove all the rollers and pin curls from the wig, beginning at the nape of the neck and working your way up to the front hairline.

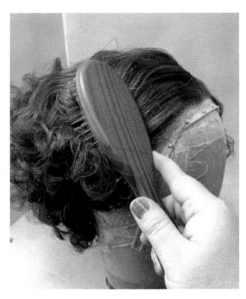

Figure 10.25 Step 11. Use a large brush to thoroughly brush through the entire wig.

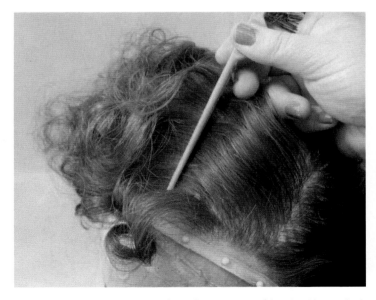

Figure 10.26 Step 12. Next, smooth out the top section of the wig with a teasing/smoothing brush. Use the pointed end of the brush to begin pushing the waves of the wig into place.

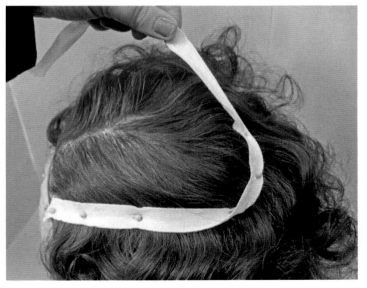

Figure 10.27 Step 13. Use a piece of bias tape of ribbon to shape the waves in place. Pin back and forth around the head to make a continuous wave pattern.

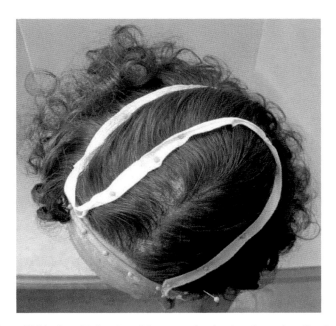

Figure 10.28 Step 14. Top view of the waves after they have been pinned in place with the ribbon. The tape should hold the waves tight to the head down to the middle of the head below the crown.

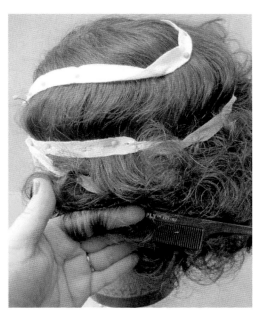

Figure 10.29 Step 15. Begin to shape the curls around the nape of the neck by brushing them up and around your finger.

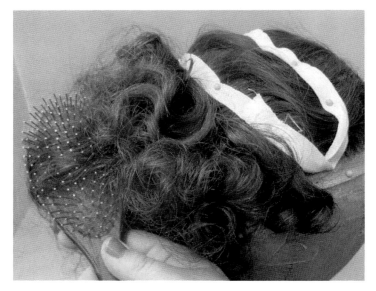

Figure 10.30 Step 16. If you wish to add some fullness to the shape of the wig, you may need to tease the lower section of curls before neatening up the locks around your finger.

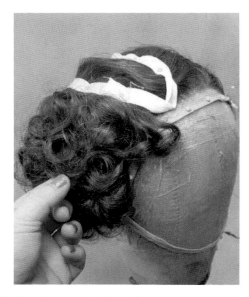

Figure 10.31 Step 17. Arrange the finished hair in a pretty way to finish off this hairstyle.

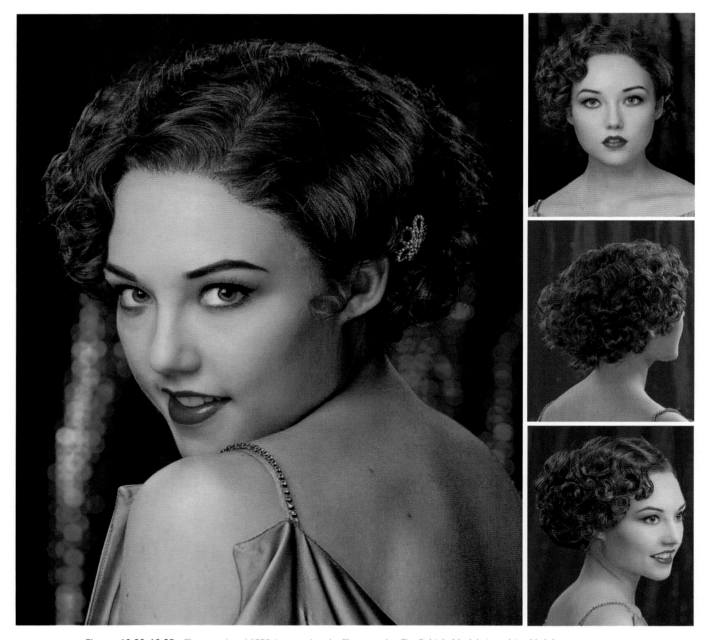

Figures 10.32–10.35   The completed 1950s' woman's style. Photography: Tim Babiak. Model: Josephine McAdam.

1950s' Woman's Poodle Updo Styling— Step by Step

This hairstyle is based on Figure 10.1.

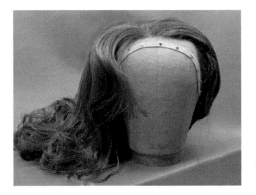

Figure 10.36 Step 1. Begin with a wig that has bangs or short layer layers around the face and is long in the back. Here, I used a fronted synthetic wig.

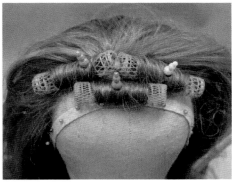

Figure 10.37 Step 2. Saturate each section of the wig with water and/or setting lotion as you work. Begin by setting the bang section of the wig on pencil rollers going forward towards the face.

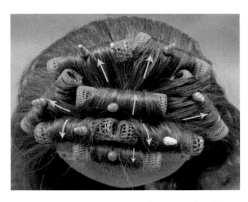

Figure 10.38 Step 3. The next five rollers should be placed rolling away from the face in a semi-circular pattern. The hair in these rollers should be no longer than six inches.

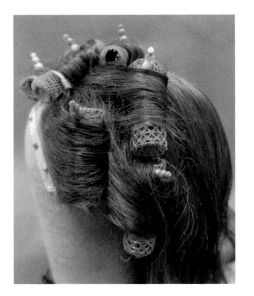

Figure 10.39 Step 4. Set the side section on nickel sized rollers with a little bit of drag going off the face. This will help the finished hairstyle to be nice and close to the head on the sides.

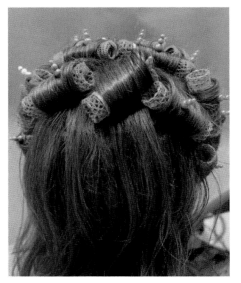

Figure 10.40 Step 5. Set the back of the wig on nickel sized rollers in diagonal rows that alternate directions.

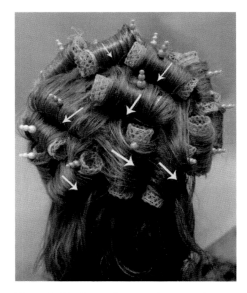

Figure 10.41 Step 6. Continue alternating the direction of the rows down the back of the wig until you reach the nape of the neck.

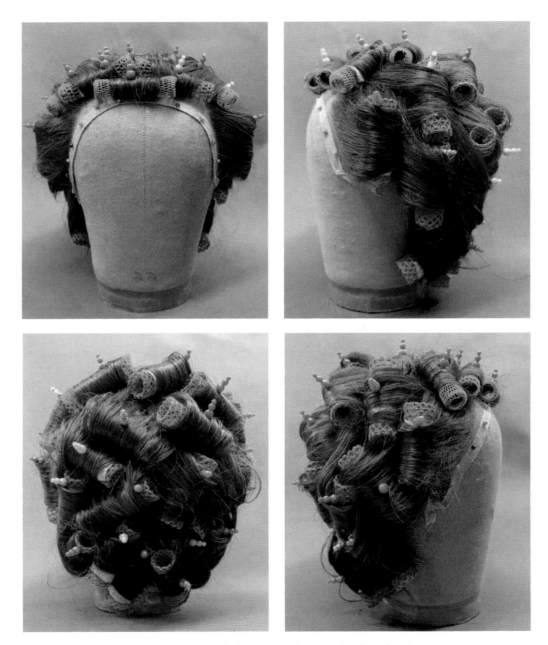

Figures 10.42–10.45   The finished 1950s' woman's Poodle Updo style set.

Once you have finished setting the wig, steam each roller thoroughly if the wig is made of synthetic hair. If the wig is human hair, soak each roller with water sprayed from a spray bottle. After steaming or wetting, place the wig in a wig dryer for 75 minutes.

To style:

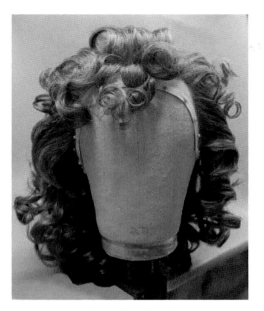

Figure 10.46 Step 7. Remove all the rollers from the wig and comb through the curls with your fingers.

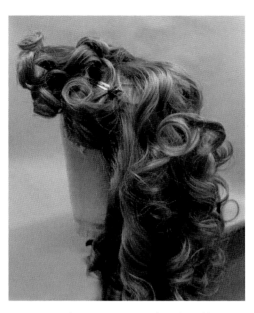

Figure 10.47 Step 8. Use clips to separate out the side and bangs sections of the hair and begin work on the back section first.

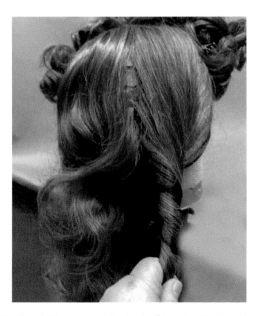

Figure 10.48 Step 9. Brush through the back of the wig with a large brush. Divide the hair in half. Take half of the hair in your hand and twist it towards the face.

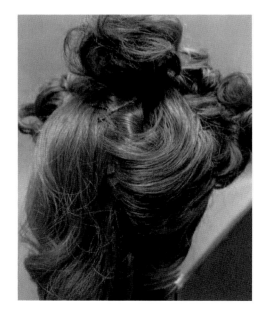

Figure 10.49 Step 10. Twist the hair up the center back, creating a sort of half French twist. Pin the ends on the top of the head with crossed bobby pins.

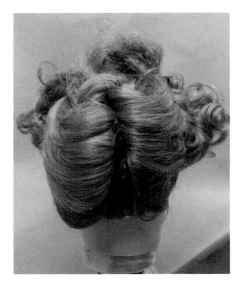

Figure 10.50 Step 11. Repeat the process on the other side of the wig, creating a double French twist.

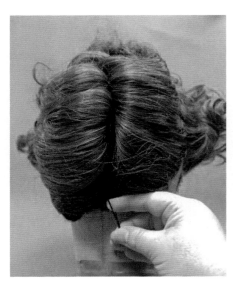

Figure 10.51 Step 12. Use bobby pins in the center of the two rolls to join them together so that they are right next to each other. Smooth the hair and make sure that the rolls are neat.

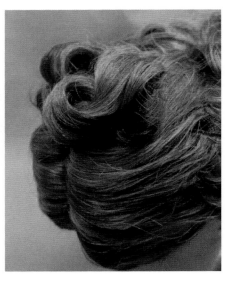

Figure 10.52 Step 13. Shape the ends of the hair in each roll into pretty curl clusters on top of the head.

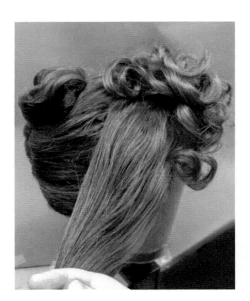

Figure 10.53 Step 14. Next, move to the side sections. (The bangs will still be held out of the styling for now.) Brush through the side section with a smoothing brush.

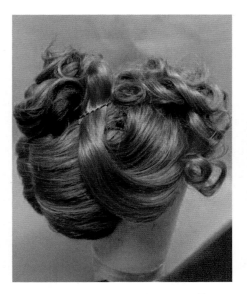

Figure 10.54 Step 15. Drape the section of hair down over the ear and then up towards the top of the head, creating a smooth wave. Pin the ends with bobby pins.

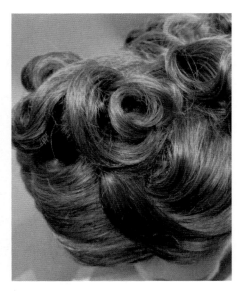

Figure 10.55 Step 16. Again, arrange the ends into pretty curls. Repeat on the other side.

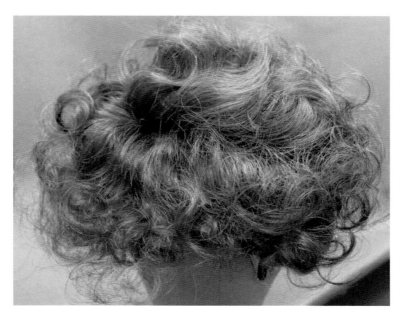

Figure 10.56 Step 17. Move to the bang section of the wig. Brush out the bang curls with a smoothing brush.

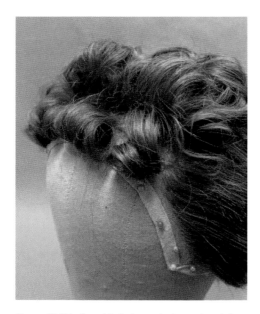

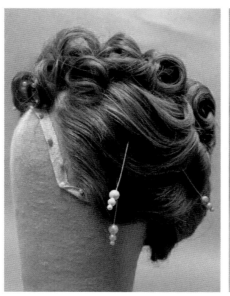

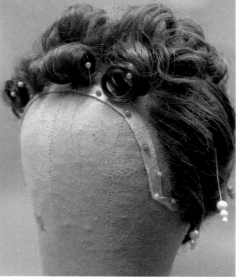

Figure 10.57 Step 18. Reshape the bangs into tight curls, working in a circle from the center point. The curls should radiate out from the center point like petals on a flower.

Figures 10.58 and 10.59 Step 19. Use pins to hold the bang curls in place. Also use pins to flatten down the sides so that the hair remains close to the head. Once the pins are in place, mist the hair with hairspray and allow it to sit overnight.

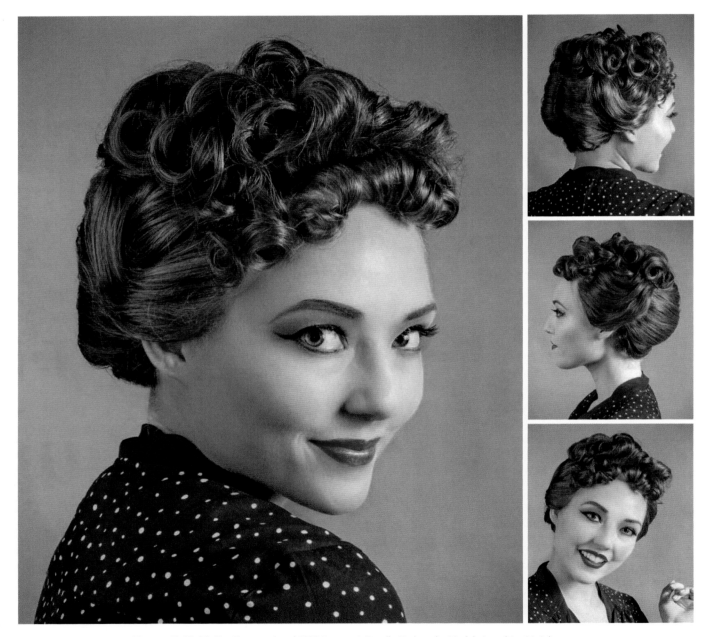

Figures 10.60–10.63   The completed 1950s' woman's Poodle Updo style. Model: Josephine McAdam.

Variations

Part of the reason short curly hair was so popular in the 1950s was its role in showing off the chic little hats that were trendy at the time (see Figure 10.64). Use period hats and fascinators to create variety in your 1950s' looks. Longer, more voluptuous versions of these softly curled hairstyles were also popular, especially in creating a glamorous pinup girl look.

Even longer hairstyles, such as the shoulder length hair made popular by Bettie Page can be used during this period. Look to the pinup girl illustrations by Gil Elvgren and Alberto Vargas for style inspirations. Some 1950s' hairstyles were so short that they had few to no curls, such as in Figure 10.5.

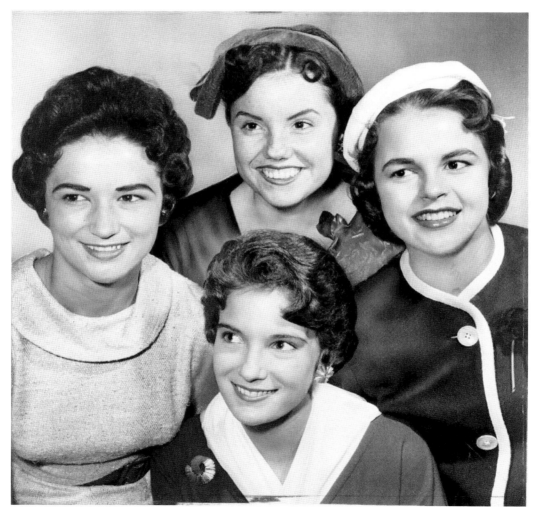

Figure 10.64   *Four Miss America candidates: Jacque Baker (Miss Iowa), Linda(?) Mead (Miss Mississippi), Sharon O'Neal (Miss Kansas), Suzie Jackson (Miss Arkansas), by Al Ravenna, 1959 or 1960, World-Telegram & Sun photo, Library of Congress Prints and Photographs Division, New York World-Telegram and the Sun Newspaper Photograph Collection.*

1950s' Makeup

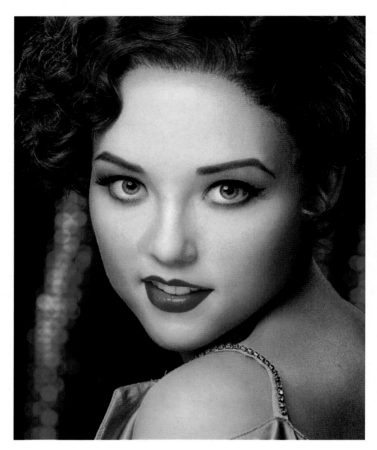

Figure 10.65 The typical arched eyebrows, true red lips, and winged eyeliner of the 1950s. Model: Josephine McAdam.

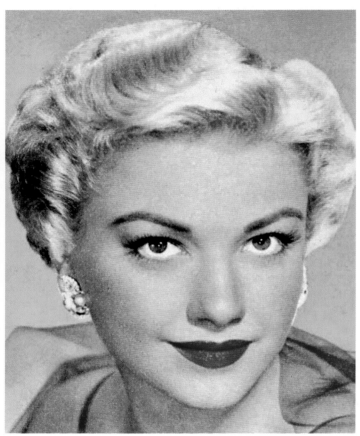

Figure 10.66 Cropped photo of Anne Baxter in a Lustre-Crème Shampoo advertisement in *Modern Screen* magazine, 1953.

1950s' makeup, much like the hair, was very classic and precise. Skin was clear and well cared for, and foundation was heavier and more powdered looking than in the 1940s. Marilyn Monroe's "bedroom eyes" and Elizabeth Taylor's famous violet eyes were accented by strong arching eyebrows and winged black eyeliner. Eye shadow was available in a variety of colors, including shimmer. Lip color was often a true red, with some younger women preferring pink lipstick.

eleven

THE 1960S

$\left(\textit{1960–1969}\right)$

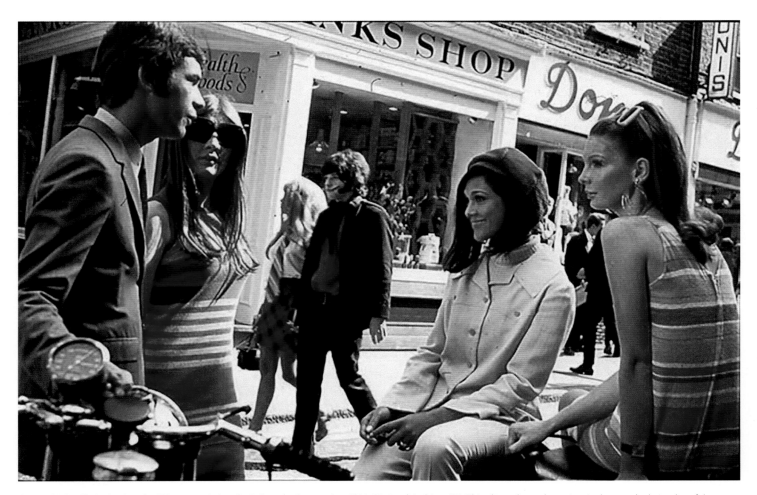

Figure 11.1   "Swinging London" Teenagers in London's Carnaby Street, circa 1966, National Archives UK. This photo shows the variety in the popular hairstyles of the 1960s.

Important Events

1960	Women's birth control pills are released in the United States
1960	Motown Record Corporation is founded
1961	Bay of Pigs Invasion
1963	President John F. Kennedy is assassinated
1964	The Beatles arrive in America, kicking off the British "invasion"
1964	Mary Quant invents the miniskirt
1968	Martin Luther King, Jr. is assassinated
1969	Woodstock music festival
1969	Astronaut Neil Armstrong walks on the moon

Important Artists/Designers

Oleg Cassini, Hubert de Givenchy, Jasper Johns, Roy Lichtenstein, Emilio Pucci, Mary Quant, Vidal Sassoon, Andy Warhol

Important People/Style Icons

Brigitte Bardot, Jane Birkin, James Dean, Audrey Hepburn, Janis Joplin, Jackie Kennedy, John Lennon, Sophia Loren, Peggy Moffitt, Diana Ross, Edie Sedgwick, Twiggy

1960s' Women

The 1960s was a time of change and upheaval, not the least of which happened in the world of fashion and hairstyles. Popular styles went spinning off in a variety of directions. In the early part of the 1960s, women were still clinging to the ideal of being the perfect woman with the perfect hair. First Lady Jackie Kennedy (Figure 11.2) helped set the trends with her teased bouffant pageboy style. (Aerosol cans, developed in World War II, made aerosol hairspray possible. This lighter weight styling product revolutionized the possibilities in hairstyles.) This teased hair was often girlish in shape and decoration—tall on top with a flip on the bottom (sometimes called the bubble flip), wrapped in a tall Beehive, or neatly teased at the crown and accented with a headband or bow.

As the 60s progressed, bringing with them new attitudes about personal and sexual freedom, these hairstyles became more tousled with long, full curls. Sex symbols such as Brigitte Bardot (as seen in Figure 11.3), Sophia Loren, and Ann-Margret led the way in this hair fashion.

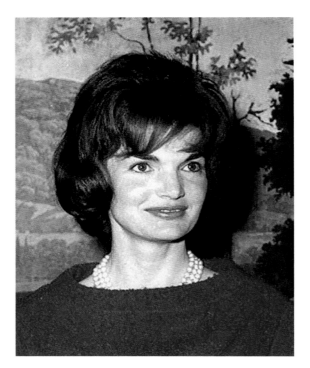

Figure 11.2 Mrs. Kennedy in the Diplomatic Reception Room, by Robert Knudson, December 5, 1961.

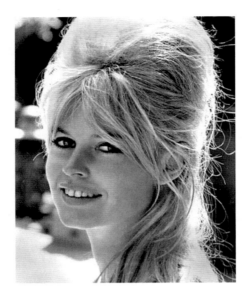

Figure 11.3 Publicity photo of Brigitte Bardot in the film *A Very Private Affair*, 1962, MGM.

Falls (long hairpieces that were meant to sit on the crown of the head and match the wearer's hair color) were often used to add height and create these long hairstyles. Hairpieces were also used to create the tall elaborately arranged hairstyles of the 60s.

Full wigs also came back into fashion in the 1960s, thanks in part to the many girl singing groups of the era. Singers, including Diana Ross and the Supremes (Figure 11.4), the Ronettes, and Patti LaBelle and the Bluebells, helped to make it fashionable to wear wigs again. (It was easier to achieve teased hairstyles with wigs, plus it was much easier on the condition of one's hair!) Wigs also made it possible for these mostly African American groups to mimic the hairstyles that were popular with white America that they would not have been able to achieve with their own hair.

In the mid-1960s, the Beatles appeared on American television and started off the British "invasion." There was a craze for all things English and fashionable. The world was looking to fashionable Carnaby Street in London for the next trends. Hair began to move again—many girls wore their hair long with sideswept bangs. Women

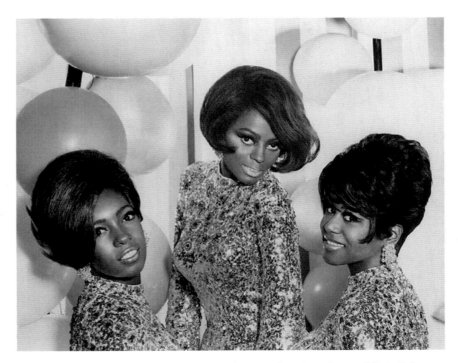

Figure 11.4 Photograph of the Supremes, 1967, General Artists Corporation. From left: Mary Wilson, Diana Ross, and Cindy Birdsong.

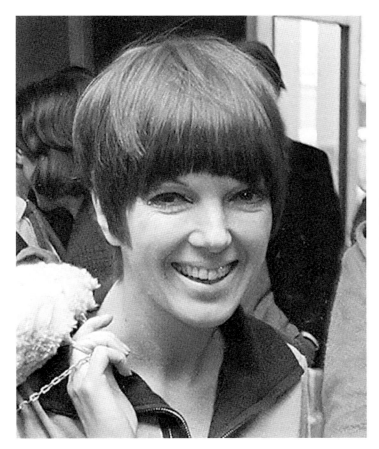

Figure 11.5 The arrival of Mary Quant, English fashion queen, at Schipol, the Netherlands, by Jac. De Nijs, 1966, Anefo. Quant's Mod hairdo was designed and cut by Vidal Sassoon.

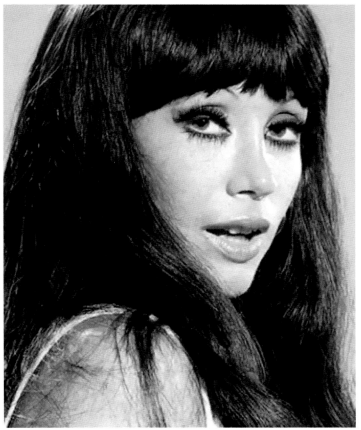

Figure 11.6 Moria Casan, circa 1969. Casan wears the straight flat look and huge eyelashes that were popular in the late 1960s.

either ironed their hair straight, or set it on large juice cans to try and achieve the long straight look they wanted. Hairdresser Vidal Sassoon revolutionized haircutting with his famous five point cut. His idea was to cut the hair geometrically, and work with the natural movement and swing of the individual woman's hair. These short haircuts were a staple of "mod" fashion, and helped launch the careers of models Twiggy and Peggy Moffitt.

Later in the 1960s, the hippie/ flower child movement picked up steam. People protested for peace and love, and looked to an ideal of a more natural beauty.

Hair was often center parted, grown long, and left loose and natural in texture. These hairstyles were sometimes accented with headbands, tiny braids, beads, feathers, and flowers. African American women also saw the rise in popularity of natural hair. After years of attempting to process their hair or wear wigs in order to conform to fashion, these women let their hair grow into Afros, a round, picked out natural hairstyle. Stars such as Cher, influenced by the beatnik movement, favored a flat straight look that was often either ironed flat or set on enormous rollers to achieve the look.

1960s' Men

At the beginning of the 1960s, men were still wearing short, conservative haircuts. Military influence could still be seen on the still popular crewcut or flattop. Clean cut teen idols were admired by many teenagers.

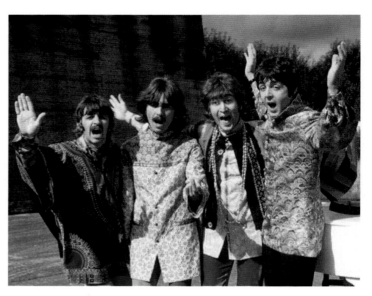

Figure 11.8   Press photo of the Beatles during the *Magical Mystery Tour*, 1967, Parlophone Music Sweden.

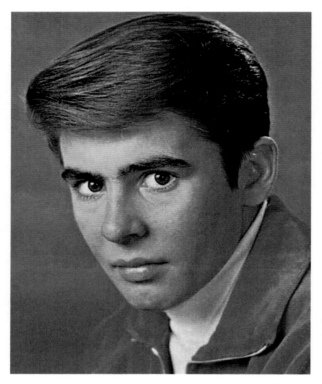

Figure 11.7   Photograph of Davy Jones from an ad for the 1965 single "What are We Going to Do?"/"This Bouquet", *Billboard* magazine, July 1965, Colpix Records.

The arrival of the Beatles and their signature "mop top" haircuts set off the trend for young men to begin growing their hair longer.

As the decade progressed, men's hair grew longer, eventually reaching their shoulders. Long sideburns were popular for a time; then the fashion turned to full beards. At the end of the decade, men looked very similar to women in terms of hairstyle. Men wore center parts, and long natural hair. African American men, like African American women, began to grow out their hair in its natural state and comb it into an Afro.

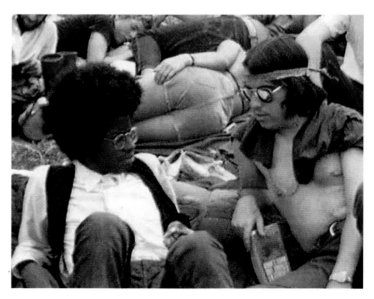

Figure 11.9   Two hippies at the Woodstock Festival, Derek Redmond and Paul Campbell, August 1969. The photo show two versions of men's hair in the late 60s—a natural Afro and a longer style worn with a headband.

1960s' Beehive Styling—
Step by Step

This hairstyle was based on the styles worn by the Motown girl group the Ronettes and also on the style worn by Brigitte Bardot in Figure 11.3.

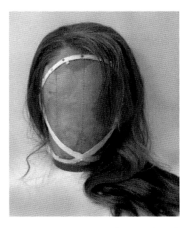

Figure 11.10 Step 1. Begin with a wig that is long and mostly one length (at least 14 inches long at the nape of the neck). It is also good if the wig has a section of bangs in the front. Hard front wigs are another good choice for 1960s' styles, because so many of them were actually wigs. Here, I used a lace front synthetic wig.

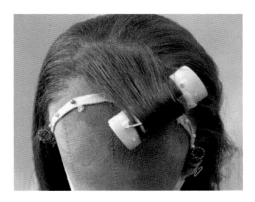

Figure 11.11 Step 2. Set the bang section on a quarter sized roller, going towards the face at an angle. If your wig does not have bangs, you can set a longer section of hair in the same manner and use it to sweep across the forehead later as part of the finished style. Also note that a tiny tendril of hair has been set in front of each ear on pencil rollers.

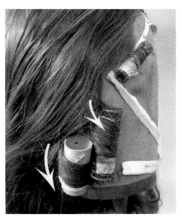

Figure 11.12 Step 3. This version of the Beehive is going to have a long curled section that comes down over one shoulder. To achieve this look, set a couple of rollers behind one ear. Use either dime or nickel sized rollers.

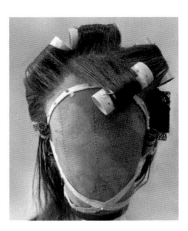

Figure 11.13 Step 4. Set several sections of hair on quarter sized rollers, going straight back away from the face. At the side of the face, use nickel sized rollers.

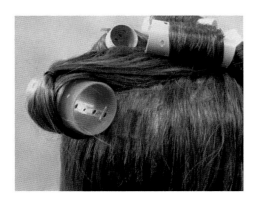

Figure 11.14 Step 5. At the crown of the head, pull a small section of hair into a loose ponytail. Begin using larger rollers (the size of a half dollar) to continue setting the hair.

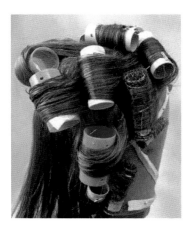

Figure 11.15 Step 6. Continue working your way around the head, setting the hair on large rollers. The rollers should be set with some drag so that they all roll inwards towards the center back of the head.

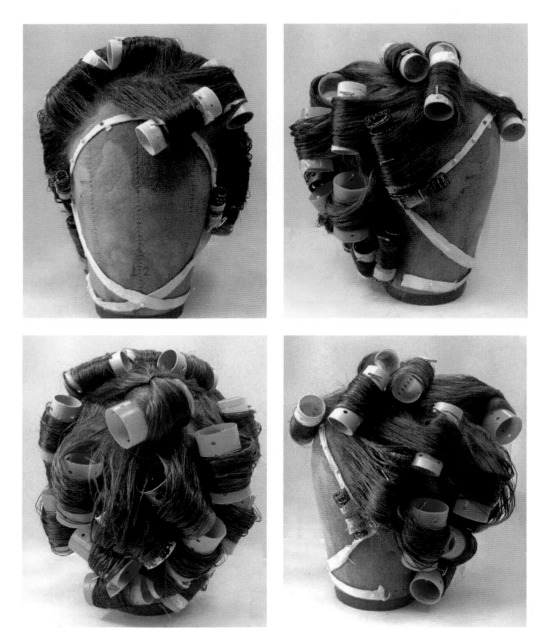

Figures 11.16–11.19   The finished 1960s' Beehive style set.

Once you have finished setting the wig, steam each roller thoroughly if the wig is made of synthetic hair. If the wig is human hair, soak each roller with water sprayed from a spray bottle. After steaming or wetting, place the wig in a wig dryer for 75 minutes.

To style:

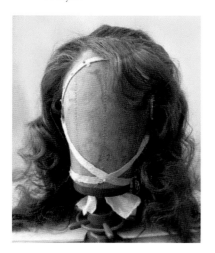

Figure 11.20 Step 7. Remove all the rollers from the wig, beginning at the nape of the neck and working your way up towards the front hairline. Brush through the hair with a large hairbrush.

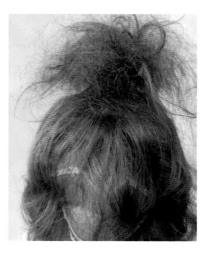

Figure 11.21 Step 8. Move to the crown of the head where you made the small ponytail. Use a teasing/smoothing brush to tease the hair in the ponytail. Make sure you tease the hair thoroughly so that this section is very dense. Spray the ponytail with hairspray periodically as you work to help all the hair stick together as a unit.

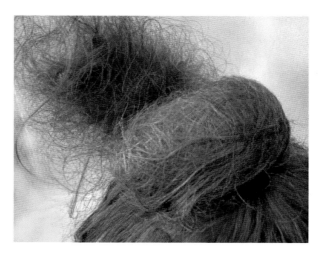

Figure 11.22 Step 9. Place a hair rat behind the ponytail and pin it in place with bobby pins.

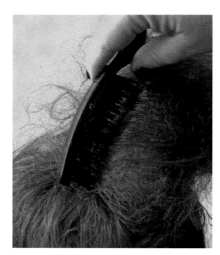

Figure 11.23 Step 10. Use the smoothing brush to smooth all the hair around the rat, forming a cone like shape. Brush the hair with a swirling motion, gently skimming/smoothing the top layer of hair, working in a circular direction around the hair rat. Pin the base of this section with hairpins to secure the hair. (Hairpins slide right into the rat, forming a firm base for the rest of the hairstyle.)

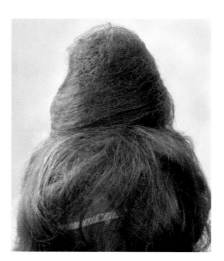

Figure 11.24 Step 11. All the hair in the ponytail should now be formed into the cone shape.

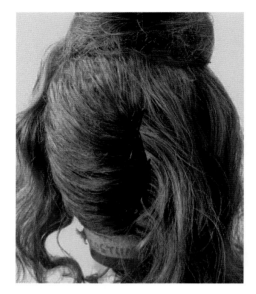

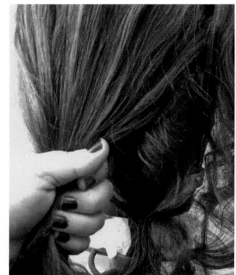

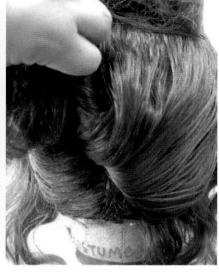

Figure 11.25 Step 12. Separate out the long lock of hair that is going to hang down over the shoulder. Continue to leave out the bangs and the pieces of hair around the face. Pull the rest of the hair in the back of the wig into a French twist by first sweeping all the hair to one side and pinning it up the center back with crossed bobby pins.

Figures 11.26 and 11.27 Step 13. Next, gather the hair into a ponytail at the nape of the wig, twist the hair, and pull it up into a twist.

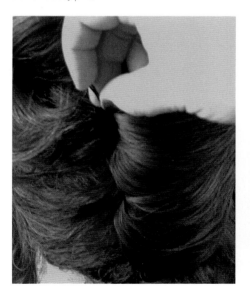

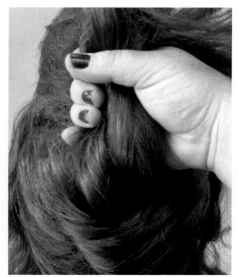

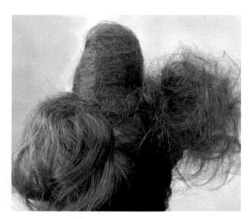

Figure 11.30 Step 16. Use the teasing brush to tease those loose ends of hair.

Figure 11.28 Step 14. Secure the twist with bobby pins.

Figure 11.29 Step 15. Brush through the loose ends of hair that are now at the top of the French twist.

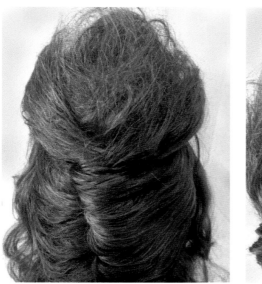 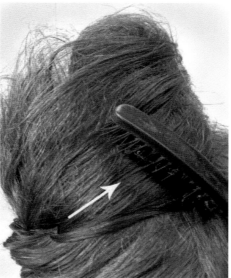

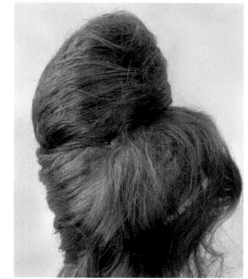

Figure 11.31 and 11.32 Step 17. Smooth the loose ends of the hair around the first cone you made, making the cone bigger as you incorporate the hair.

Figure 11.33 Step 18. At this point, you should have a good sized Beehive.

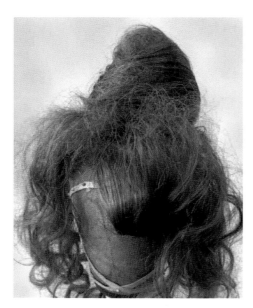

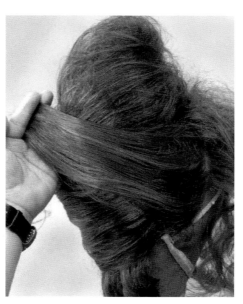

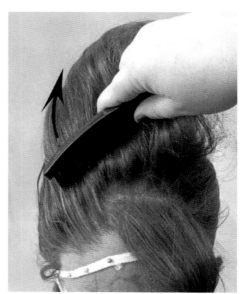

Figure 11.34 Step 19. Tease the hair around the face and in the bangs.

Figure 11.35 Step 20. Pull up the section of hair at the sides of the face and incorporate them into the Beehive.

Figure 11.36 Step 21. Brush the center front section of hair just behind the bangs into the Beehive and use it to complete the teased cone.

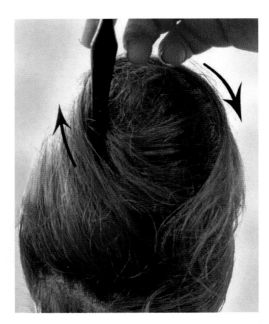

Figure 11.37   Step 22. Smooth this last section of hair over and around the cone, tucking the ends in so that the Beehive has a smooth, finished look.

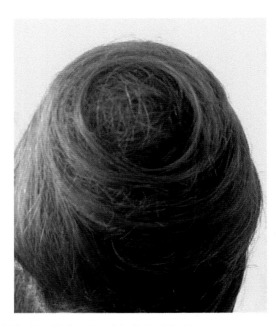

Figure 11.38   Step 23. Top view of the finished Beehive.

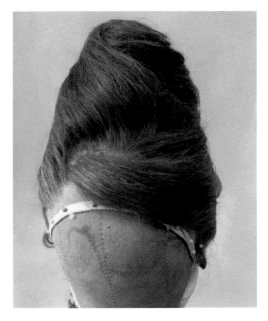

Figure 11.39   Step 24. Tease and smooth the bangs, smoothing them over to one side of the forehead.

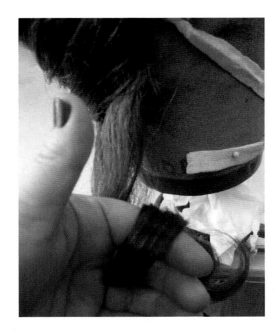

Figure 11.40   Step 25. Brush the long lock of hair that is going to hang over the shoulder around two fingers in order to make the curl neat.

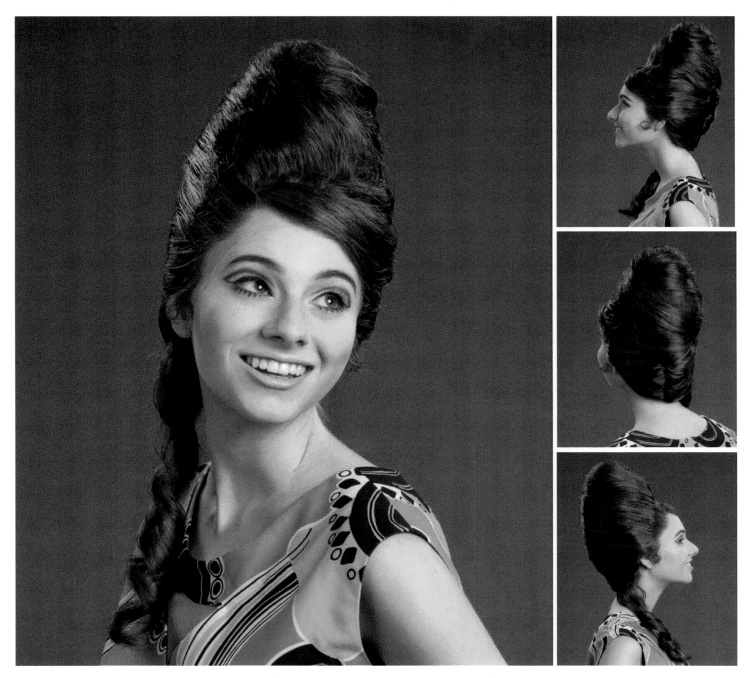

Figures 11.41–11.44 The completed 1960s' Beehive style. Photography: Tim Babiak. Model: Ariel Livingston.

1960s' Bubble Flip Styling— Step by Step

This hairstyle was inspired by the wigs worn by the Supremes in Figure 11.4.

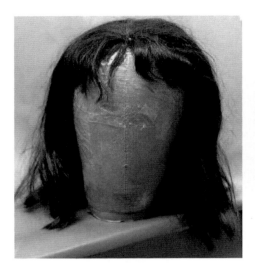

Figure 11.45   Step 1. For this hairstyle, I used a shoulder length hard front synthetic wig with bangs.

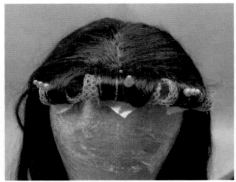

Figure 11.46   Step 2. Begin by setting the bangs on quarter sized rollers.

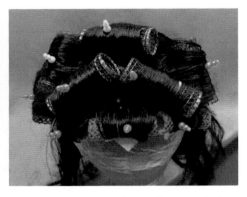

Figure 11.47   Step 3. Use large rollers to set the hair behind the bangs, rolling away from the face.

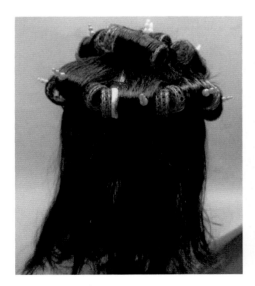

Figure 11.48   Step 4. Set another layer of rollers curling under at the level of the tops of the ears.

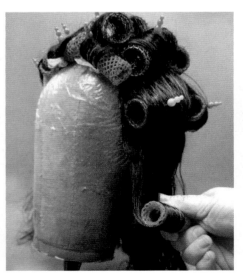

Figure 11.49   Step 5. To create the flip, use quarter sized rollers. Roll the hair up instead of down and under.

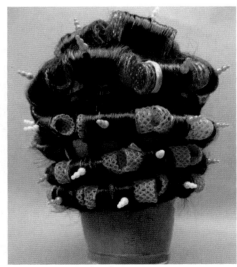

Figure 11.50   Step 6. Set the entire back of the wig below the ears on quarter sized rollers rolled upwards.

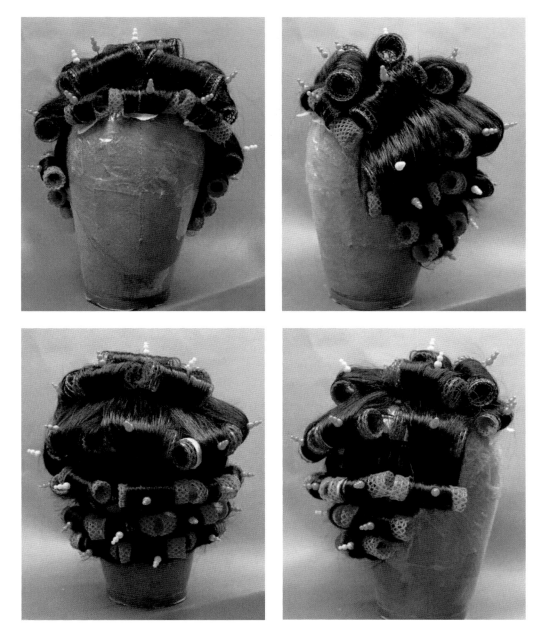

Figures 11.51–11.54   The finished 1960s' Bubble Flip style set.

Once you have finished setting the wig, steam each roller thoroughly if the wig is made of synthetic hair. If the wig is human hair, soak each roller with water sprayed from a spray bottle. After steaming or wetting, place the wig in a wig dryer for 75 minutes.

To style:

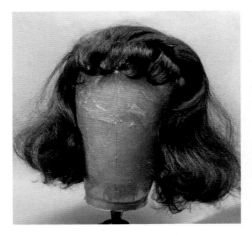

Figure 11.55 Step 7. Remove all the rollers and brush through the entire wig with a large brush.

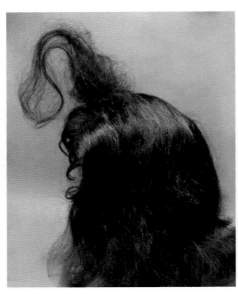

Figure 11.56 Step 8. Beginning at the center front (ignore the bangs for now), begin teasing the hair in small sections. Make sure to hairspray each section in order to create a solid foundation for the style.

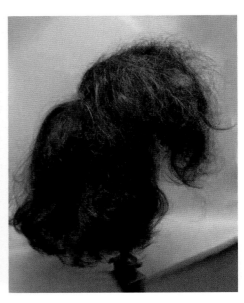

Figure 11.57 Step 9. Continue working your way around the wig, teasing and spraying each section.

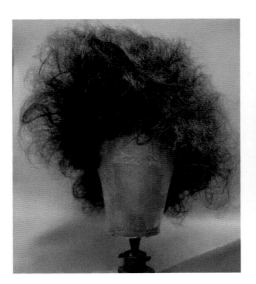

Figure 11.58 Step 10. The fully teased wig will be quite large!

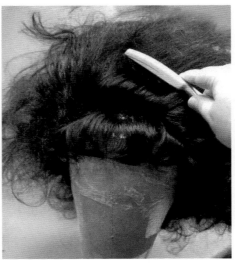

Figure 11.59 Step 11. Use a teasing/smoothing brush to begin gently smoothing the top layer of hair into the shape you want.

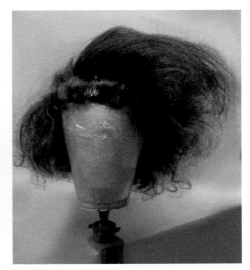

Figure 11.60 Step 12. Because I have chosen an asymmetrical style, I have swept the majority of the hair to the right.

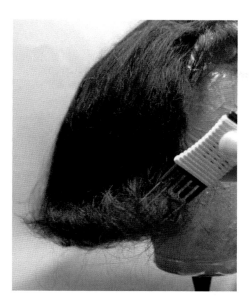

Figure 11.61 Step 13. Once the hair on the top and back have been smoothed, begin to work on the flip section. Use a teasing pick to flip the ends of the hair up.

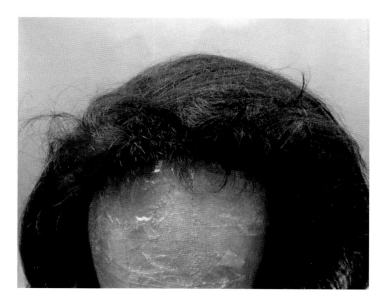

Figure 11.62 Step 14. Tease the bangs into one solid section.

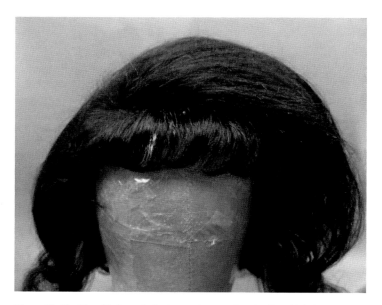

Figure 11.63 Step 15. Smooth the bangs down and under. Set with hairspray.

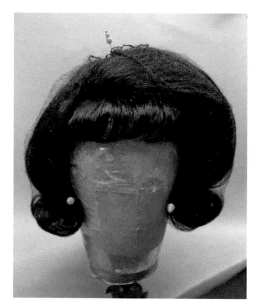

Figure 11.64 Step 16. To reinforce the flip shape, use a hairnet. Pin the hairnet in place so that it shapes the flip and pulls it up. Mist with hairspray and let it set until it is time for the wig to be worn.

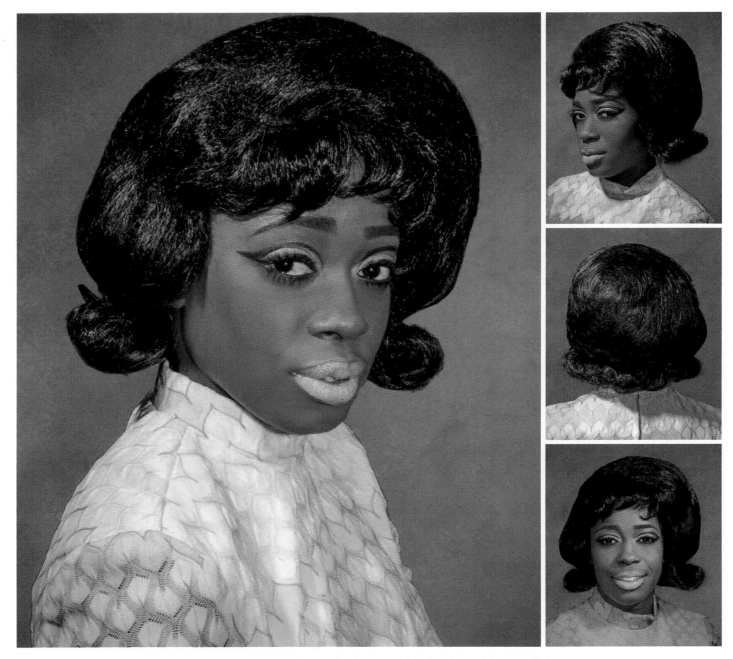

Figures 11.65–11.68   The completed 1960s' Bubble Flip style. Model: Antonia Taylor

Variations

1960s' teased hairstyles come in all shapes and sizes. Some of these hairstyles were short and flippy; others were much longer with the teasing concentrated at the crown. These hairstyles were often accented with small bows and headbands, such as those seen in Figures 11.45 and 11.46. The styles in both Figure 11.45 and 11.46 have been created using hard front synthetic wigs.

You can also choose to focus on the more natural looks of the later 1960s. Long flowy hairstyles can be created by setting a wig with large rollers or in braids to create the texture. Once the set has dried, the wig can simply be brushed through in order to create a natural look, à la Janis Joplin.

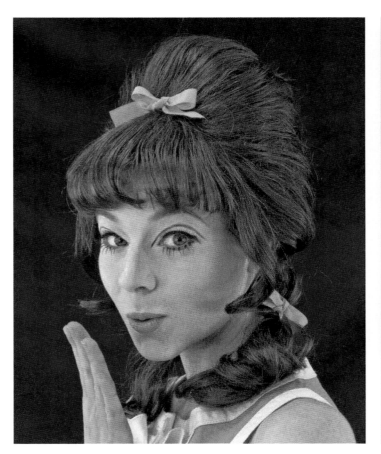

Figure 11.69   Maur Sela's Beehive wig that has been modified with small curled ponytails and accented with orange bows. Model: Ariel Livingston.

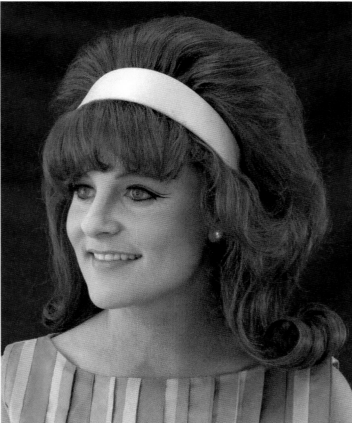

Figure 11.70   Thumper Gosney's Bubble Flip wig has been accessorized with a head band.

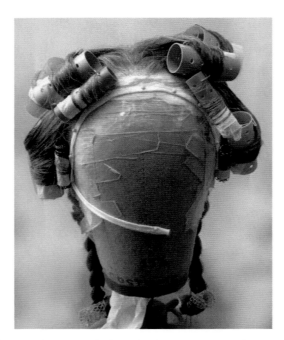
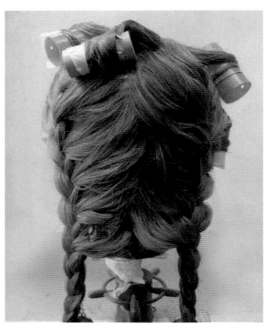

Figures 11.71 and 11.72   This "Hippie Chick" wig has been set using a combination of rollers and French braids.

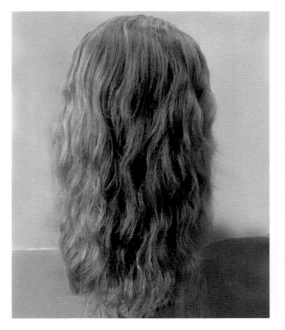
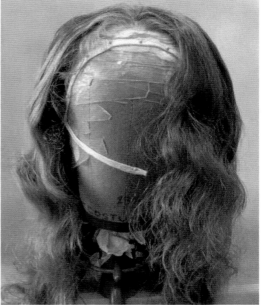

Figures 11.73 and 11.74   The finished "Hippie Chick" wig, after it has been brushed through. A lace front synthetic wig was used for this style.

1960s' Makeup

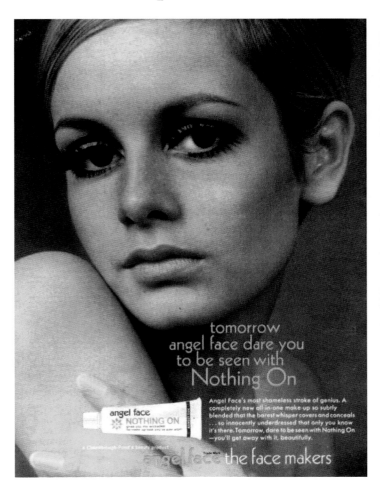

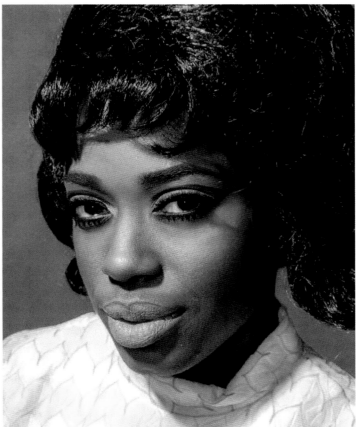

Figure 11.76 A graphic makeup look with false lashes, dramatic eyeliner, and a pale pink lipstick. Model: Antonia Taylor.

Figure 11.75 This cosmetic ad featuring British model Twiggy shows off her drawn-on eyelashes, pale blue eye shadows, and pale lip color, Twiggy/Bridgeman Images.

Makeup in the 1960s, like the hairstyles, shifted dramatically away from 1950s' looks. The focus moved from the lips to the eyes. Huge doll eyes with big eyelashes became the fad, popularized by fashion models such as Twiggy and Peggy Moffitt. False eyelashes were essential for achieving this look, and might be worn on both the top and bottom lashes. The bottom lashes might also be simply drawn on. Eyes were often defined with a sharp back line in the crease. Winged cat eye eyeliner shapes became popular. Eye shadow colors were often either black and white or pastel—this complemented the graphic mod fashion colors. Lipsticks were pale frosty pinks and peaches, flesh toned, or even white in color. Lots of powder was used to set and complete the look.

twelve

THE 1970S

$\left(1970-1979\right)$

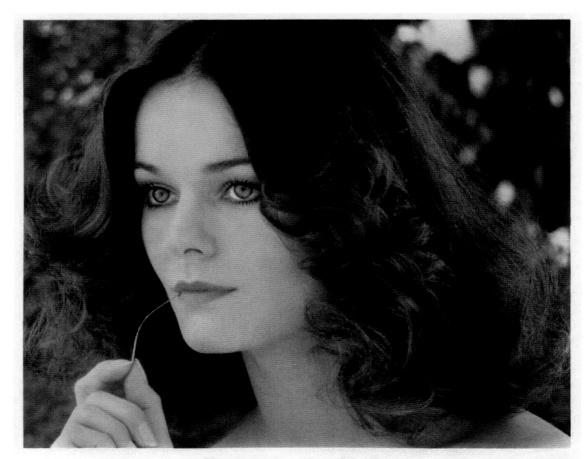

Shampooings doux Ecoflor.
Dans les plantes,ce sont les huiles essentielles qui font de beaux cheveux.

Dans les plantes, ce sont les huiles essentielles qui agissent. Ce sont elles qui ont le pouvoir de traiter la beauté de vos cheveux, en douceur et en profondeur.

Avec les huiles essentielles de plantes, Ecoflor a fait trois shampooings doux à usage fréquent, qui embellissent vos cheveux, sans agressivité ni accoutumance.

Trois shampooings doux pour chaque nature de cheveux, car Ecoflor a sélectionné des huiles essentielles : de verveine pour adoucir les cheveux secs, de cèdre et de citron pour purifier les cheveux gras, de genévrier pour assainir les cheveux à pellicules.

Ecoflor. Trois shampooings doux pour retrouver naturellement de très beaux cheveux.

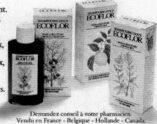

Demandez conseil à votre pharmacien.
Vendu en France - Belgique - Hollande - Canada.

Ecoflor,3 shampooings doux aux huiles essentielles de plantes.

Ogilvy & Mather

100

Figure 12.1   French advertisement for Ecoflor shampoo, 1977, PVDE/Bridgeman Images.

Important Artists/Designers

Jean-Michel Basquiat, Biba, Halston, Keith Haring, Jeff Koons, Yves Saint Laurent, Diane von Furstenberg, Vivienne Westwood

Important People/Style Icons

David Bowie, Farrah Fawcett, Debbie Harry, Lauren Hutton, Iman, Bianca Jagger, Beverly Johnson, John Travolta

1970s' Women and Men

Women in the 1970s were still embracing the more natural look that became popular in the late 1960s. Rather than being completely natural, however, the prevailing look was a more styled and "done" version of natural. Hot rollers were used on hairstyles to add volume and large curls. Actress Farrah Fawcett, one of the stars of the television show *Charlie's Angels*, was greatly admired for her feathered, sun streaked, and curled blonde hair.

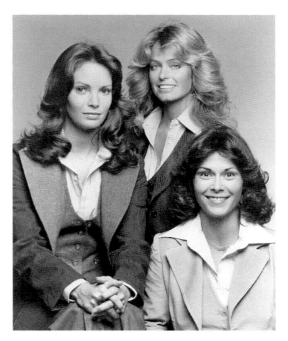

Figure 12.2   Publicity photo of the cast of the television program "Charlie's Angels", 1976. From left: Jaclyn Smith, Farrah Fawcett-Majors, and Kate Jackson. All three actresses wear the voluminous curled hair that was popular in the 1970s.

Men in the 1970s were also wearing their hair in feathered haircuts. Feathered haircuts had the hair layered on the sides and brushed back by the ears, which gave the hair a feathered appearance rather like a bird wing. This style could be worn with either a center or a side part.

Androgyny was another prevalent theme in 70s' fashions. Stars such as David Bowie (Figure 12.4) and Grace Jones helped make glam rock popular by wearing androgynous hairstyles, makeup, and elaborate

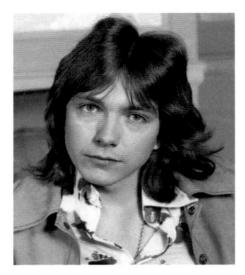

Figure 12.3   Portrait of David Cassidy taken at the Plaza Hotel New York, by Allan Warren, 1974. Pop idol Cassidy wears his hair in a feathered haircut.

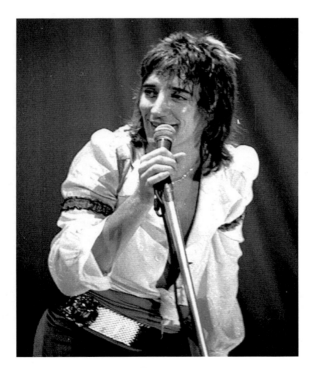

Figure 12.5   Rocker Rod Stewart, performing in Oslo, Norway, by Helge Overas, 1976.

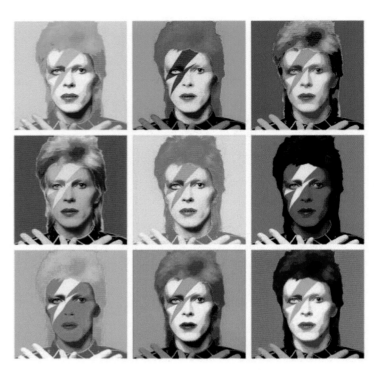

Figure 12.4   David Bowie Pop Art, by Gil Zetbase. This artistic interpretation shows off David Bowie's androgynous "Ziggy Stardust" look from 1970s.

costumes when performing. The popularity of disco and disco fashion, inspired by John Travolta in the film *Saturday Night Fever*, was another part of the androgynous look.

One particular unisex haircut was the Shag. The Shag haircut was a style that was layered all over the head and brushed forward at the crown so that the layers frame the face. Stars including Rod Stewart (Figure 12.5) and Jane Fonda wore their hair in a Shag.

The 70s was also a time in which punk fashion was gaining strength. This style originated in London and was influenced by bands such as the Sex Pistols and the New York Dolls. The idea of punk was the rebellion against established norms. Because it was based in the idea of creation amid poverty, punk looks often had a do-it-yourself quality. Hair was often dyed bright colors and styled into spiked Mohawks and Liberty Spikes.

African American women and men still favored the Afro hairstyle in the 1970s. Afros were larger than ever—the hair was allowed to grow long and a hair pick was used to pick the hair out to its full volume.

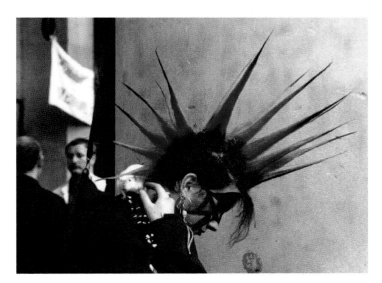

Figure 12.6 Punk girl, © by Odile Nöel, 1984, Bridgeman Images. This photograph shows an example of a punk hairstyle and fashion.

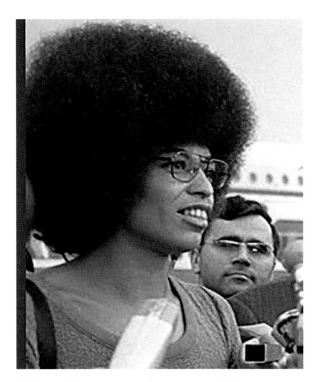

Figure 12.7 Angela Davis in Moscow, by Yuriy Ivanov, 1972.

1970s' Woman's Hot Roller Styling—Step by Step

This style is inspired by Farrah Fawcett's hairstyle, seen in Figure 12.2.

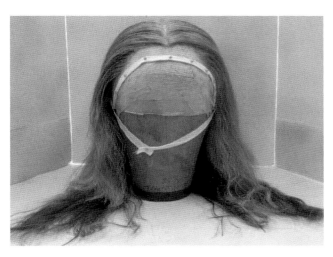

Figure 12.8 Step 1. Begin with a wig that is long in the back (at least ten inches long at the nape) with layers around the face (the layers should be four to eight inches in length). I used a fully ventilated human hair wig.

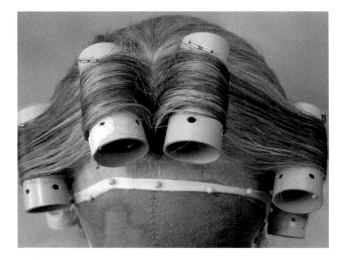

Figure 12.9 Step 2. Part the wig in the center. Wet the hair with a combination of water and setting lotion. Use quarter sized rollers to set curls on either side of the part. Continue setting rollers straight down the sides of the wig on either side of the face. If you are using a human hair wig, you could create this set with hot rollers, but I prefer the longer lasting set created by using water and heat to style the hair.

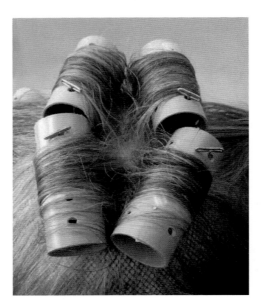

Figure 12.10 Step 3. Set two more rollers behind the ones on either side of the center part. These rollers have been set with drag at the roots in order to help create the "wing" shape at the front of the wig.

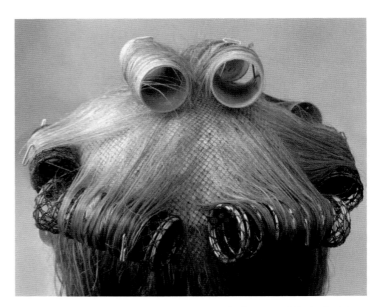

Figure 12.11 Step 4. Continue using quarter sized rollers around the back of the wig, setting them horizontally at the crown of the head.

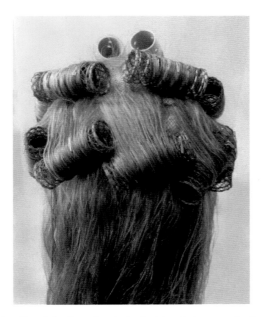

Figure 12.12 Step 5. Begin setting the back of the wig in rows going in alternating diagonal rows. The first row should be set on quarter sized rollers.

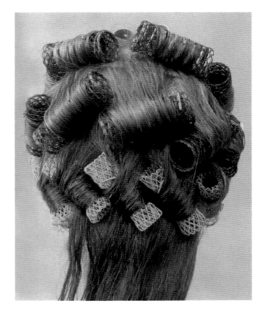

Figure 12.13 Step 6. The rest of the wig should be set on nickel sized rollers. Continue setting the hair in alternating diagonal rows.

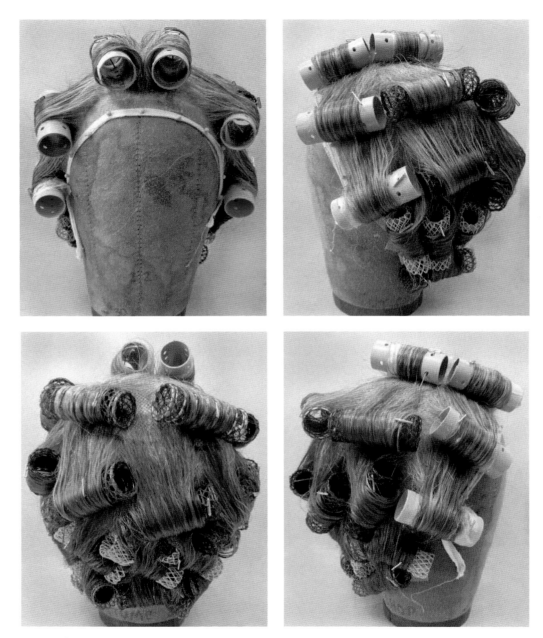

Figures 12.14–12.17   The finished 1970s' woman's Hot Roller style set.

Once you have finished setting the wig, steam each roller thoroughly if the wig is made of synthetic hair. If the wig is human hair, soak each roller with water sprayed from a spray bottle. After steaming or wetting, place the wig in a wig dryer for 75 minutes.

To style:

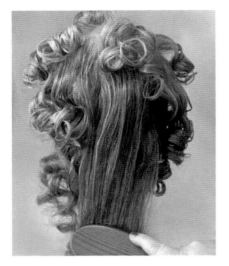

Figure 12.18 Step 7. Remove all the rollers, beginning at the nape of the neck. Brush through the entire wig with a large hairbrush. Be sure to brush very thoroughly, making sure to get the underside of the wig as well as the top side.

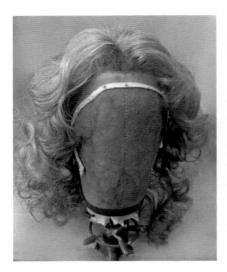
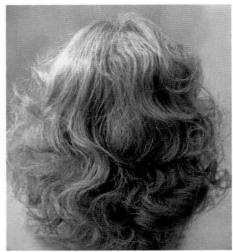

Figure 12.19 and 12.20 Step 8. Once it has been brushed out, the wig should have very soft curls all over.

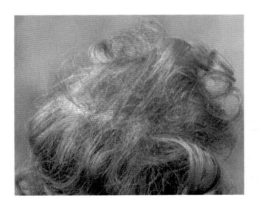

Figure 12.21 Step 9. Tease the hair at the front section of the wig on either side of the center part, and also at the crown of the wig.

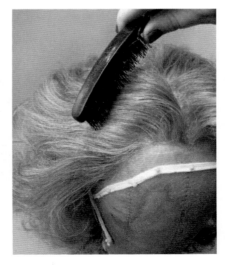

Figure 12.22 Step 10. Use a teasing/smoothing brush to smooth the teased hair back away from the face. Use your fingers to shape the waves on top. Spray with hairspray once the waves and feathers look the way you want them to.

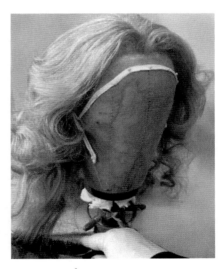

Figure 12.23 Step 11. Shape the curls at the bottom of the wig by brushing them around your fingers. Be careful not to overwork the bottom of the wig—it should still look soft.

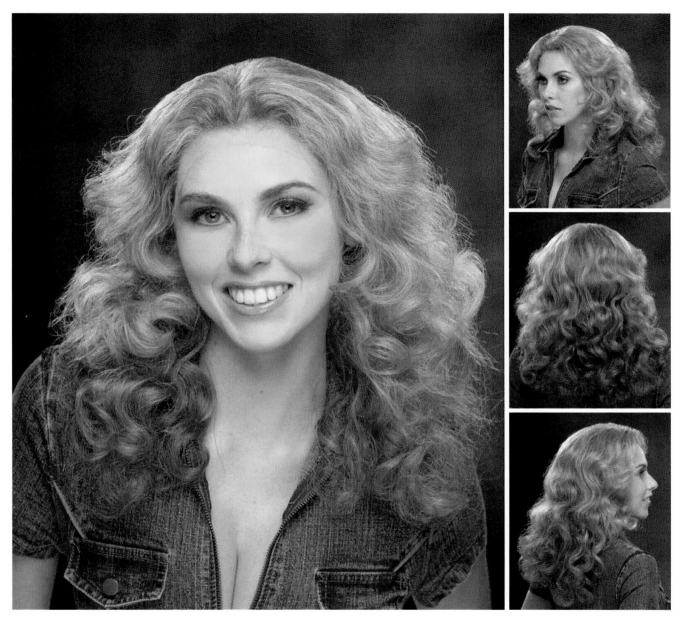

Figures 12.24–12.27 The completed 1970s' woman's Hot Roller style. Photography: Tim Babiak. Model: Emma Dirks.

1970s' Afro Styling—
Step by Step

This style was inspired by the Afro look seen in Figure 12.7.

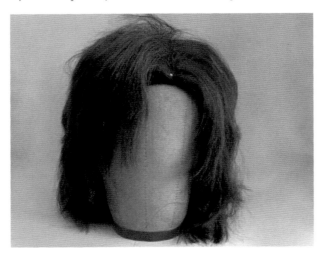

Figure 12.28   Step 1. Begin with a wig that is layered to be about the same length all over. The longer the hair is, the larger your finished Afro will be. I used a synthetic hard front wig with layers that were about five inches long all over the head.

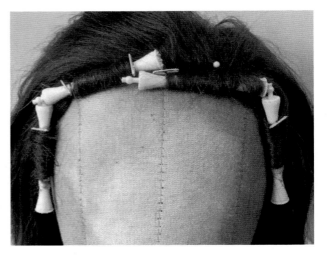

Figure 12.29   Step 2. Set the front of the wig going forwards towards the face on the tiniest perm rods you can find. This will help conceal the hard front edge of the wig.

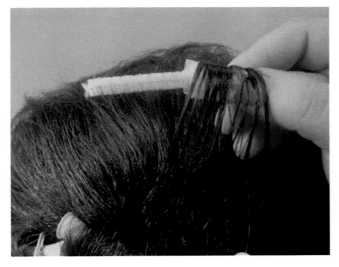

Figure 12.30   Step 3. After setting the front row of curls going towards the face, set the rest of the wig with the rollers going away from the face. If you do not have perm rods, you can also set the wig using pipe cleaners as rollers. Use an endpaper and roll the hair onto the pipe cleaner just like you would roll it on a perm rod.

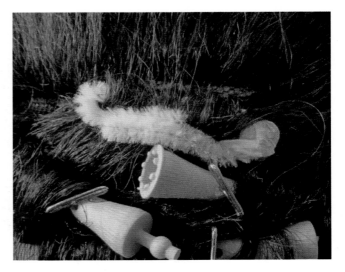

Figure 12.31   Step 4. Once you have rolled the pipe cleaner all the way to the roots, simply bend the ends of the pipe cleaner in towards the center. This will anchor the pipe cleaner roller in place.

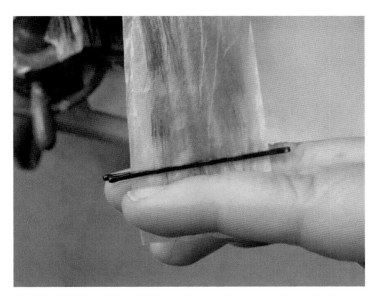

Figure 12.32 Step 5. Yet another setting method you can use is to set the hair on bobby pins. This produces the tiniest possible curl, and it especially useful around the edges of the wig. I find large size bobby pins easier to use as rollers, but regular sized ones are excellent for making very tight curls. Use an endpaper to hold the ends of the hair together. Slide the endpaper and hair inside the bobby pin and roll it up as you would a regular roller.

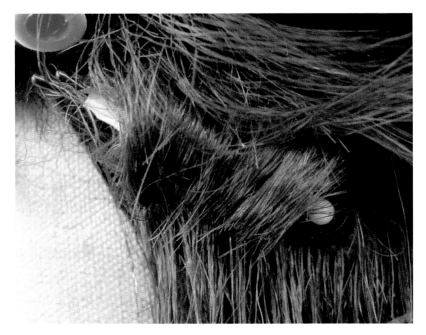

Figure 12.33 Step 6. Once you have rolled the hair to the root on the bobby pin, pin it in place with a blocking pin.

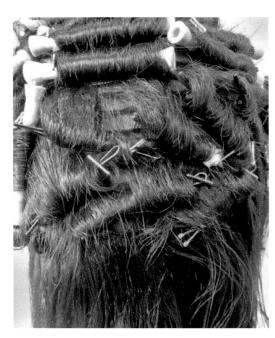

Figure 12.34 Step 7. Large bobby pins have been used to set part of the back of this wig.

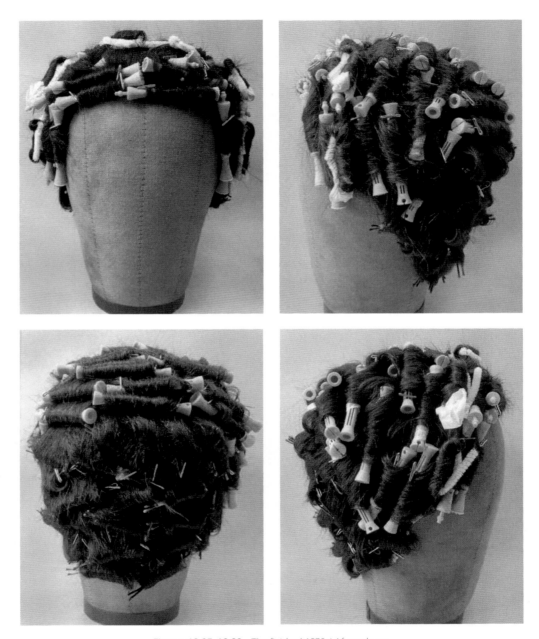

Figures 12.35–12.38   The finished 1970s' Afro style set.

Once you have finished setting the wig, steam each roller thoroughly if the wig is made of synthetic hair. If the wig is human hair, soak each roller with water sprayed from a spray bottle. After steaming or wetting, place the wig in a wig dryer for 75 minutes.

To style:

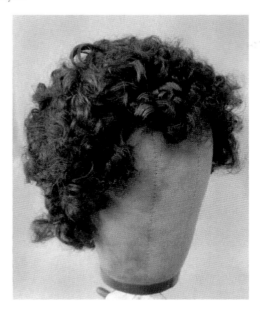

Figure 12.39 Step 8. Remove all rollers, pipe cleaners, and bobby pins from the wig, beginning at the nape of the neck. Take your time doing this—rollers this small can sometimes be tricky to unroll without tangling the hair.

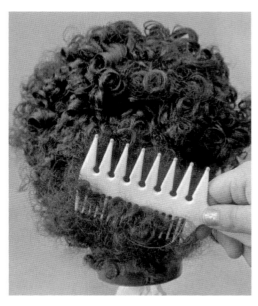

Figure 12.40 Step 9. Use a wide toothed comb to begin picking out the curls. Again, take your time and be sure that you comb through every curl.

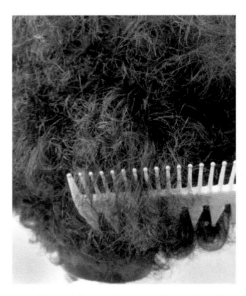

Figure 12.41 Step 10. Comb from both the top of the curl and from the underside. This will make sure that the curls are completely fluffed out.

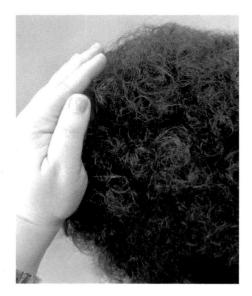

Figure 12.42 Step 11. Once you have the entire wig picked out, mist it with hairspray and pat the hair in place, working to create a round shape.

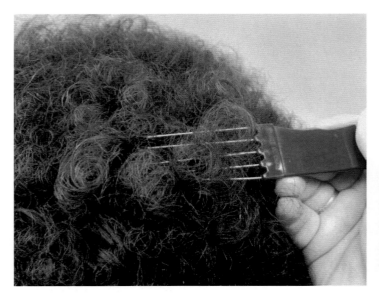

Figure 12.43   Step 12. Use a wire pick to create extra lift in the wig where you need it.

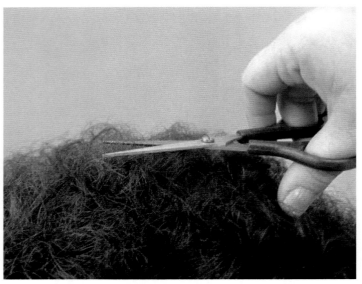

Figure 12.44   Step 13. You may need to trim some hairs in the wig in order to create the perfect round Afro shape.

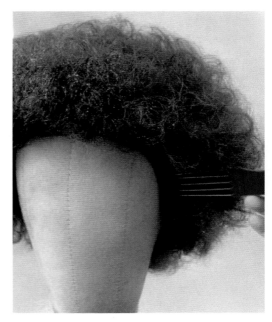

Figure 12.45   Step 14. Integrate that hair that was set going towards the face with the hair that was set going away from the face by combing through both sections with the wire pick. When the wig is the overall shape that you desire, thoroughly spray it with hairspray.

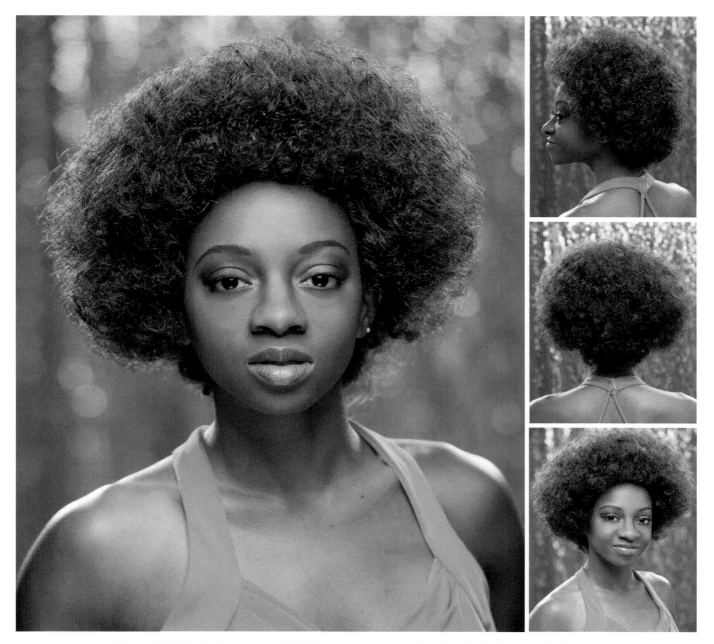

Figures 12.46–12.49 The completed 1970s' Afro style. Photography: Tim Babiak. Model: Marsherrie Madkins.

Variations

For your 1970s' styles, you can create different looks by adding bangs to some of your wigs. You can also use accessories to help establish the period. For example, silk scarves were very popular in the 70s, so you can add head wraps to change up your looks.

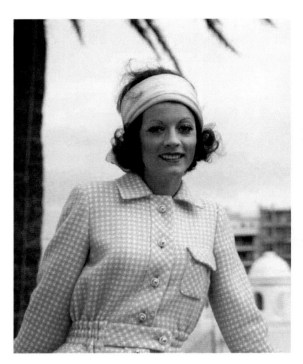

Figure 12.50   A fashion model photographed in Spain, Canary Islands, 1973. Fortepan photograph. This model shows off the popular 1970s trend of wearing a head scarf.

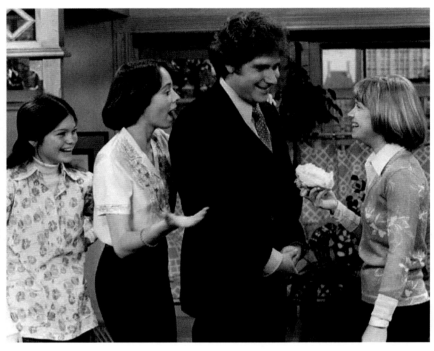

Figure 12.51   A photo of the main cast of the television program One Day at a Time. From left-Valerie Bertinelli (Barbara), MacKenzie Phillips (Julie), Richard Masur (David Kane), Bonnie Franklin (Ann Romano). Masur played Romano's boyfriend in the show's first season. 2 April 1976, CBS Television. Phillips and Franklin both wear examples of shorter 1970s hairstyles.

1970s' Makeup

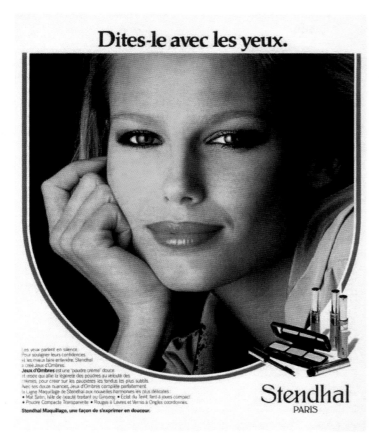

Figure 12.52 French advertisement for Stendhal make up, Paris, 1977,/ PVDE/ Bridgeman Images.

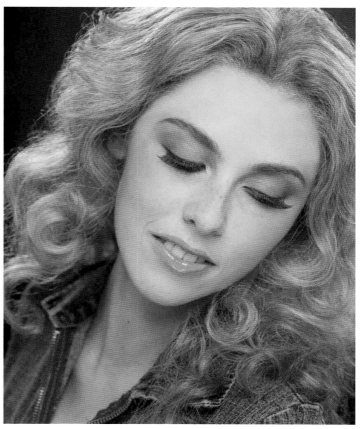

Figure 12.53 The blue eye shadow and orange lipstick made popular in the 1970s. Model: Emma Dirks.

In the 1970s, psychedelic colors and graphic shapes were replaced with warm colors and gloss. A tanned, sun kissed look became extremely popular. Blush, lip gloss, and lipstick were often found in tones of orange, bronze, coral, and tangerine. Frosty blue eyeshadow dominated other colors in popularity. False eyelashes were still worn to give the wearer the appearance of large, bright eyes, but they became a bit more natural in shape. The rise of disco fashion also brought with it glittery makeup.

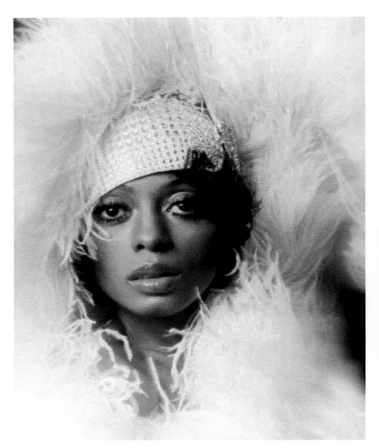

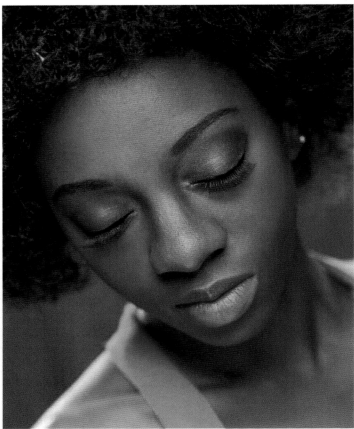

Figure 12.54 Photograph of Diana Ross in the film *Mahogany*, 1975, © Motown Productions/Nikor Productions/Paramount Pictures/Diltz/Bridgeman Images. In the photo, Diana Ross wears blue eye shadow, large wide eye lashes, and a glossy lip.

Figure 12.55 A close up of the bronzed 1970s' look. Model: Marsherrie Madkins.

thirteen

THE 1980S
TO THE PRESENT

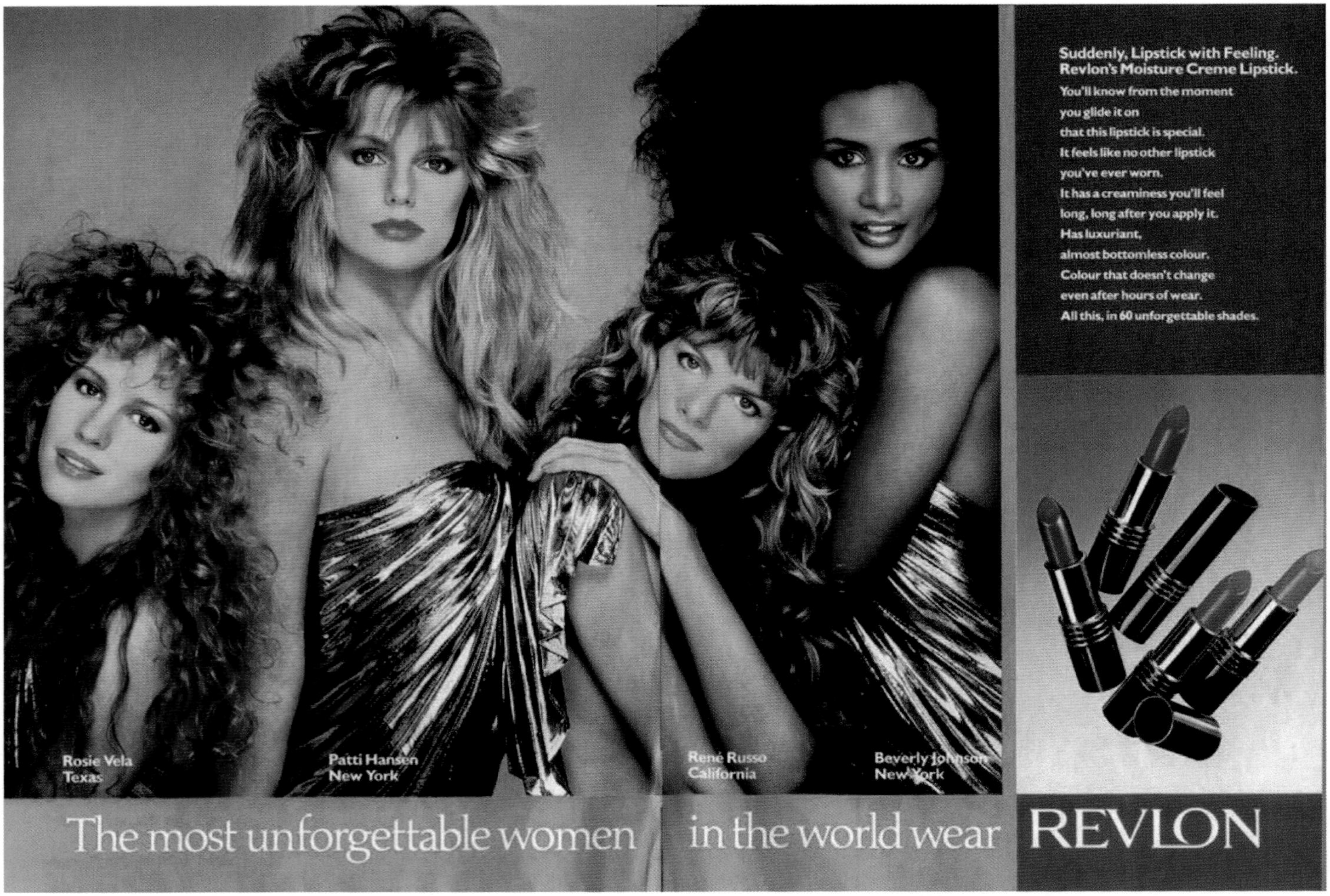

Figure 13.1 Advertisement in *Revlon* magazine advert, 1980s, © Advertising Archives/Bridgeman Images. The models in this ad wear a great variety of big 1980s' hairstyles.

Important Events

1980	John Lennon is assassinated
1981	MTV is launched
1989	The Berlin Wall is torn down
1990	Nelson Mandela is released from prison in South Africa
1998	Apple introduces the iMac computer
2001	Jets crash into and destroy the World Trade Center
2008	Barack Obama is the first African American elected as President of the United States
2015	US Supreme Court allows same sex marriage

Important Artists/Designers

1980s:	Jean Paul Gaultier, Calvin Klein, Ralph Lauren, Donna Karan
1990s:	John Galliano, Tommy Hilfiger, Michael Kors, Stella McCartney, Alexander McQueen, Gianni Versace, Vera Wang
2000s:	Banksy, Tom Ford, Marc Jacobs, Yayoi Kusama, Karl Lagerfeld, Takashi Murakami

Important People/Style Icons

1980s:	Princess Diana, Linda Evangelista, Jane Fonda, Michael Jackson, Madonna, Brooke Shields
1990s:	Jennifer Aniston, Cindy Crawford, Kate Moss, Gwyneth Paltrow, Julia Roberts
2000s:	Victoria Beckham, Beyoncé, Gisele Bundchen, Lady Gaga, the Kardashian/Jenner sisters, Jennifer Lopez, Rihanna

1980s' Women and Men

The 1980s was decade of excess, of money and power, and of artificial glamor. Women's hairstyles continued to grow bigger and curlier. Permed hair became common as many women pursued curly hair that they were not born with. Figure 13.01 is an example of the full, curled 1980s' styles. Pop stars such as Madonna were famous for their wild, unkempt hair, often featuring obvious color at the roots. Color was an important part of 1980s' hair look—people were bleaching their hair lighter or adding unnatural colors to create a mainstream look influenced by punk. Singer Cyndi Lauper is a good example of this trend.

1980s' hairstyles also often required teasing in addition to perming. Bangs, in particular, were subject to curling, teasing, and spraying in order to achieve the desired look. Curly side ponytails had their moment in fashion, influenced by the popularity of aerobics inspired fashion.

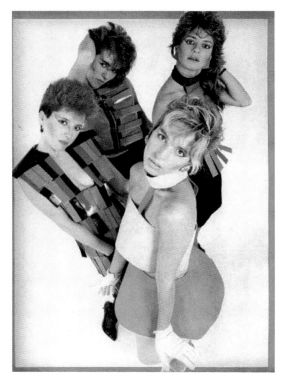

Figure 13.2   Musicians in the Argentinian rock band Viuda e Hijas de Roque Enroll (Widow and Daughters of Roque Enroll), *Pelo* magazine, 1986. The band members wear a variety of wild hair and makeup looks.

Short hairstyles became popular in the 1980s, inspired partly by Princess Diana's short, thick, feathered hairstyle. Some women, influenced by the idea of 80s' power dressing and the trend of menswear for women, took short hairstyles to the extreme and created, stiff, sprayed masculine looks.

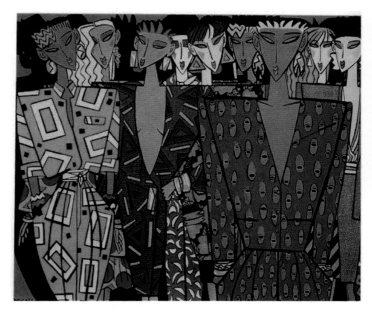

Figure 13.3   This illustration by Joel Resnicoff from 1985 shows the short spiky hairstyles, bright colors, and wide shoulder pads that made up 1980s' androgynous power dressing.

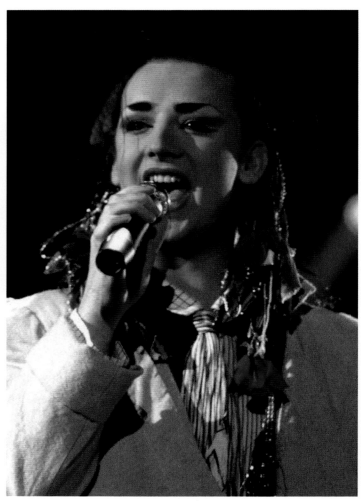

Figure 13.4   Boy George singing, © by Lynn McAfee/Bridgeman Images.

1980s' men's hair was not that different from women's hair wore at that time. Men were also using hair products like mousse and getting perms in order for their hair to be as big and curly as possible. The idea of androgyny in appearance was still going strong, featured by musicians such as Culture Club lead singer Boy George (Figure 13.04), who performed in full makeup and elaborate hairstyles. The popularity of "hair bands"—Poison, Mötley Crüe, Def Leppard—also helped make long permed hair a trend for men. Bands such as Flock of Seagulls made asymmetrical hairstyles with sweeping waves and a heavy sprayed bang popular. Other men wore shorter versions of the 1980s' fluffy, waved styles. Actor Tom Selleck, from the television show *Magnum P.I.*, helped make the heavy mustache popular for men.

1980s' Permed Hair Styling— Step by Step

The reference picture for this wig was the hair on the models in Figure 13.1.

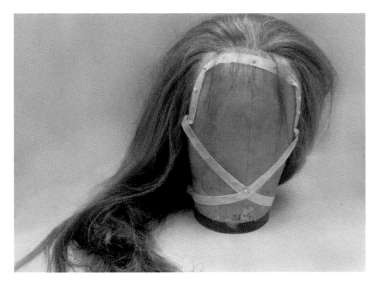

Figure 13.5 Step 1. Begin with a wig that is long in the back (at least 12 inches long at the nape of the neck) with bangs in the front. I used a long lace front synthetic wig with bangs.

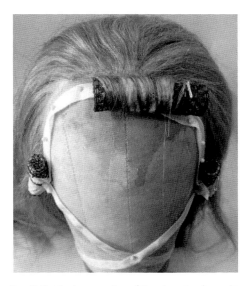

Figure 13.6 Step 2. Set the bang section of the wig going forward towards the face on a nickel sized roller. Small tendrils of hair have also been set in front of each ear.

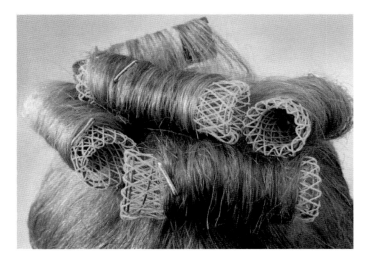

Figure 13.7 Step 3. Continue using nickel sized rollers to set the hair just behind the bangs going back away from the face. Make sure to offset the rollers so that there will not be gaps when you brush out the wig later.

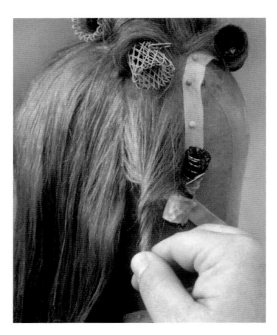 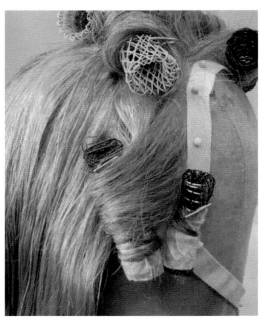

Figures 13.8 and 13.9 Step 4. The rest of the wig will be set using the spiral curl setting technique. Twist each section of hair before rolling it onto a dime sized roller. Begin with the hair at the bottom of the roller and spiral it up around the roller as you set the hair.

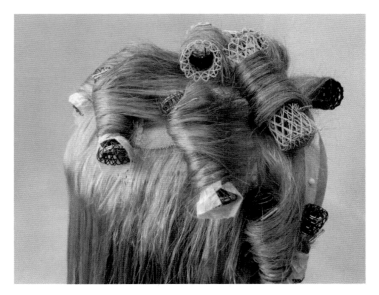 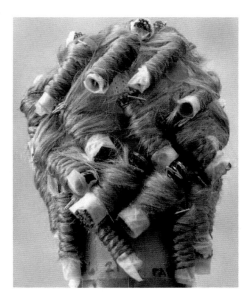

Figure 13.10 Step 5. Continue setting the spiral curls up over the crown of the wig.

Figure 13.11 Step 6. Set the rest of the wig in spiral curls going in alternating diagonal rows. Use pencil sized rollers to create extra tight curls at the crown of the wig and around the nape of the wig.

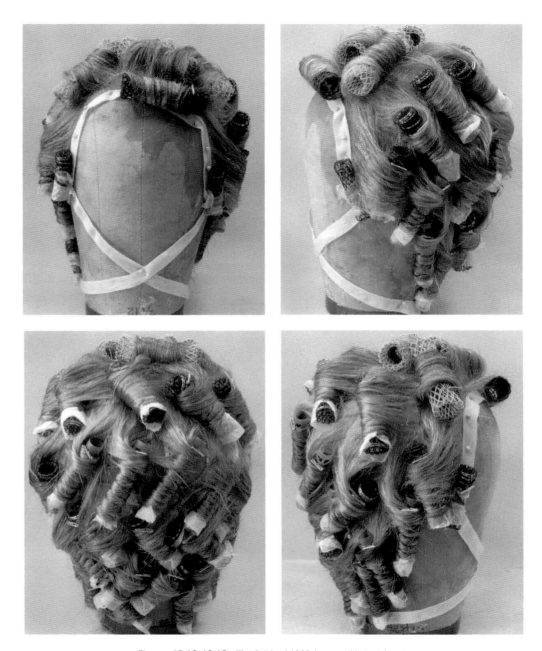

Figures 13.12–13.15 The finished 1980s' permed hair style set.

Once you have finished setting the wig, steam each roller thoroughly if the wig is made of synthetic hair. If the wig is human hair, soak each roller with water sprayed from a spray bottle. After steaming or wetting, place the wig in a wig dryer for 75 minutes.

To style:

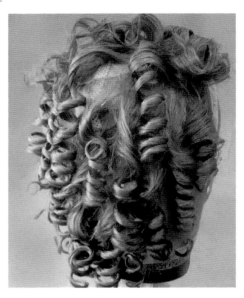

Figure 13.16   Step 7. Remove all the rollers from the wig, beginning at the nape. Be sure the carefully unwind each of the spiral curls.

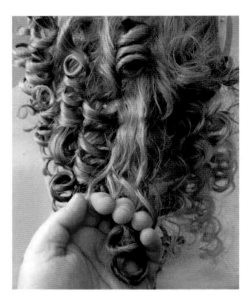

Figure 13.17   Step 8. Use your fingers to gently comb through each spiral curl.

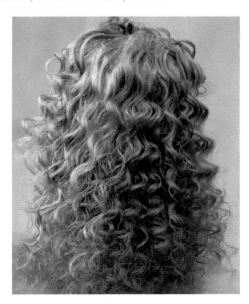

Figure 13.18   Step 9. The back of the wig, after each spiral curl has been finger combed. If there are any breaks in between the curls, use a very wide toothed comb to blend the curls together. This should only be done at the roots of the hair—do not comb all the way down to the ends of the hair. Spray with hair spray.

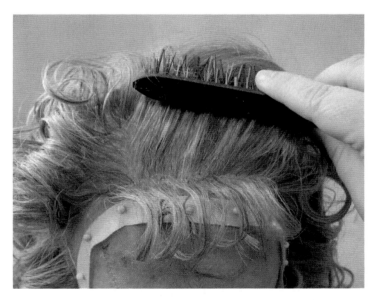

Figure 13.19   Step 10. Move to the front of the wig and brush out the front section with a teasing/smoothing brush.

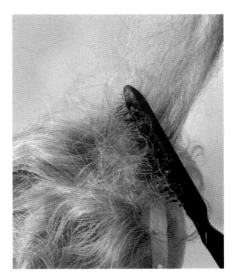
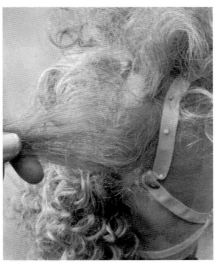

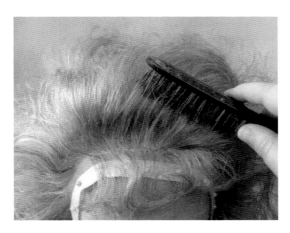

Figure 13.22   Step 12. Smooth the hair back away from the face with the brush. Again, mist the front with hairspray.

Figures 13.20 and 13.21   Step 11. Tease the front and side front sections of the wig. Mist with hairspray.

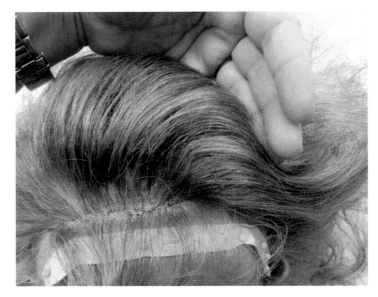

Figure 13.23   Step 13. Use your hand to push a large wave into the front of the wig.

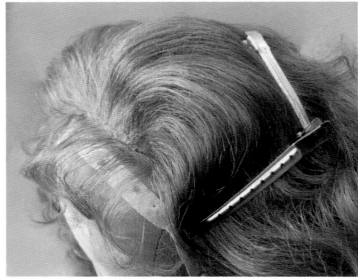

Figure 13.24   Step 14. Hold the waves in place with duckbill clips.

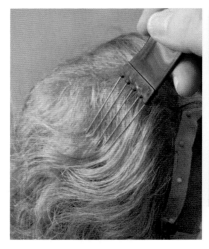

Figure 13.25 Step 15. Use a wire pick to help you shape the waves on the side of the wig around the face.

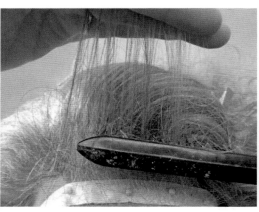

Figure 13.26 Step 16. Tease the bangs of the wig.

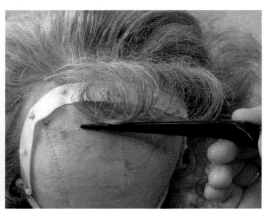

Figure 13.27 Step 17. Smooth the teased hair forward onto the face. Use the end of your brush to push the curls into place.

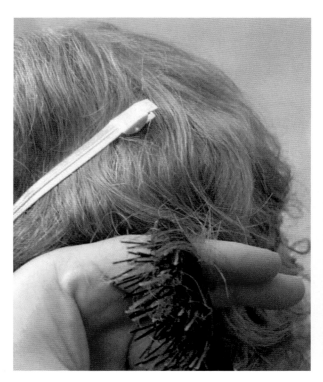

Figure 13.28 Step 18. If necessary, finish off the hair in the front section by brush the curls around your finger.

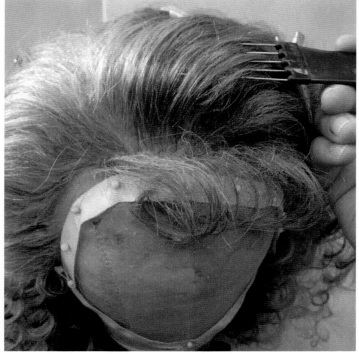

Figure 13.29 Step 19. If you want extra lift in the wig, use a wire pick to lift the hair up front the root. Spray the wig liberally with hairspray when you are done.

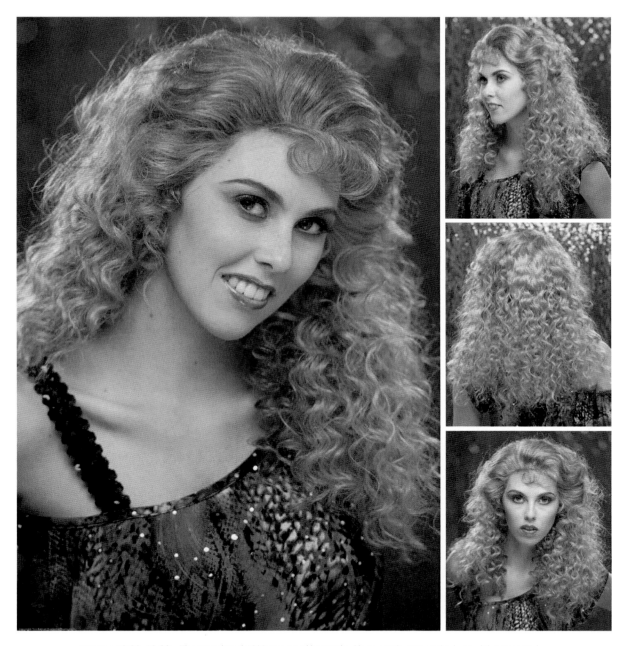

Figures 13.30–13.33   The completed 1980s' permed hair style. Photography: Tim Babiak. Model: Emma Dirks.

Variations

For your 1980s' styles, once again accessories can help you create variety. Accent your wig with brightly colored scrunchies, black lace hair bows, or colorful headbands. Pull part of the wig up into a small ponytail for a half up/half down look. You could pull all the hair into a side ponytail. Vary the texture of your 1980s' wig by combing through the entire wig to create a much frizzier overall look. You can also add roots to a light colored wig using markers in a dark brown color to color in the first few inches of the hair. You can add more extreme colors to your wigs by using temporary colored hairsprays, available at many beauty supply stores.

There are many premade wigs available at wig stores that are great versions of 1980s' and 1990s' hairstyles straight out of the box. Adding accessories to the readymade styles help add individual character to each look. Visit cosplay supply websites for ready to wear versions of popular character hairstyles. Wigs are also becoming more widely available in a rainbow of wild colors, so it is easy to find whatever wild color combo you want without having to dye the wig yourself. Yet another way you can add bright colors to wigs is to sew in streaks of brightly colored wefting. This is especially useful when you only want sections of color in a wig, not color all over the head.

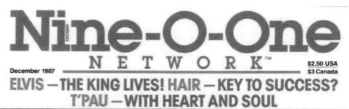

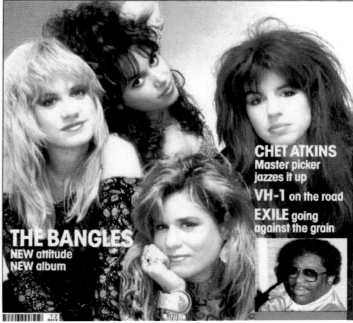

Figure 13.34 Musician Lisa Lisa performs with Full Force and Cult Jam in Ithaca New York, 1987. Photograph by Kenneth C. Zirkel. Her headband and spiky permed hair are very typical of 1980s hair

Figure 13.35 Nine-O-One Network Magazine Cover featuring the Bangles, December 1987.

1980s' Makeup

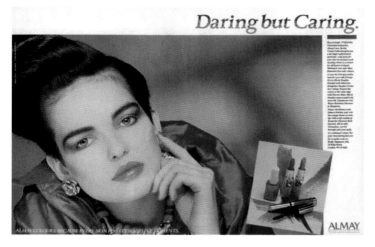

Figure 13.36 Advertisement in *Almay* magazine, 1980s, © Advertising Archives/ Bridgeman Images. This ad is a great example of the bold colors used in 1980s' makeup.

1980s' makeup was bold and colorful. All the features of the face were given equal attention. Blush was very popular and often applied in bold stripes on the cheeks in colors like coral and hot pink. Every color of the rainbow was available in eye shadow, with neon colors being especially popular. This application was not subtle either— the eye shadow was often applied winging past the eye into the temples. Black eyeliner was still popular, but colors such as teal and purple were also commonly seen. Lips were usually brightly colored and glossy.

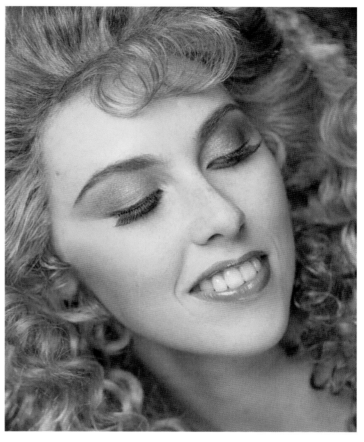

Figure 13.37 A 1980s' look featuring bright tropical colors. Model: Emma Dirks.

1990s'–Present Women and Men

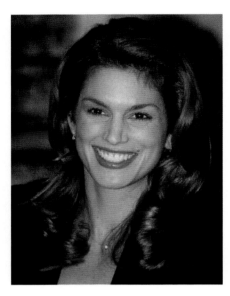

Figure 13.38   Supermodel Cindy Crawford in Washington DC, 1995.

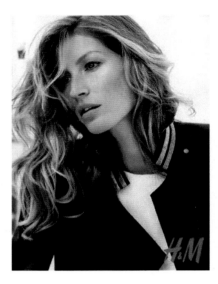

Figure 13.39   Model Gisele Bundchen in an advert in *Hennes* magazine, 2010s, © Advertising Archives/Bridgeman Images.

Far and away, the most popular 1990s' haircut for women was "the Rachel," as worn by Jennifer Aniston's character in the television show *Friends*. This haircut featured dramatic face framing layers, accented by the actress's blonde highlights. The 1990s was the era of the supermodel. Supermodels were some of the most important style setters at this time. Models including Cindy Crawford (Figure 13.37) and Linda Evangelista were wearing curled, sculpted hairstyles that still bore some influence from the 1980s. Long, straight center parted hair was also popular in the 1990s. Made popular by stars such as Gwyneth Paltrow and Naomi Campbell, this look often required a flat iron to achieve. Women would painstakingly straighten their hair so that it would lie perfectly flat with no hint of wave or curl. Later in the 1990s, supermodel Kate Moss gained great popularity modeling for Calvin Klein. She helped usher in the "grunge" era in fashion, where hair was worn very simply and a bit unkempt, often with obvious roots. 1990s' makeup shifted dramatically, partly due to the influence of makeup artist Kevyn Aucoin. He helped create the neutral colored look, full of flesh tones, greys, raisin, and tawny browns that dominated the face of this decade.

In the 2000s, fuller hair regained popularity, inspired by models such as Gisele Bundchen (Figure 13.39) and the Victoria's Secret

Angels. The idea was for hair to have a sexier and more natural look, as though the woman had spent a day at the beach and her hair just happened to end up looking full and glamorous. Many texturing salt sprays were created to help women achieve this look.

Hip-hop music greatly influenced men's hairstyles in the 1990s. The hi-top fade (an African American men's style that was shaved almost to the skin on the sides and allowed to grow very tall on top and then sculpted into a geometric shape) was made popular by the band Kid-n-Play. Grunge hairstyles, long unkempt hair, were worn by rock stars such as Kurt Cobain. Men in the 1990s and 2000s often wore their hair in cornrows and dreadlocks. (These styles were traditionally African, but were worn by people of all races at this time.)

In the present day, contemporary hair features a lot of razor cutting (for jagged edges), and extreme hair colors. New hair dyes make it possible for hair to be any color of the rainbow. "Emo" rock bands such as My Chemical Romance helped create a dark, dyed black spiky Gothic inspired look for hair (Figure 13.41). Rockabilly fashions for both men and women feature hairstyles that are a throwback to the 1940s and 50s, with women wearing their hair in Victory rolls and Bettie Page bangs, and men wearing sculpted pompadours. Pop stars such as Lady Gaga (Figure 13.42), Nicki Minaj (Figure 13.43), and Beyoncé have made the wearing of outrageous wigs popular again. Hipster men of today often wear scraggly longish hair with beards. There is a strong Japanese influence in fashion as well, with anime inspired looks, cosplay, and extreme looks worn in the harajuku district of Tokyo inspiring fashion around the world.

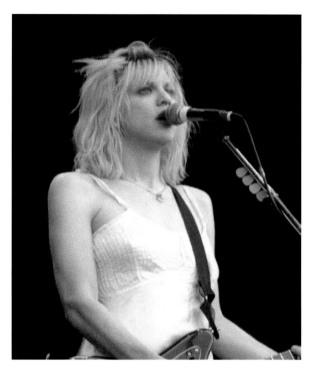

Figure 13.40 Courtney Love, lead singer of Hole, singing and playing electric guitar at Phoenix Festival, © by Toby Jacobs/Bridgeman Images. Love is an example of grunge fashion.

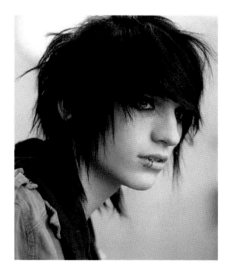

Figure 13.41 Emo hairstyle, by DanielRo9696, April 2018.

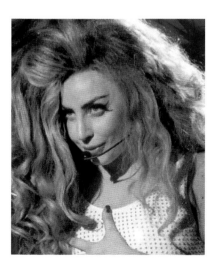

Figure 13.42 Closeup of Lady Gaga in concert at Roseland, by Aphrodite-in-NYC, 2014.

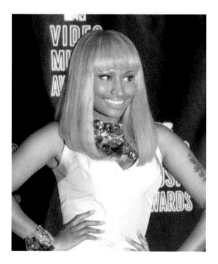

Figure 13.43 Nicki Minaj at the MTV Video Music Awards, by Philip Nelson, 2010. Nicki is wearing one of her trademark colorful wigs.

1990s'–Present Makeup

Contemporary makeup has swung back around to being a full face of makeup. As we enter the era of the selfie and social media, people feel the need to be camera ready at all times. A full face of foundation, with heavy contouring to emphasize or transform the shape of the face can been seen all over Instagram. Elaborate eye makeup designs feature a dramatically defined crease line, liberal use of color, glitter highlighting, and a heavy false eyelash. Even lips are contoured, with new shapes being drawn in using highlights, shadow, and accenting gloss.

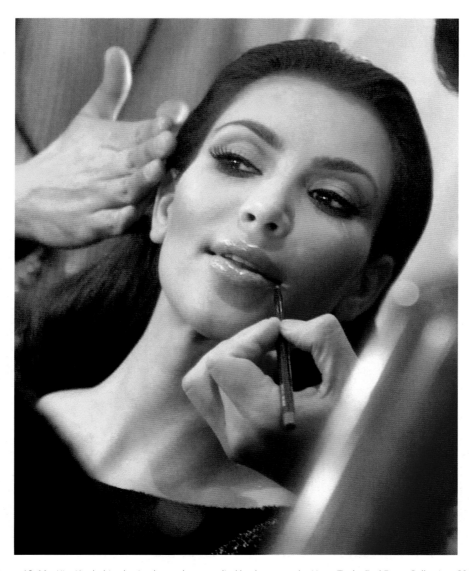

Figure 13.44   Kim Kardashian having her makeup applied backstage at the Heart Truths Red Dress Collection, 2010.

fourteen

NON-WESTERN HAIRSTYLING

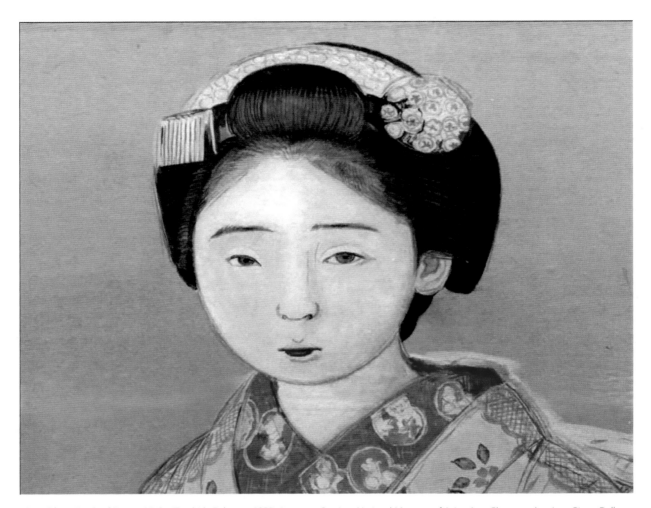

Figure 14.1   Detail from *Study of Dancer Maiko*, Tsuchida Bakusen, 1923, Japanese Section, National Museum of Asian Arts. Photography: Jean-Pierre Dalbera.

Non-Western Hair

For the purposes of this book, I have been focusing primarily on Western fashion, hair, and history. There are obviously many other cultures all over the globe that have their own unique traditions in hairstyles, dress, and culture. This could be another whole book in and of itself! Some of the hairstyles of these cultures are very elaborate; other styles are much simpler and might consist of simple braids or loose hair. Still others are much more focused on headdresses or other hair coverings, leaving the hair itself very simple. There is a wealth of research out there available to assist you in creating a global look for your characters (or for inspiring unique fictional cultures). I have chosen to discuss in detail two non-Western looks that come up often when I am working on plays and operas: the geisha hairstyle, and African tribal hairstyles.

Important Events

2070 BC	Yu the Great establishes the Xia Dynasty in China
660 BC	Supposed date of the accession of Jimmu, the mythical first emperor of Japan
550 BC	Foundation of the Persian Empire by Cyrus the Great
202 BC	Han Dynasty established in China; the Silk Road opens in this period, establishing trade between China and the West
570	Muhammad, the Islamic prophet, is born
1099	First Crusade, in which Jerusalem is retaken from the Muslims
1206	Genghis Khan is elected Khagan of the Mongols and the Mongol Empire is established
1258	Siege of Baghdad, considered the end of the Islamic Golden Age
1325	Tenochtitlan, the capital of the Aztec Empire, is founded
1502	First reported African slaves in the New World
1548	The Ming Dynasty in China issues a decree banning all foreign trade
1707	Mount Fuji erupts in Japan
1828	Shaka, king of the Zulus, is assassinated
1859–1869	The Suez Canal is built in Egypt
1872	Western dress is prescribed for official ceremonies in Japan
1994	Nelson Mandela becomes president of South Africa

Geisha Hairstyles

Geisha are traditional, female Japanese entertainers. (Interestingly, some of the first geisha were men, who entertained customers waiting to see popular courtesans.) Geisha specialize in many fine arts, including dance, calligraphy, classical music performance, poetry, and performing many traditional Japanese ceremonies. By the 1830s, geisha style began to be emulated by fashionable women throughout society. World War II brought a huge decline to the geisha arts, because many women had to go to work to rebuild their war torn country.

There are multiple stages and ranks within geisha culture. A *maiko* is an apprentice geisha and is bonded under contract to her *okiya* (geisha house). The *okiya* supplies the *maiko* with food, shelter, clothing, and other tools of the trade. Traditional *maiko* hair and makeup is often what people think of when they think of the image of the geisha. *Maiko* wear a version of the *shimada*, a hairstyle that is similar to a chignon. This hairstyle is pulled back in the center front, sticking out wide on the sides of the face before it is pulled back and elaborately dressed in the back, depending on the age and rank of the geisha. Wax or pomade was used to give the hair a perfectly smooth appearance.

Maiko also wear traditional white makeup, with two or three bare strips left at the nape of the neck, considered to be a highly erotic area (visible in Figure 14.3).

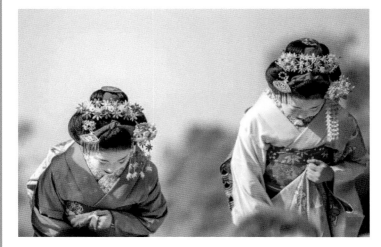

Figure 14.2 Chion-in maiko, by Norio Nakayama. The elaborate hairstyles can be clearly seen in this photograph.

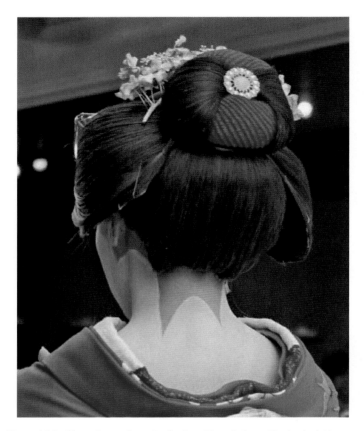

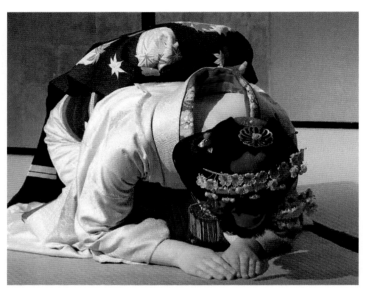

Figure 14.4   Detail of the wareshinobu hairstyle from the top, by Elmarte74.

Figure 14.3   The makeup of a maiko, by Jean-Pierre Dalbera. The back of this hairstyle is simple and shows off the back of the neck and the makeup on the nape of the neck.

One hairstyle, called *momoware*, or "split peach," is worn only by *maiko* (Figure 14.4). Traditionally, a geisha's own hair was dressed in these styles at least once a week; modern geishas often wear wigs instead. (The tight heavy hairstyling led many geishas to develop bald spots.)

Shimada are decorated with *kanzashi*, elaborate hair combs and hairpins (see Figures 14.2 and 14.5). These come in an enormous variety—sometimes the decorations are chosen to be appropriate to the season of the year. Others signify what house and area a geisha is from by their colors and styles.

As a geisha gains experience, she moves up in rank. Once she becomes a geisha, her hairstyle and makeup become much more subdued.

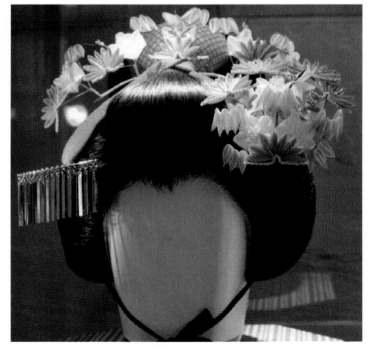

Figure 14.5   January kanzashi for maiko (geisha apprentice) with pine, bamboo, plum, Kanawa Kuniko, Atelier Kanawa.

Geisha Styling— Step by Step

This hairstyle is inspired by the traditional *maiko* hairstyle.

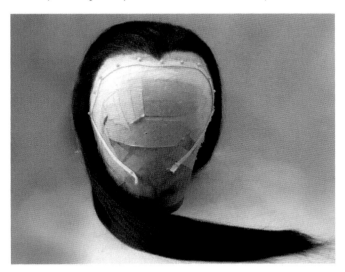

Figure 14.6 Step 1. Begin with a long, thick, black lace front wig (at least 16 inches long at the nape of the neck). I used a wig made from synthetic hair. Unlike most other hairstyles, a geisha wig does not need to be set on rollers. You can go directly to the styling process.

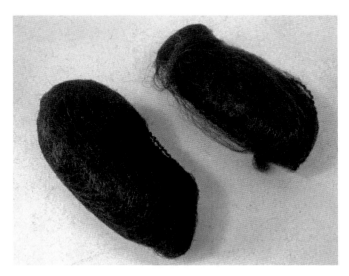

Figure 14.7 Step 2. You will also need some black hair rats or pads (at least three inches long and one and a half inches wide) to create this style.

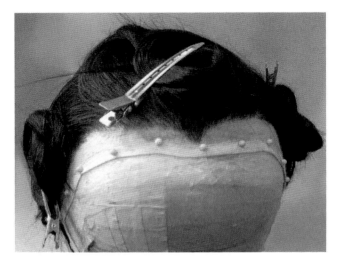

Figure 14.8 Step 3. Divide the front of the wig into three sections—the center front, and right and left sides.

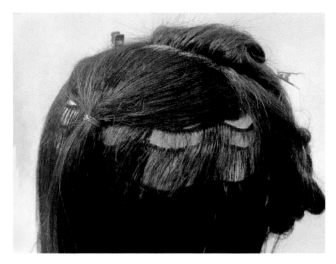

Figure 14.9 Step 4. Pull a section of hair at the crown of the head into a small ponytail.

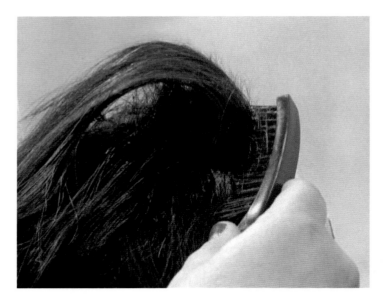

Figure 14.10   Step 5. Move to the center front section of the wig. Tease the hair at the roots.

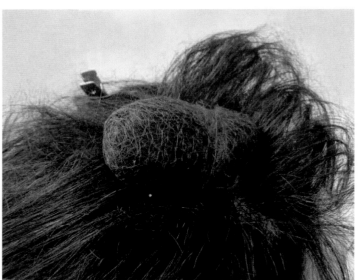

Figure 14.11   Step 6. You may also need to use a small hair pad under this section, depending on the size and shape you wish to create in the finished style.

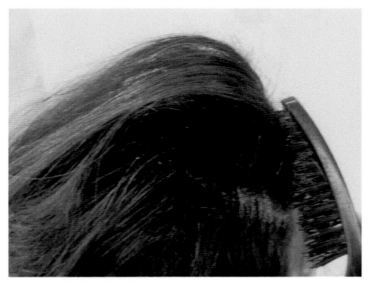

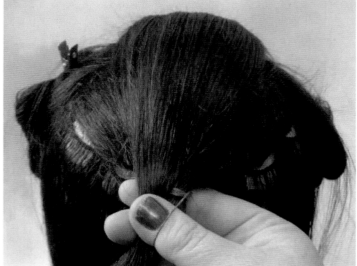

Figures 14.12 and 14.13   Step 7. Once you have created volume in this section, smooth the hair with your smoothing brush back towards the first ponytail you created. Add the hair to the ponytail, putting a second rubber band around the first.

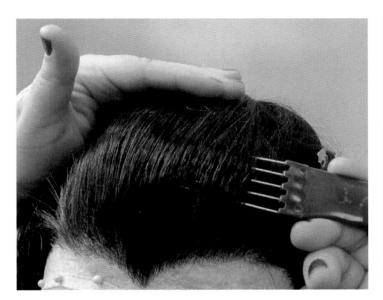

Figure 14.14 Step 8. Use your wire lifting comb to add more height to this section if desired.

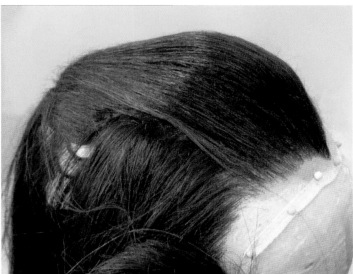

Figure 14.15 Step 9. Side view of the finished center front section.

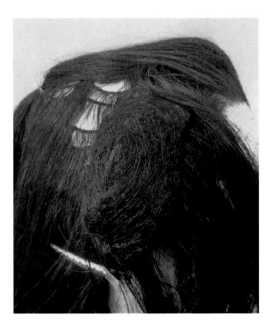

Figure 14.16 Step 10. Comb the hair in one of the side sections forward onto the face. Tease the section at the roots. Place one of your larger hair pads vertically along this section and pin it in place with bobby pins.

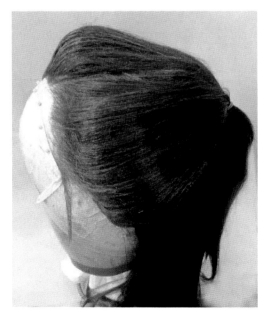

Figure 14.17 Step 11. Pull this section of hair back over the hair pad towards the ponytail at the crown of the head, covering the hair pad completely. Use another rubber band to join this hair to the original ponytail. Spray the section with hairspray and smooth it with your teasing/smoothing brush until the hair is lying very neatly.

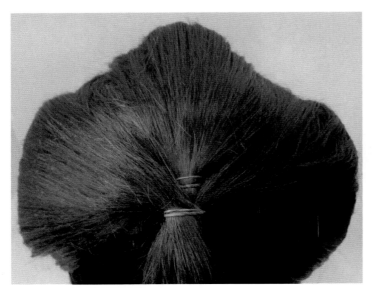

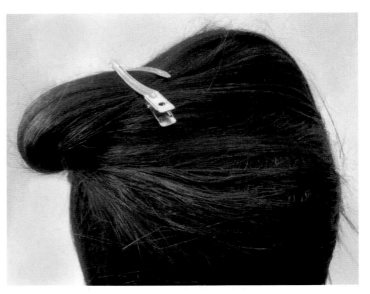

Figure 14.18 Step 12. Repeat this process on the other side front section. From the back, all the hair should be joined to the original ponytail—just keep adding small rubber bands on top of the ponytail as you add in sections of hair.

Figure 14.19 Step 13. Use duckbill clips to pin the hair in the ponytail out of the way.

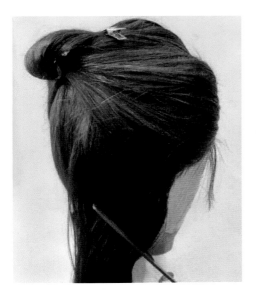

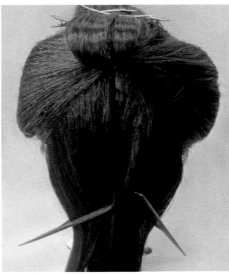

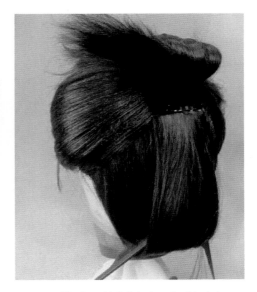

Figure 14.20 Step 14. You are now going to style the lower back of the wig. Comb through the back section and firmly wedge a rattail comb into the hair. (The comb is going to serve as a tool to hold the section of hair in place.)

Figure 14.21 Step 15. Add a second comb even with the first comb on the other side of the wig.

Figure 14.22 Step 16. Pull the length of the hair up towards the crown ponytail and anchor it in place with crossed bobby pins.

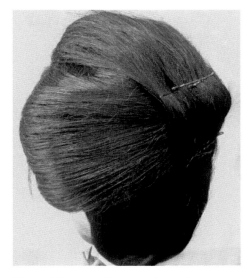

Figure 14.23 Step 17. Remove the rattail combs from the wig. Smooth the back and spray with hairspray so the hair is free from flyaway hairs. Place a second row of bobby pins a couple of inches above the first row, just underneath the base of the ponytail at the crown.

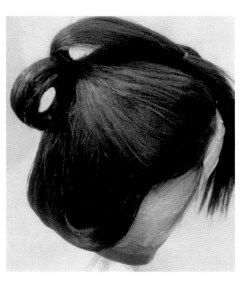

Figure 14.24 Step 18. Roll the pinned section of hair under into a small loop. You can either fold the hair or use a dowel rod to help create a uniform shape. You can also see that I place a second rubber band in the ponytail at the crown. This wig had some long layers, so I used the second rubber band to hold all the pieces together.

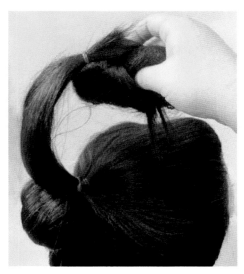

Figure 14.25 Step 19. Roll the hair in the crown ponytail around a rat. Roll all the hair under until you reach the base of the ponytail.

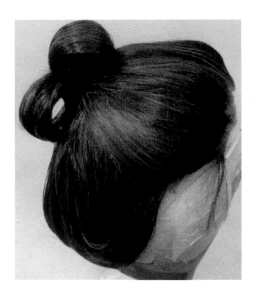

Figure 14.26 Step 20. Pin the second roll you have created to the top of the wig with bobby pins. Go over the entire wig once more, spraying it with hairspray and smoothing the hairs until the wig looks perfect.

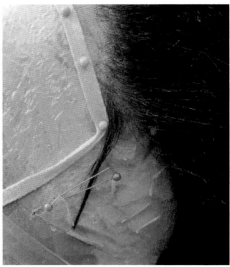

Figure 14.27 Step 21. I added a small straight piece of hair in front of each ear in order to help conceal the edge of the wig. This step is optional.

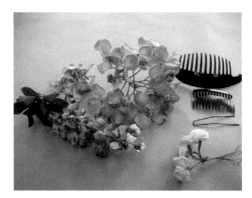

Figure 14.28 Step 22. You are now ready to decorate your wig. You can buy premade ornaments, or you can assemble your own. You can create your own by using artificial flowers, premade combs, large hairpins—there are many options.

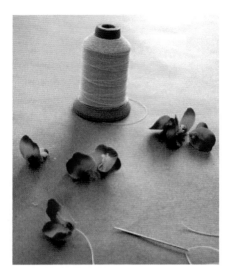

Figure 14.29 Step 23. Many Japanese hair ornaments feature strings of dangling flowers. I created my own ornament by taking apart an artificial flower made up of small individual blossoms. I used a sewing needle and heavy weight thread. I made a knot in the base of the thread to hold the lowest blossom on.

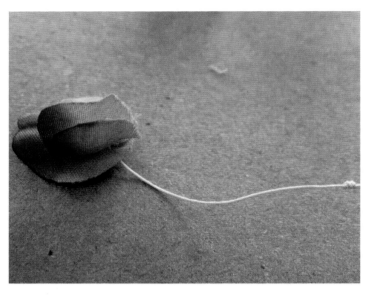

Figure 14.30 Step 24. Next, make a knot and in or two up on the thread, where you want the next blossom to sit.

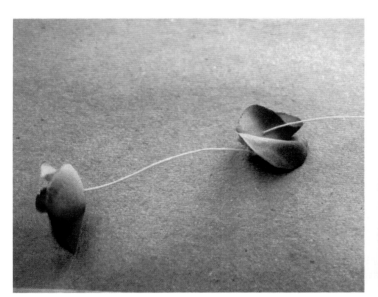

Figure 14.31 Step 25. Continue stringing the blossoms, making sure to space them evenly.

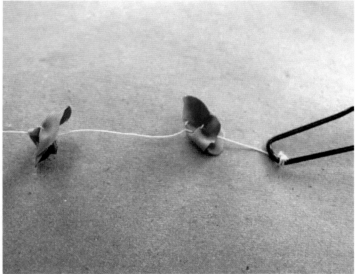

Figure 14.32 Step 26. Sew each string onto a large size wig pin. Because I did not want the strings to slide around on the comb, I added a small dab of latex at the base of each string to hold it in place. Once all the strings were in place and the latex was dry, I added larger flower blossoms to the top of the comb by stitching them on with thread. I also added a small drop pearl at the base of each flower string to add weight to help the strings hang properly.

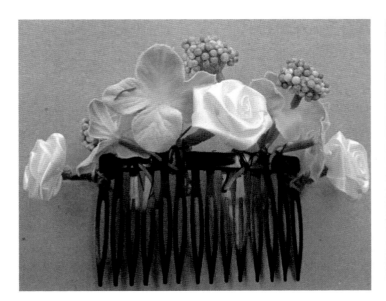

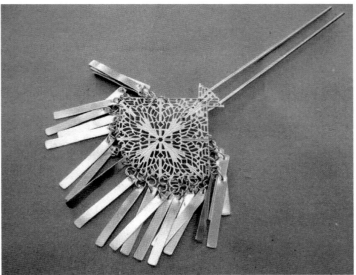

Figure 14.33 Step 27. You can create a decorative comb by wind wired flowers around the flat part of the comb. Flowers that are not on wires can be stitched in place. I have chosen flowers and colors that are appropriate to a springtime decoration.

Figure 14.34 Step 28. Tanya Olalde, craft supervisor in the Texas Performing Arts costume shop, created this *ogi-bira kanzashi* (sometimes called a rain ornament) out of found objects. She used a piece of wire coat hanger to create the base. She then added a piece of jewelry making filigree to create the fan shaped base. She then straightened brass brads and pounded them straight to make the dangling bits of metal. A hole was made in each metal piece and they were each attached to the filigree with jump rings. Finally, the entire thing was sprayed with silver spray.

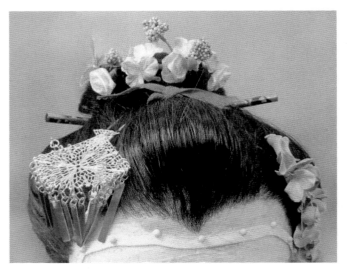

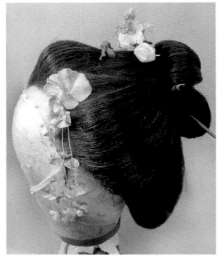

Figures 14.35 and 14.36 Step 29. The ornaments have been placed in the wig. Note the place of the *ogi-bira*. A traditional red cord has been added to the front section. Painted chopsticks with a butterfly motif have been added to the back of the wig, and a small decorative butterfly has also been added.

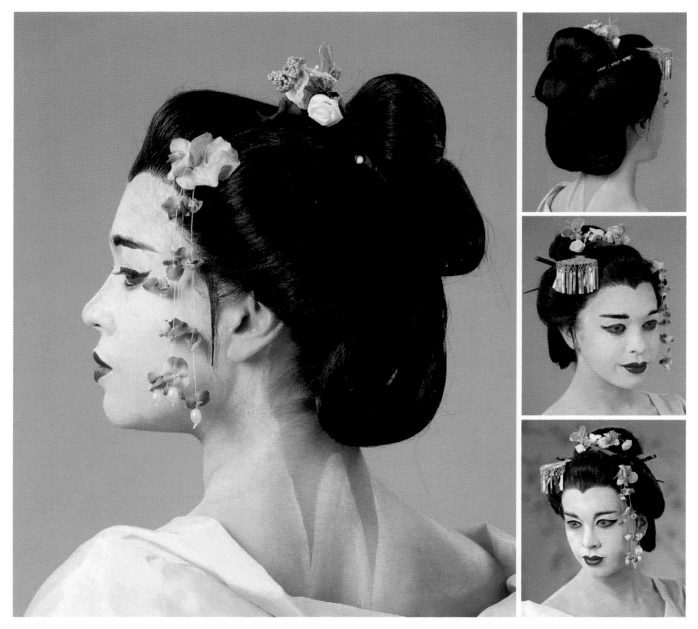

Figures 14.37–14.40   The completed Geisha style. Photography: Tim Babiak. Model: Anna Fugate.

Variations

So many different looks can be created for geisha simply through variety in your ornaments. You can also vary the sculptural shapes in the back of the wig to create different looks.

Geisha Makeup

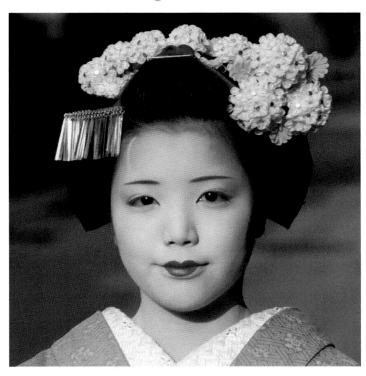

Figure 14.41   Maiko Ayano wearing June kanzashi, by Joe Baz.

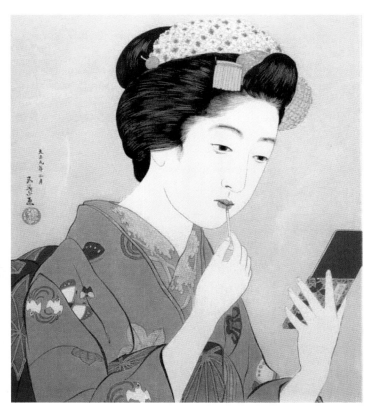

Figure 14.42   Woman applying color to her lips (*Portrait of Chiyo, a Maiko of Gion, Kyoto*), Goyo Hashiguchi, Walters Art Museum.

The traditional geisha makeup process begins with the application of a special waxy formula called *bintsuke-abura* to smooth the skin. Special white powder is mixed with water and applied to the skin using a bamboo brush. The hairline is not painted so as to give the impression of a mask being worn. *Maiko* have red makeup around their eyes and eyebrows. The eyebrows are drawn on in black with a very straight shape (no arch). The lips are filled in with red paint; the shape of the lip is determined by the geisha's status. The lips are usually drawn in smaller than their natural shape—the idea is to give the impression that the mouth is like a flower bud. Some geishas blackened their teeth (the white of the face paint makes the teeth look yellow in contrast).

African Tribal Hairstyles

Because Africa is such a large and varied continent, the countries within this continent have wildly varied look to their culture. Natural African hair texture can be manipulated into many shapes—tribal hairstyles might be made up of braids, twist, dreadlocks, cornrows, or knots. These hairstyles might be ornamented with cowries; beads; pins made of wood, bone, or ivory; medals; pieces of silver; amber balls; or metal rings. African hairstyles are often specific to status, age, ethnicity, wealth, rank, marital status, or religious beliefs. It was a common practice for the head female of the family to groom her family's hair.

Hair grooming was considered an intimate and spiritual event. Hair was often groomed with black soap, shea butter, palm oil, or argan oil. Some Africans colored their hair with red, earth, red ocher, and grease; others used mud and clay in a range of colors in order to stiffen and color their hair.

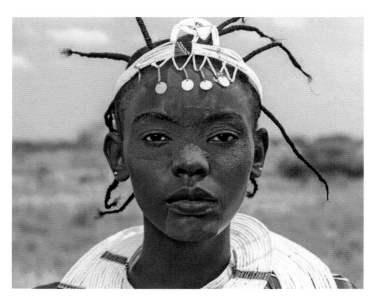

Figure 14.43 The maasai lady from Tanzania, by Dauupicha.

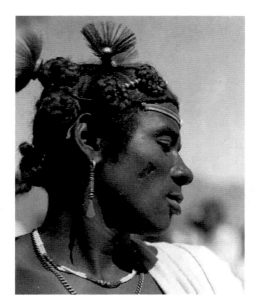

Figure 14.44 Dancer and medicine man from the Antadroy tribe, Nordisk Film's Paul Fejo's expedition to Madagascar, 1936, National Museum of Denmark.

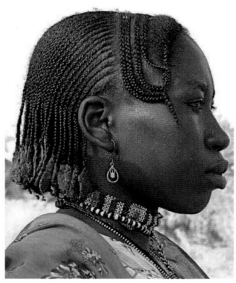

Figure 14.45 A nuba woman in Nyaro village, Kau, Nuba mountains, Sudan, by Rita Willaert. Notice how the ends of the braids have been dressed with mud or clay.

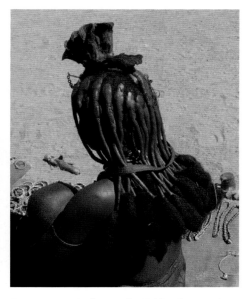

Figure 14.46 Coiffure Himba (Otkikandero Namibie), by Ji-Elle. This extremely elaborate hairstyle has been dressed with red mud/clay.

African Tribal Styling—
Step by Step

This hairstyle is made up of elements of several traditional African styles, which can be seen in Figures 14.43, 14.44, and 14.45.

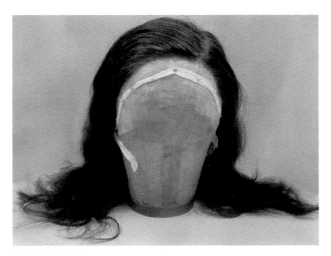

Figure 14.47   Step 1. Begin with a wig that has at least shoulder length hair. I used a fully ventilated lace wig made out of synthetic hair. It is difficult to create this hairstyle on a wig that is not fully hand tied because the braiding techniques expose so much of the inner foundation of the wig.

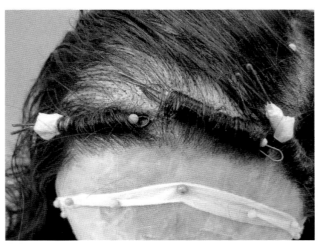

Figure 14.48   Step 2. You must thoroughly texturize the hair in the wig in order to create a successful African style. Set the hair around the hairline of the wig on large bobby pins. Use the bobby pins just as you would a roller—use an endpaper to control the ends of the hair and to assist you with rolling the hair on the bobby pin (see the 1970s' Afro style in Chapter 12 for more detailed instructions and pictures of how to use bobby pins to set hair).

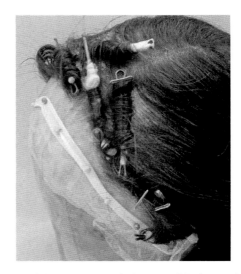

Figure 14.49   Step 3. Continue setting the hair around the face on the bobby pins.

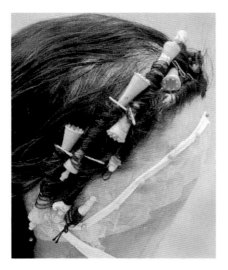

Figure 14.50   Step 4. Set another row of hair on tiny sized perm rods.

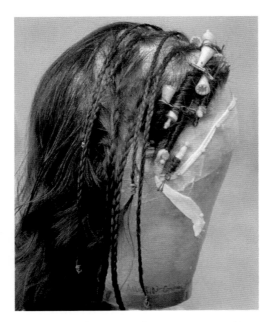

Figure 14.51   Step 5. Behind the perm rods, you are going to add texture to the hair by creating many small braids. Secure each braid with a tiny rubber band.

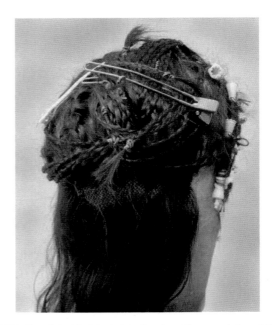

Figure 14.52   Step 6. Braid all the hair in the wig until you reach the mid back of the head. Pin all the braids up and out of the way with a duckbill clip.

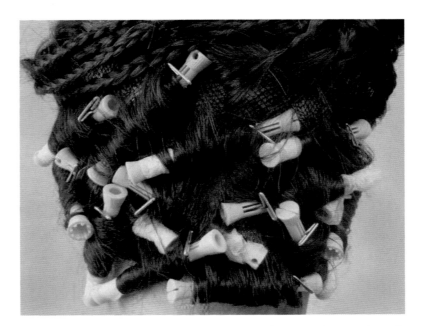

Figure 14.53   Step 7. Set the back of the wig on small perm rods going in alternating diagonal rows.

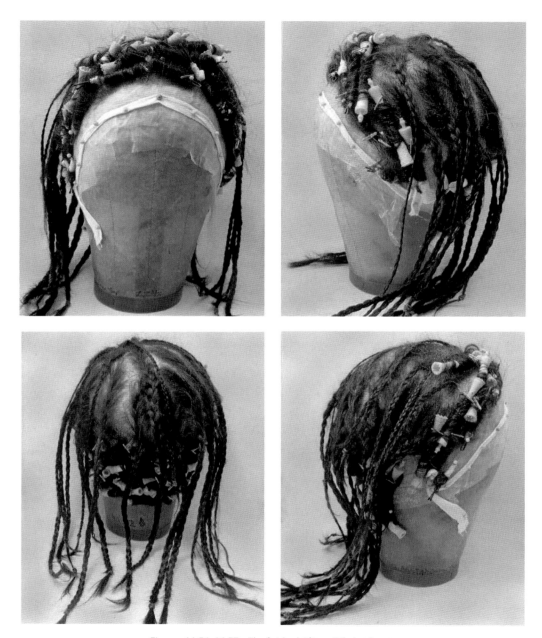

Figures 14.54–14.57   The finished African Tribal style set.

Once you have finished setting the wig, steam each roller and braid thoroughly if the wig is made of synthetic hair. If the wig is human hair, soak each roller with water sprayed from a spray bottle. After steaming or wetting, place the wig in a wig dryer for 75 minutes.

To style:

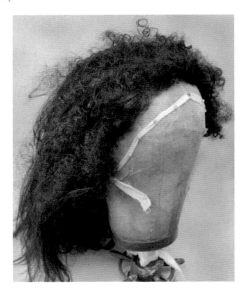

Figure 14.58 Step 8. Remove all the rollers and braids from the wig, beginning at the nape of the neck and working your way up to the front hairline.

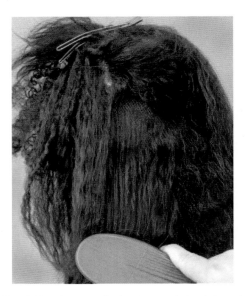

Figure 14.59 Step 9. Use a large wooden brush to gently brush through the entire wig, beginning at the nape of the neck.

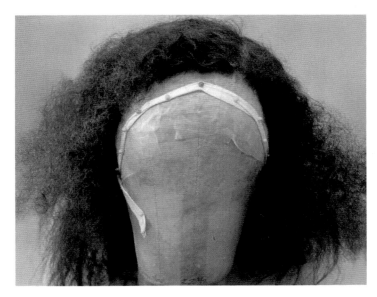

Figure 14.60 Step 10. The brushed out wig should look very soft and full.

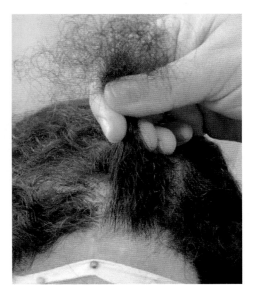

Figure 14.61 Step 11. I dressed the front section of this wig in Zulu Knots (also called *Bantu* Knots). Cleanly divide out a square or triangular section of hair with the end of your rattail comb.

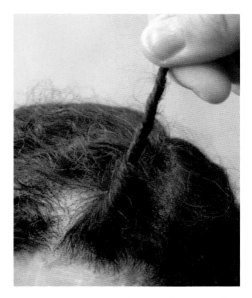

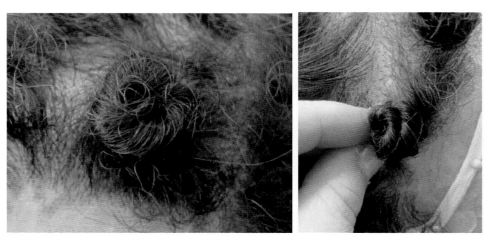

Figures 14.63 and 14.64 Step 13. Once the hair begins to twist back on itself, continue the turning movement and wind the hair into a circular knot. (The process is not unlike putting a thread shank on a button.) Tuck the ends of the hair under the knot to secure it. You can also place a small rubber band around the base of the knot if you desire more security.

Figure 14.62 Step 12. Tightly twist the section of hair until it begins to twist back on itself. For a sleeker, neater knot, you could coat the section in hair product before you twist it.

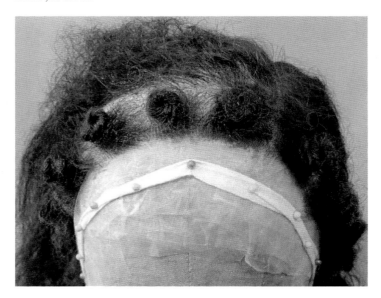

Figure 14.65 Step 14. Continue making Zulu Knots all along the hair line of the wig.

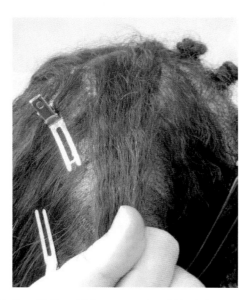

Figure 14.66 Step 15. The middle crown section of this wig is going to be styled in cornrows. Because the wig I used had a built in part, I used that as the starting point for the cornrows. To make a cornrow, first separate out a long narrow section of hair. I used clips to hold the hair away from either side of the section to keep from accidentally picking up additional hair as I braid.

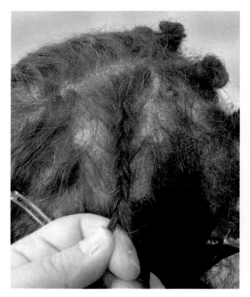
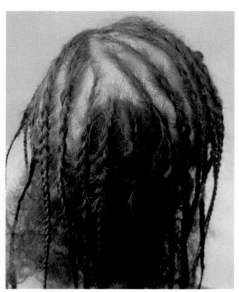
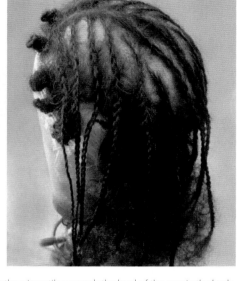

Figure 14.67   Step 16. Make a small reverse French braid in the section of the hair. It is very important to work very close to the scalp, picking up very tiny pieces of hair as you braid. This will help the cornrow to be very tight when you finish.

Figure 14.68 and 14.69   Step 17. Cornrow all the hair in the wig until you reach the level of the ears in the back.

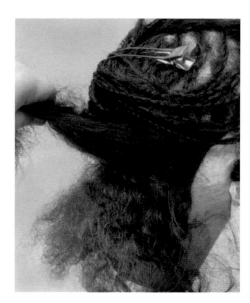
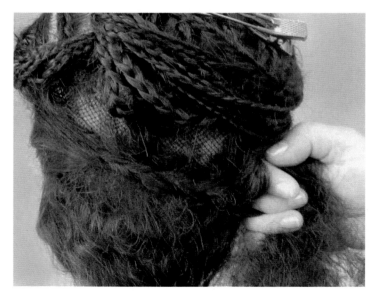

Figure 14.70   Step 18. Pin the cornrows up and out of the way with a duckbill clip. Separate the remaining hair into two horizontal sections.

Figure 14.71   Step 19. Create a larger, horizontal reverse French braid in the bottom of the wig.

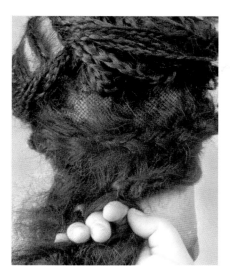

Figure 14.72 Step 20. Create a second reverse French braid, braiding from the opposite side from the first braid.

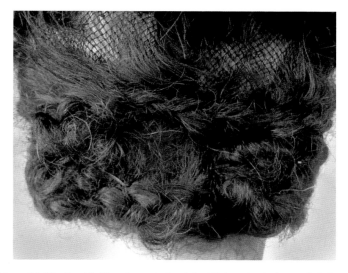

Figure 14.73 Step 21. Wrap the end of each braid into a circular bun and pin in place with bobby pins.

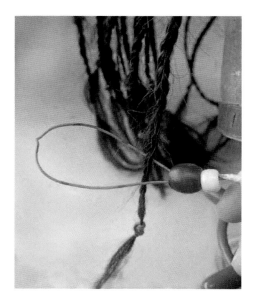

Figure 14.74 Step 22. I chose to decorate the ends of the cornrows with beads and used a variety of wooden beads in bright colors. Make a beading tool by forming a loop out of fine gauge wire. Finish off the end of the wire by wrapping masking tape around the end. (Be careful not to use too much tape—the beads still need to fit over it.) Place the beads on the tool. Thread the end of the braid through the loop.

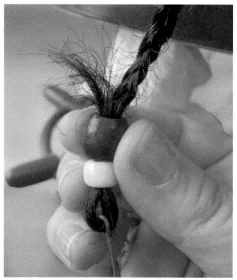

Figure 14.75 Step 24. Slide the beads off the end of the wire loop onto the braid. Use the tool to gently pull the ends of the hair through the beads.

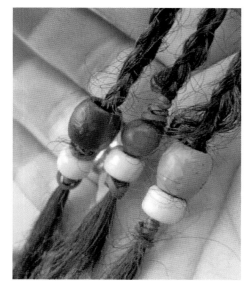

Figure 14.76 Step 25. Place a small rubber band underneath the beads on the end of each braid to keep them from sliding off.

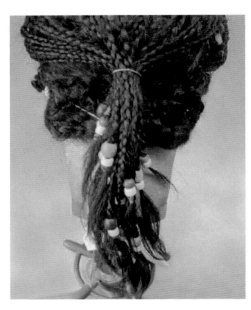

Figure 14.77 Step 26. Once you have finished beading all the braids, gather them into a ponytail at the back of the head.

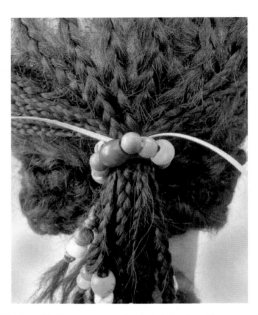

Figure 14.78 Step 27. Create a decorative hair tie by threading more of the beads onto a strip of leather lacing. Knot off the ends. Knot the beaded cord around the base of the ponytail.

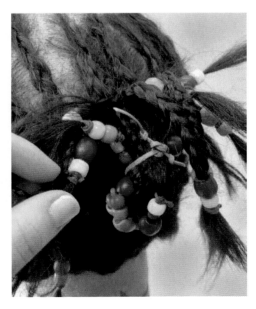

Figure 14.79 Step 28. Fold the ponytail up towards the crown of the head. Knot the leather lacing around the ponytail again so that it holds the braids up.

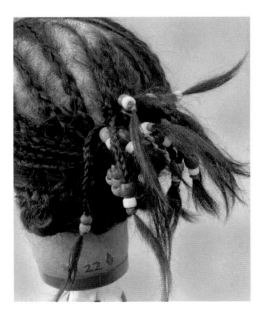

Figure 14.80 Step 29. Arrange the braids so that they have a natural, splayed look. You may need to use bobby pins to hold some of the braids where you want them.

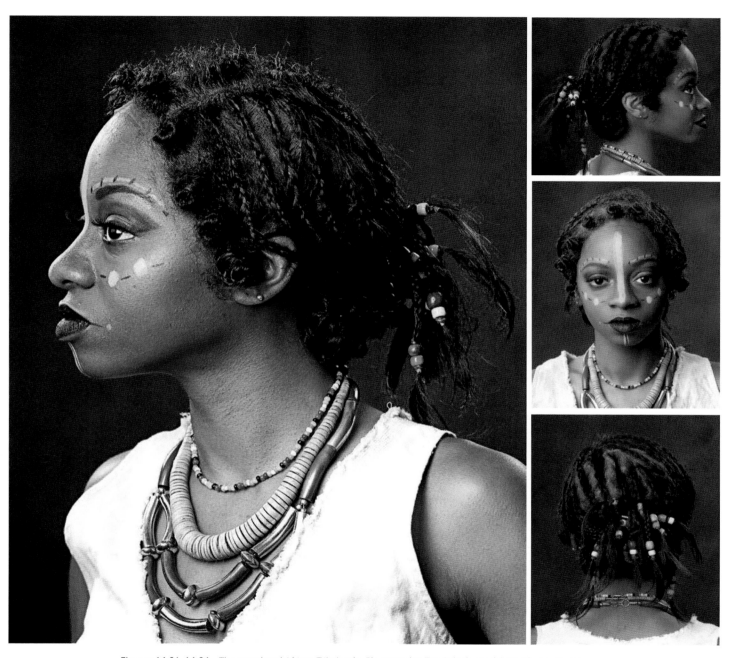

Figures 14.81–14.84 The completed African Tribal style. Photography: Tim Babiak. Model: Marsherrie Madkins.

Tribal Makeup

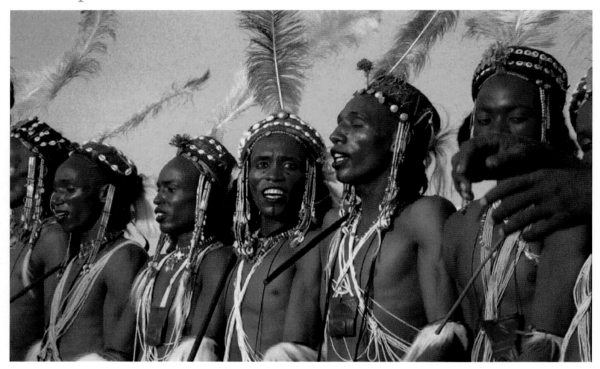

Figure 14.85 Contestants from the Wodaabe ethnic group sing and dance at the Gerewol Festival in Niger, while flaunting the whiteness of their eyes and teeth, by Dan Lundberg, 1997. These men are painted for a cultural beauty pageant featuring the men of this tribe. The makeup is used to make their faces more attractive and symmetrical.

Tribal makeup has always been used for many different purposes. Some face paint, like that pictured in Figure 14.85, was meant to enhance the beauty of the wearer's face. Other types of face paint were worn for religious rituals, to look fierce while hunting, or to show the wearer's status. There are many different symbols and colors that can be found through research. The paints themselves are usually made of natural substances such a red clay, red and yellow ochers, and various colors of mud.

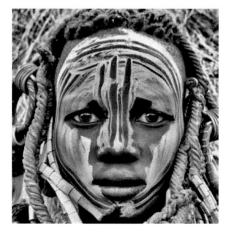

Figure 14.86 Girl, Mursi tribe, Ethiopia, by Ron Waddington.

Cultural Variations

There are volumes of unique cultures around the world with fascinating traditions in hairstyling and face painting. They are interesting to study and all cultures deserve to be honored, respected, and portrayed on stage and screen. I have included a very small section here for inspiration.

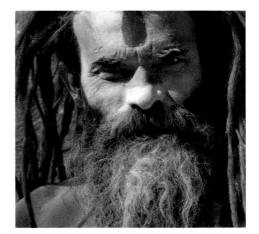

Figure 14.87 A sadhu from Pashupatinath, Kathmandu, in the morning, by Sukanto Debnath.

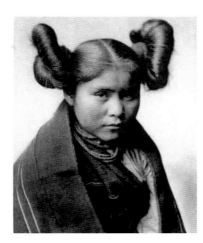

Figure 14.88 Chaiwa—Tewa peoples, from *The North American Indian*, by Edward S. Curtis.

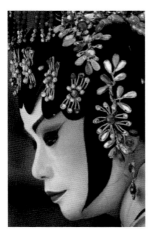

Figure 14.89 Vancouver Cantonese opera singer Connie Mah, by Darren Stone.

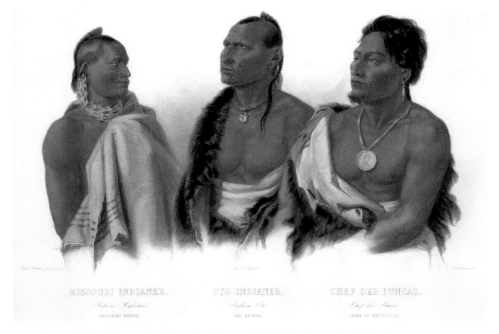

Figure 14.90 Lithograph of Missouria, Otoe, and chief of the Puncas, by Karl Bodmer.

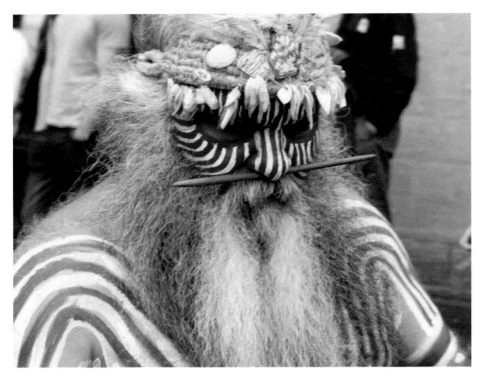

Figure 14.91   Smoking ceremony 2 Major Sumner, a Ngarrindjeri elder, in a smoking ceremony, as part of the repatriation of Old People remains, by Kevin Walsh.

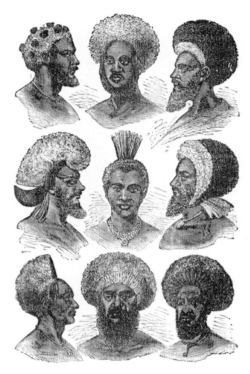

Figure 14.92   Fijian hair dressing modes, author unknown, 1874, *Popular Science Monthly*.

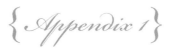

Glossary of Hairstyling and Makeup Terms

AFRO—a hairstyle, originating on people of African descent, in which naturally curly hair is allowed to grow and become bushy in a round fashion on the head.

AGGRAVATORS—short men's curls, seen in the 19th century, that were combed right to the outer corner of each eye.

ALEXANDRA CURL—a long spiral curl that is usually worn behind one ear.

ALLONGE—a long curly men's wig, worn during the Restoration period, that is styled in high curls above the forehead.

ANTIMACASSAR—a small piece of cloth placed on the arm or back of a chair to prevent soiling or staining; often used to prevent furniture from being stained by macassar hair oil used by men to give their hair shine.

APOLLO KNOT—a piece made of artificial hair that is looped and coiled and stiffened to stand up on the crown of the head as part of a popular hairstyle of the 1830s.

BAG WIG—an 18th century wig where the hair in the back is contained in a fabric bag.

BANDEAU—an artificial hairpiece that was worn on the front of the head and secured at the nape of the neck with a ribbon. A bandeau could be styled in a variety of ways. It is similar to a TRANSFORMATION.

BANGS—a fringe of hair, usually brushed forward onto the forehead.

BANTU KNOTS—a traditional African hairstyle where sections of hair are coiled into small, tight buns close to the scalp; also sometime called Zulu Knots.

BAROQUE—a style characterized by extravagant ornament and detail; originated in Europe in the early 17th century.

BARREL CURL—a hollow curl that is rolled up on itself and pinned in place. This was very commonly seen on wigs in the mid- to late 18th century.

BARRISTER'S WIG—the traditional wig worn by barristers in British courts. The wig consists of frizzy loops on top, rows of barrel curls, and two tails with tiny curls at the bottom.

BASIN OR BOWL CUT—any haircut where a bowl or basin is placed on the head and the hair is cut to the edges of the bowl. It appears in nearly all ages of history.

BEATLE CUT/MOP TOP—a hairstyle popularized in the 1960s by the Beatles. The style consisted of hair that was brushed forward onto the forehead and roughly the same length all around the head. This hairstyle was considered radical because of its length after the very short men's haircuts of the 1950s.

BEEHIVE—a 1960s' hairdo where the hair is pulled on top of the head, teased, and smoothed into a dome that resembles a beehive.

BINTSUKE-ABURA—a soy based wax used to coat the skin before applying the white face makeup of a geisha.

BOB—a short hairstyle for women, popularized in the 1920s, where the hair was chopped off at chin level. The bob has continued its popularity to the present day, where many different variations of the bob have been created.

BOB WIG—a 17th and 18th century wig with short curls at the bottom. There was both a long bob wig and a short bob wig. These wigs were most frequently worn by laborers and tradesmen.

BOUFFANT—any hairstyle that is teased around the face for volume.

BRAID—a length of hair where the strands are woven or twisted together. Three sections of hair is the most common braid, but braids can be made with many more sections.

BRILLIANTINE—scented oil used on men's hair to make it look glossy.

BRUTUS STYLE—a short tousled hairstyle popularized by French Revolutionaries.

BUN—any tightly wound arrangement (usually circular in shape) of hair on the back of the head.

BUZZ CUT—also called a crew cut. A haircut where the hair is shaved evenly around the head, at a short length very close to the scalp.

CADOGAN—a knot of hair at the nape of the neck that was folded back onto itself and tied around the middle. This was a popular style in the late 18th century.

CAESAR HAIRCUT—a short layered men's haircut with short bangs that are brushed onto the face.

CAGE—a wire frame used to support large, structural hairstyles.

CARMINE—a vivid crimson pigment made from cochineal.

CASCADE—an artificial hairpiece with long falling curls.

CAT EYE—an eyeliner shape where the upper line extends past the outside corner of the eye and wings up at an angle.

CAULIFLOWER WIG—a short, white, curled bob wig that was worn by clergymen and physicians in the 18th century.

CHIGNON—a smooth twist, knot, or roll of hair, worn on the back of the head.

CHONMAGE—a traditional Japanese men's hairstyle where the top of the head is either shaved or slicked down; the rest of the hair is pulled into a small ponytail and folded up onto the crown of the head.

CLUB—see CADOGAN.

COIF—can refer to either a close fitting cap, or the act of creating a hairstyle.

COIL—a type of bun where the hair is wound in concentric circles and pinned.

CONTOUR—a makeup technique where makeup in shades lighter than the natural skin and darker than the natural skin are used to visually sculpt or reshape the face.

CORNROWS—a type of braid where a narrow strip of hair is braided tightly against the scalp.

CORONET—a hairstyle that mimics a crown, usually consisting of braids wrapped around the head.

COXCOMB—a hairstyle where the hair at the center of the forehead is swept up and back into a curl. This hairstyle got its name from its resemblance to the crest of a rooster.

CRESPINE—a jeweled net for securing the hair, used in the 15th century; sometimes called crespinette.

CRIMPING—the act of pressing hair between shaped metal plates to create texture.

CUPID'S BOW—an upper lip shape said to resemble the double curved bow carried by Cupid in mythology. Popularized in the 1920s.

CUT CREASE—an eye shadow application technique where eye shadow is applied only in either the natural crease or drawing a line (cutting) just above the crease that is very defined and sharp, creating a separation between the actual lid and the upper eye area; the line is then blended outward towards the brow.

CYPRIOTE CURL—a sculptural curl that was piled onto a frame around the face on some Roman women's hairstyles.

DREADLOCK—a hairstyle that forms over time when naturally curly hair is allowed to wind around itself, eventually forming a solid lock of hair.

DUCKTAIL—a men's haircut, popular in the 1950s, where the hair was parted in the center back like a duck's tail. The hair on the sides was combed back and the hair in the front was intentionally disarrayed so that some pieces hung down.

FADE—a haircut that originated in the military in the 1940s, where the hair was cut short on top and tapering down to the skin on the sides.

This haircut was then widely embraced and elaborated on by the black community.

FALL—a hairpiece used to add thickness and length to the back of the head. It generally sits at the top of the head and covers to the nape of the neck.

FAVORITES—locks of curly hair that dangle at the temples.

FEATHERED HAIR—a haircut where the layers are tapered, especially around the face. This hairstyle was very popular in the 1970s.

FINGER WAVE—a method of setting wave into hair by using the fingers to mold the waves in place.

FLAT TOP—a haircut that is similar to a crew cut, except the hair is cut into a flat plane on top.

FLIP—a hairstyle where the bottom ends are curled or flipped up. A popular hairstyle in the 1960s.

FONTANGE—a women's hairstyle of the Restoration period where the hair over the forehead is dressed in wired curls. This was often topped by the Fontange headdress which was made of stiffened, pleated lace. This hairstyle is named after the Duchesse du Fontanges, who created the style after her original hairstyle fell down. She tied her hair up off her forehead with ribbons, and the hairstyle caught on after Louis XIV admired it on her.

FRENCH BRAID—a method of braiding where hair is gradually added to the braid in sections, instead of braiding all the hair together at once. This allows the braid to lie extremely close to the head.

FRENCH DOT—a tiny goatee that sits directly under the bottom lip.

FRENCH ROLL—a hairstyle where the hair arranged in a vertical roll on the back of the head. Also called a French twist.

FRENCH TWIST—see FRENCH ROLL.

FRINGE—short hair brushed forward. Fringe is sometimes used as another word for bangs.

FRISETTE—a fringe of curled or frizzed hair worn of the forehead. Usually an artificial piece.

FRIZZLE—a short, crisp curl.

FULL BOTTOM WIG—a type of wig, popular in the 18th century, that was very large and elaborately curled, with a section of curls falling in front of each shoulder.

GAMINE—a term used for a girl with attractively boyish beauty; this term also came to mean the short haircuts worn by women in the 1950s such as Audrey Hepburn.

GORDIAN KNOT—an intricate, figure of eight knot of hair.

GRECIAN KNOT—a style where the hair at the nape of the neck was coiled and knotted to resemble the hairstyle of ancient Greek women.

HANDLEBAR MUSTACHE—a mustache style where the ends stick out past the lips and turn up at the ends. These ends are often waxed into points.

HEDGEHOG—a name for hairstyles worn by both men and women in the late 18th century. For men, this was a hairstyle where the hair was short all around the face and worn spiked out. For women, the Hedgehog hairstyle consisted of a shorter cloud of curls around the face, with long ringlets hanging down in the back.

HENNA—the powdered leaves of a tropical shrub, used as a dye to color the hair and decorate the body.

HIME CUT—an Asian hairstyle that consists of long straight hair with blunt bangs and a section of hair that is cut to shoulder length.

HOLLYWOOD BEARD—a short full beard where the section of hair under the lower lip and on the front of the chin area has been shaved away.

HURLUBERLU—a women's hairstyle of the late 17th century, where the hair is usually center parted, and worn very curly all around the head, with a few long ringlets hanging down the back. The term roughly translates from the French to "screwball" "cabbage head," or "scatter brain."

KANZASHI—hair ornaments used in traditional Japanese hairstyles.

KISS CURL/SPIT CURL—a small short curl that is worn curling onto the face.

KOHL—a black powder, usually antimony sulfide or lead sulfide, used as eye makeup.

LADYKILLER—also referred to as Dundreary Whiskers or Piccadilly Weepers. Long drooping sideburns that nearly touch the shoulders.

LAPPET—a longer curl that hangs loose on the face or neck.

LIBERTY SPIKES—a hairstyle popularized by the British punk culture of the 1970s where the hair was styled into wide pointed spike that stuck out all over the head. This hairstyle often requires the use of extreme styling products, including glue, egg whites, gelatin, starch, and hairspray, in order to keep its stiff shape.

LION WIG—the term can refer either to an 18th century wig that resembles the mane of a lion, or, more commonly, a style of Kabuki wig. A Lion Kabuki wig is usually white in color and consists of long bangs brushed forward onto the forehead and three long full tails of hair (one over each shoulder and one hanging down the back).

LOCK OF HORUS—a lock of hair that was left uncut over the right ear of young Egyptian boys. (The rest of the head was shaved.)

LOVELOCK—a long curl or ringlet of hair that is pulled forward to hang over the shoulder. These were worn by both men and women in the Cavalier period.

MACARONI—a male dandy or fop of the late 18th century. The term Macaroni also refers to the wig style worn by these dandies where the hair in the front was dressed very tall and sometimes pointy. A small hat was often perched on this tall section of hair. The hair in the back of this wig style was usually pulled into a queue and clubbed.

MADDER—a red dye or pigment obtained from the root of the madder plant, or a synthetic dye resembling it.

MAQUILLAGE—a French term for makeup.

MARCEL WAVE—a method of waving the hair where the hair was pressed with hot waving irons. It is similar method of hairstyling to crimping the hair. It was invented by French hairdresser Marcel Grateau in 1872.

MASCARA—a cosmetic for darkening and thickening the eyelashes.

MOHAWK—a hairstyle where the entire head is shaved to the skin except for a strip of hair down the center that is spiked up.

MOMOWARE—a Japanese hairstyle worn by maiko (apprentice geisha). This style is also known as the "divided peach."

MULLET—a hairstyle where the hair is cut short in the front and side and left long in the back.

MUTTON CHOP—a type of sideburn that is narrow near the temple and wide at the jaw line.

ODANGO—a hairstyle, inspired by Japanese anime, where the hair is arranged in two buns on top of the head that resemble animal ears.

OGI-BIRA KANZASHI—a metal, fan-shaped kanzashi with aluminum streamers, worn by maiko/geisha apprentices. Sometimes called a rain ornament.

ORNATRIX—a Roman term for a woman who adorns another; a hairdresser.

PAGEBOY—a long bobbed hairstyle, usually just touching the shoulders, with the ends turned under. This hairstyle first came into being as a style used on medieval boys serving under knights. It later gained popularity as a woman's hairstyle in the 1930s and 40s.

PANCAKE MAKEUP—makeup in cake form applied to the face with a damp sponge in order to cover up imperfections and even out skin tone.

PENCIL MUSTACHE—a mustache made up of a very thin line of hairs.

PERIWIG—another term for a wig from the 17th century. This term was especially used by the British.

PERM—a slang term for a permanent wave. This is a process where the hair is rolled onto tiny rollers and treated with chemicals so that the hair takes on a "permanent" curl.

PERRUKE/PERRUQUE—the French word for wig.

PIGTAIL—long hair that is pulled back, cinched, and braided; in modern usage, this can also refer to a ponytail on each side of the head.

PIGTAIL WIG—a men's wig with a long queue that is bound all the way to the tip by a ribbon.

PIN CURL—a flat curl held in place by a hairpin while it is being set.

PIXIE CUT—a short women's hairstyle that has wispy layered bangs.

PLAIT—another word for braid. There are many varieties of plait.

POMPADOUR—a hairstyle where the hair is not parted and brushed straight back off of the forehead with some height. Originally named for the Marquise de Pompadour. This term later became associated with a men's hairstyle in the 1950s where the hair above of the forehead was styled extremely high and pouffed.

PONYTAIL—long hair that is pulled close to the head, cinched, and allowed to hang loose.

PROFESSIONAL BEAUTIES—Society ladies in the 1880s who had their portraits painted. These portraits were then publicly displayed and copies were sold to collectors.

PSYCHE KNOT—a style where the hair is divided into two sections. The two sections are coiled and one coiled is pulled through the center of the other coil. This knot is usually placed on the back of the head just below the crown.

QUEUE—a long tail of hair, usually referring to a men's hairstyle. A queue can be curled or braided.

QUIFF—a hairstyle, similar to the pompadour, where the hair over the forehead is shaped into a sculpted curl or wave.

RATTAIL—a small section of hair, usually at the nape of the neck, that is allowed to grow much longer than the rest of the hair.

RINGLET—any long, vertical hanging curl.

ROUGE—a red powder or cream used for coloring the cheeks or lips.

ROUNDHEAD—a name applied to the Puritans who supported parliament against Charles I in England. The name came from their rounded bowl cuts.

SAUSAGE CURL—a long vertical curl that has an uninterrupted tube shape.

SHAG—a hairstyle where all of the hair is cut into layers of various lengths. This style was first popularized in the 1970s.

SHAITTEL/SHEITEL—the Yiddish word for the wigs worn by married Orthodox Jewish women. These wigs allow the women to follow the Jewish law requiring them to keep their hair/head covered.

SHIMADA—a Japanese women's hairstyle, usually worn by geisha.

SHINGLE—a version of the 1920s' bob haircut where the hair was cut to the occipital bone; the hair remaining underneath was cut into a "V" shape.

SIDEBURN—a short side whisker, worn without a beard. The style was named for American Civil War General Ambrose Burnside.

SNOOD—an ornamental net that holds or contains part of the hair.

SPADE BEARD—a beard that is cut into a rounded or pointed blade shape.

TENDRIL—a small wisp of curly hair, usually found in front of the ear.

TIEBACK—another term for a man's 18th century wig that was pulled back into a queue.

TITUS—a short layered women's hairstyle seen in the 19th century. This was one of the rare instances of a short women's hairstyle before the 20th century.

TONSURE—a hairstyle seen on monks where the hair at the crown of the head is shaved.

TRANSFORMATION—an artificial hairpiece that goes all the way around the circumference of the head, but does not have a crown.

UPDO—any hairstyle where all of the hair is pulled up and away from the neck.

VAMP—a term used to describe a seductive woman. This term was used in the 1920s to describe femmes fatales in the movies; they were often known to wear extremely dark eye makeup.

VAN DYKE BEARD—a small pointed goatee. The style gets its name from the beards that frequently appeared in the portraits painted by Sir Anthony Van Dyke.

VERMILION—a brilliant red pigment made from mercury sulfide (cinnabar).

VICTORY ROLL—a 1940s' hairstyle where the hair on the sides of the head is swept up into hollow rolls and pinned. A true victory roll has the rolls going all the way down the head until they meet in a point at the nape of the neck, forming a "V" for Victory.

WALRUS MUSTACHE—a large mustache that hangs over the lips and drops down at the outer corners of the mouth.

WEDGE—a haircut, popularized in the 1970s, that uses a weight line and tapered layer to create the illusion of extra fullness. This is sometimes referred to as a stacked haircut.

ZULU KNOT—an African hairstyle where the hair is divided in triangular or rectangular sections and each section is tightly twisted into a knot.

List of Historical Films and Television Shows Set in Each Era (Early Victorian–Present)

These films can be used as a good reference for the period in question. Primary research is direct research from a historical period, and is always the most authentic reference and the one you should look to first. Primary research includes actual wigs from the period (very rare due to their rapid deterioration), portraits painted during a period, and photographs. Interpretations of other time periods, including films, are secondary research. Keep in mind that the look of a film is always visually affected by the year the film was made, so while the looks portrayed in the film may not be 100 percent authentic, they are still great for giving you a feel for the period and a place to begin brainstorming ideas and inspiring your research. There is no substitute for authentic period research, but these films make for excellent supplemental material.

Early Victorian Era

Amistad (1997)
Angels and Insects (1995)
Gangs of New York (2002)
Jane Eyre (2011)
The Young Victoria (2009)

Mid-/Late Victorian

12 Years a Slave (2013)
A Christmas Carol (several versions)
The Four Feathers (2002)
Gettysburg (1993)
Glory (1989)
Gone With the Wind (1939)
An Ideal Husband (1999)
The King and I (1956)
Lincoln (2012)
Little Women (several versions)
Mrs. Brown (1997)
The Piano (1993)
Topsy Turvy (1995)

The Gay Nineties (1885–1901)

The Age of Innocence (1993)
The Importance of Being Earnest (2002)
Moulin Rouge (1952 and 2001)
O Pioneers! (1992)
The Prestige (2006)

Edwardian Era/Gibson Girls

The House of Mirth (2000)
Iron Jawed Angels (2004)
Meet Me in St. Louis (1944)
Ragtime (1981)
A Room with a View (1986)
Wings of the Dove (1997)

The Teens

All Quiet on the Western Front (1979)
Doctor Zhivago (1965)
Downton Abbey (2010–present) (covers the Teens and the 1920s)
A Night to Remember (1958)
Titanic (1997)

The Roaring Twenties

Boardwalk Empire (television series 2010–2014)
Cabaret (1972)
Chicago (2002)
Grand Hotel (1932)
Metropolis (1927)
Ninotchka (1939)
Some Like it Hot (1959)
Wings (1927)

The 1930s

Atonement (2007)
The Blue Angel (1930)

Road to Perdition (2002)
The 39 Steps (1935)
The Women (1939)

The 1940s

A League of Their Own (1992)
Casablanca (1942)
Darkest Hour (2017)
His Girl Friday (1940)
L.A. Confidential (1997)
The Philadelphia Story (1940)

The 1950s

All About Eve (1950)
Funny Face (1957)
I Love Lucy (television series 1951–1957)
Leave it to Beaver (television series 1957–1963)
On the Waterfront (1954)
Pillow Talk (1959)
The Seven Year Itch (1955)
Where the Boys Are (1960)

The 1960s

The Apartment (1960)
The Avengers (television series 1961–1969)
Beach Blanket Bingo (1965)
Gidget (television series 1965)
Hairspray (1988 and 2007)
The Help (2011)
Hidden Figures (2016)
Mad Men (television series 2007–2015)
The Mod Squad (television series 1968–1973)
Selma (2014)

The 1970s

American Hustle (2013)
Annie Hall (1977)
Bohemian Rhapsody (2018)
Charlie's Angels (television series 1976–1981)

The Jeffersons (television series 1975–1985)
Klute (1971)
The Mary Tyler Moore Show (television series 1970–1977)
Saturday Night Fever (1977)
Taxi Driver (1976)
Velvet Goldmine (1998)
Xanadu (1980)

The 1980s

Back to the Future (1985)
The Cosby Show (television series 1984–1992)
Dynasty (television series 1981–1989)
Girls Just Wanna Have Fun (1985)
Heathers (1988)
Miami Vice (television series 1984–1989)
Pretty in Pink (1986)
Straight Outta Compton (2015)
This is Spinal Tap (1984)
The Wedding Singer (1998)

The 1990s

American Beauty (1999)
Beverly Hills, 90210 (television series 1990–2000)
Clueless (1995)
The Fresh Prince of Bel-Air (television series 1990–1996)
Friends (1994–2004)
Pretty Woman (1990)
Pulp Fiction (1994)
Reality Bites (1994)
Saved by the Bell (television series 1989–1993)

2000s to the Present

Desperate Housewives (television series 2004–2012)
The Devil Wears Prada (2006)
Eternal Sunshine of the Spotless Mind (2004)
The Girl with the Dragon Tattoo (2011)
Gossip Girl (television series 2007–2012)
Mean Girls (2004)
Sex and the City (television series 1998–2004)

List of Wig and Hair Suppliers

This is a listing of the suppliers I use most frequently in wig making projects. I like the products they sell and have had good luck with their service.

Amid Beauty
www.amidbeauty.com

A great source for wig making materials and supplies.

Arda Wigs
348 N Ashland Ave
Chicago IL 60607
(312)918-0648
www.arda-wigs.com
*by appointment only

Carries a wide variety of both natural and party colors of wigs and wefting.

Atelier Bassi
www.atelierbassi.com

A European based company with extensive wig making materials, supplies, wigs, hair, makeup, wig stands, and tools you don't know how you were living without.

Banbury Postiche
0 1295 757406
www.banburypostiche.co.uk

A UK based source for all things wig related.

Frends Beauty
5244 Laurel Canyon Blvd
North Hollywood CA 91607
(818) 769-3834
www.frendsbeauty.com

A source for makeup, wig, and hair supplies; has a great customer loyalty program.

Hair Boutique
(866) 469-4247
http://mp.hairboutique.com

This website carries an extensive variety of hair accessories.

Hairess Corporation
880 Industrial Blvd
Crown Point IN 46307
(219)662-1060
www.hairess.com

Hairess is an excellent one stop shopping place for wig styling needs. It carries everything—wig steamers, canvas heads, wig clamps, Styrofoam heads, combs, brushes, scissors, pins, elastics, wig caps, wig styling products—really, almost everything you could need. Be aware that there is a minimum order and that some items can only be purchased in bulk.

Hats by Leko
P.O. Box 170
Odell OR 97044
www.hatsupply.com

This hat supply store is a good source for millinery wire (for making wig frames), horsehair, hat bases, tiaras, ribbons, veiling/netting, and flowers (really lovely ones for hair decoration purposes).

His and Her Hair Goods Co.
5525 Wilshire Blvd
Los Angeles CA 90036
1-800-421-4417
www.hisandher.com

An excellent source for weaving and braiding hair. They also carry a decent selection of wig laces and nets. Their textured hair for African-Americans is particularly good.

I Kick Shins
www.ikickshins.net

This website is a great source of all manner of funky hair things. They carry artificial dreadlocks, tubular crin for making cyberlox, strips of foam, feather extensions, and everything else you might need to make a custom anime, cosplay, or cyber look.

International Wigs
Hairs to Wigs
848 N. Rainbow Blvd, suite 4557
Las Vegas NV 89107
1-800-790-5013
www.internationalwigs.com

International Wigs has a *huge* selection of wigs and hairpieces. I really like their selection of weaving and braiding hair and use it quite frequently to both add to existing wigs and to build wigs from scratch.

Japanese Style
1-877-226-4387
www.japanesestyle.com

This website has a small but nice selection of kanzashi (Japanese hair ornaments).

M&J Trimming
1008 Sixth Avenue
(Between 37th and 38th)
New York NY 10018
www.mjtrim.com

This trimming store is a good place to buy beads, ribbons, braids, and all sorts of other decorative object that can be used to make hair decorations.

Manhattan Wardrobe Supply
245 West 29th St, 8th Floor
New York NY 10001
(888) 401-7400
www.wardrobesupplies.com

Manhattan Wardrobe carries everything—wigs, wig supplies, hairpins, styling products, laundry supplies, craft supplies, makeup supplies, labelling supplies, storage supplies, and shoe supplies.

Sally Beauty Supply
Stores nationwide
www.sallybeauty.com

Sally's carries a broad selection of combs, brushes, styling products, styling tools, hair nets, pins, colored hairsprays, and hair dyes.

Wilshire Wigs
5241 Craner Ave
North Hollywood CA 91601
1-800-927-0874
www.wilshirewigs.com

Wilshire Wigs is an excellent source for all manner of wigs. They carry a huge variety of brands, and carry many synthetic and human hair wigs. They also carry many hairpieces (good for taking apart and making into other things), and some extension hair/wefting. I buy the Giant, Wig America, and Look of Love brands most often. Specific wigs that I find most useful are:

- the "Ashley" wig by Giant. This wig comes in a huge range of colors, including white, several different colors of gray, and bright party colors.

- the "Angela" wig by Giant. A nice shoulder length wig, again available in a ton of colors.

- "Cassie" and "Christine" by Wig America. This is a reasonably priced long wig (Cassie is curly and Christine is straight) that comes in a nice range of colors. (These come in white, but not in gray.)

- "Dolly" by Wig America is a great base wig to create the Hedgehog style because it has lots of long, fluffy layers.

- "Lily" by Wig America. This wig is a good wig that is shoulder length, good for styles like the 1940s' women and Cavalier men that require a medium length wig.

- the "Fingerwave Wig" in the 1920's, 30's, and 40s' Costume category is a nice little classic wig that comes styled and works great in a pinch.

Wow Wigs
P.O. Box 3054
Cerritos CA 90703
1-714-228-9627
www.wowwigs.com

Wow Wigs is another company with a huge range of wigs, hairpieces, and weaving/braiding hair.

The wigs I order most often are from the Sepia brand:

- the "Ashley" wig is reasonably priced and comes in a nice range of colors.

- the "Nicole" wig is a bit longer than the Ashley wig, and also comes in a nice range of colors, especially blonds.

- the "LA4000" is a good quality, waist length wig. The color range is limited, but it does come in white.

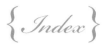

{Index}